Local Antibiotics in Arthroplasty

State of the Art from an Interdisciplinary
Point of View

Edited by Geert H. I. M. Walenkamp

With Contributions by

J.-N. Argenson
K. Bargiotas
S. J. Breusch
S. K. Bulstra
H. J. Busscher
M. Drancourt
L. B. Engesæter
C. Foucault
L. Frommelt
P. Gaston
K. Ibrahim
T. S. Karachalios
K.-D. Kühn
H. Malchau
K. N. Malizos
F. Matl

E. Meani
H. C. v. d. Mei
M. Mulier
D. Neut
S. Parratte
L. A. Poultsides
M. Rößner
N. T. Roidis
C. L. Romano
J. Schwabe
P. T. J. Spierings
A. W. Stemberger
J. Stuyck
S. Vogt
G. H. I. M. Walenkamp
E. Witsø

83 figures in 105 single illustrations
30 tables

Georg Thieme Verlag
Stuttgart · New York

Bibliographic Information published by
Die Deutsche Bibliothek

Die Deutsche Bibliothek lists this publication
in the Deutsche Nationalbibliographie;
detailed bibliographic data is available on
the internet at http://dnb.d-nb.de.

This book has been sponsored by Heraeus Medical,
a subsidiary of Heraeus Kulzer GmbH, Hanau, Germany.

Editor:
Prof. Geert H. I. M. Walenkamp, MD, PhD
Professor and Chairman of the Clinic
for Orthopedics of the University of Maastricht
Department of Orthopedic Surgery
University Hospital Maastricht
P. Debyelaan 25
P.O. Box 5800
6202 AZ Maastricht
gwa@sort.azm.nl
The Netherlands

© 2007 Georg Thieme Verlag,
Rüdigerstrasse 14
70469 Stuttgart, Germany
http://www.thieme.de
Thieme New York, 333 Seventh Avenue,
New York, NY 10001, USA
http://www.thieme.com

Printed in Germany

Cover: A false-color SEM image of vacuum-mixed, poly-
merized antibiotic-loaded bone cement (Palacos R+G),
showing a homogeneous cement matrix (green) without
air voids, the imbedded gentamicin (red), and the radiographic contrast medium zirconicum dioxide (blue).
Image: Heraeus image archive.
Typesetting by Sommer Druck, Feuchtwangen
Printing and bookbinding by Grafisches Centrum Cuno, Calbe

ISBN 978-3-13-134641-4 (TPS)
ISBN 978-1-58890-607-6 (TPN)   1 2 3 4 5 6

Important Note: Medicine is an ever-changing science
undergoing continual development. Research and clinical
experience are continually expanding our knowledge, in
particular our knowledge of proper treatment and drug
therapy. Insofar as this book mentions any dosage or application, readers may rest assured that the authors, editors,
and publishers have made every effort to ensure that such
references are in accordance with **the state of knowledge
at the time of production of the book.**

Nevertheless, this does not involve, imply, or express any
guarantee or responsibility on the part of the publishers in
respect to any dosage instructions and forms of applications stated in the book. **Every user is requested to examine carefully** the manufacturers' leaflets accompanying
each drug and to check, if necessary in consultation with a
physician or specialist, whether the dosage schedules mentioned therein or the contraindications stated by the
manufacturers differ from the statements made in the
present book. Such examination is particularly important
with drugs that are either rarely used or have been newly
released on the market. Every dosage schedule or every
form of application used is entirely at the user's own risk
and responsibility. The authors and publishers request
every user to report to the publishers any discrepancies or
inaccuracies noticed.

IV

Preface

In 1960 John Charnley reported how the anchorage of a femoral head prosthesis could be improved by the use of a "cold curing" acrylic cement. The fluid was self sterilising and the powder had to be exposed to formalin vapour for several weeks. His article in the British Journal of Bone and Joint Surgery was only 3 pages long. It was illustrated with a photo and X-rays of a cemented Moore hemi hip prosthesis. The version familiar at that time contained a stem with 'self-locking windows' where, however, bone ingrowth often failed to fix the prosthesis. He published his article having used the cement for just one year in a series of 29 patients.

Since then, this improved fixation of the prosthesis has been the main reason for the worldwide success of joint replacements, the most frequently performed operation with the highest success rate, as well as the medical intervention with one of the highest QALY (quality of adjusted life years) improvements.

The admixture of antibiotics to commercial bone cement was invented by the other pioneer in this field, Hans Wilhelm Buchholz. He developed his concept in collaboration with the German companies Merck and Kulzer, starting in 1969. The use of PMMA as a drug carrier with sustained release of gentamicin proved to be a perfect combination. The combination was strong enough to fix prostheses and was able to kill bacteria during 6 weeks postoperatively.

Although some reservations were expressed regarding the increased local use of antibiotics, this protracted release of antibiotics made it possible to re-implant prostheses in infected cases. Another and even more successful indication was prophylactic use in primary prostheses implantation. Smaller randomised series were able to prove the preventive effect on deep postoperative infections, but the enormous number of prostheses evaluated in the Swedish and Norwegian hip registers showed not only the prophylactic effect to deep infections, but also a protective effect against loosening probably due to non diagnosed low grade infections.

The therapeutic properties of PMMA as an antibiotic delivery system were improved by the development of PMMA beads: more porous cement, an increased amount of gentamicin and above all the increase in the total releasing surface resulted in a potent local antibiotic instrument. These gentamicin beads came on the market in 1976, and have thus had one of the longest lives as a pharmaceutical product, and are still considered the gold standard in local antibiotic treatment. Since then, numerous other local drug release systems and many applications have been developed, combining local high effective drug concentrations with the absence of systemic side effects.

Many bone cements entered the market, and also many antibiotic bone cement combinations. Many, however, have not survived. Only a few cement antibiotic combinations appear to have offered the requisite high quality.

The need for antibiotic protection of non cemented prostheses and other implants made it necessary to research into the binding of antibiotics to metal and polymer. Although many forms of binding to biomaterial surfaces are possible, protracted release after implantation is difficult to achieve. It is even more difficult considering that the ideal release pattern required for prevention or therapy is not fully known.

Concerns surrounding the increased use of antibiotics, often expressed in the initial period of local application, have proved unfounded. Only indirect evidence of increased resistance of bacteria to the antibiotics was obtained, and both the clinical relevance and the causal relationship remained uncertain. In view of these reports, however, the limitations of antibiotics should be borne in mind. Growing resistance of bacteria such as

MRSA and especially MRSE is making it increasingly difficult to combine antibiotics and bone cements commercially. There is a clear need for customized admixtures of antibiotics with bone grafts or bone substitutes and their use will increase.

New positioning in the market of bone cement producers prompted us to organize an international congress in Maastricht in April 2006 to update our knowledge about local antibiotic treatment. We succeeded in inviting prominent European experts in this field, and the meeting was held under the patronage of the "European Bone and Joint Infection Society". This Society has now for 25 years been the platform for orthopaedic surgeons, traumatologists, infectiologists and bacteriologists interested in infections of the musculoskeletal system. All important aspects of antibiotic loaded bone cement, as mentioned above, were discussed, as well as new and upcoming developments. We were also able to review existing practices in the treatment of infected prostheses in most of the European countries.

This congress and the publication of this book was only possible with assistance from many quarters. First of all, the authors who attended the Maastricht congress and who were willing to write their contribution despite their busy work schedules.

The help provided by Dr. Klaus Dieter Kühn, a well known expert on bone cement, was invaluable. In 2000, Dr. Kühn – representing the company Heraeus Kulzer GmbH – wrote the standard work "Bone cements" which brought all the available information on bone cement up to date. Heraeus Kulzer GmbH was ever the producer of the original Palacos – with and without antibiotics like gentamicin – which was the starting point for all the subsequent developments.

Ms. Angelika Rückle of the Thieme Verlag publishing house was very helpful in preparing the manuscripts and providing editorial support to the authors. She understood that the combination with other, often clinical work was not always self-evident.

I hope that those who read this book, who are likely to be interested in the fascinating subject of local antibiotic prophylaxis and treatment, will find what they are looking for: a clear and comprehensive presentation of the state of the art.

March 2007,
Maastricht   Geert Walenkamp

Adresses

Editor:

Prof. Geert H. I. M. Walenkamp, MD, PhD
Professor and Chairman of the Clinic
for Orthopedics of the University of Maastricht
Department of Orthopedic Surgery
University Hospital Maastricht
P. Debyelaan 25
P.O. Box 5800
6202 AZ Maastricht
gwa@sort.azm.nl
The Netherlands

Contributors (first-mentioned):

Prof. Steffen J. Breusch, MD, PhD, FRCSEd
Department of Orthopedic Surgery
University of Edinburgh
New Royal Infirmary of Edinburgh
Little France
51 Little France Crescent
Old Dalkeith Road
EH16 4SA Edinburgh
steffen.breusch@ukonline.co.uk
Scotland

Prof. Lars B. Engesæter, MD, PhD
Department of Orthopedic Surgery
Haukeland University Hospital
5021 Bergen
lars.engesaeter@helse-bergen.no
Norway

Lars Frommelt, MD
Holstenstr. 2
22767 Hamburg
lars.frommelt@t-online.de
Germany

Paul Gaston, FRCSEd (Orth)
Department of Orthopedic Surgery
University of Edinburgh
New Royal Infirmary of Edinburgh
Little France
51 Little France Crescent
Old Dalkeith Road
EH16 4SU Edinburgh
pgaston@staffmail.ed.ac.uk
Scotland

Klaus-Dieter Kühn, MSc, PhD
Heraeus Kulzer GmbH
Philipp-Reis-Str. 8/13
61273 Wehrheim
klaus-dieter.kuehn@heraeus.com
Germany

Prof. Konstantinos N. Malizos, MD
Orthopedics School of Health Sciences
University of Thessalia
P.O. BOX 1425
P.C 41110
Larissa
kmalizos@ortho-uth.org
Greece

Prof. Michiel Mulier, MD, PhD
Department of Orthopedic Surgery
University Hospital K.U. Leuven
U. Z. Pellenberg
Weligerveld 1
3212 Pellenberg
michiel.mulier@uz.kuleuven.ac.be
Belgium

Daniëlle Neut, MSc, PhD
Department of Biomedical Engineering/
Orthopedic Surgery
University Medical Center Groningen
Antonius Deusinglaan 1
9713 AV Groningen
d.neut@med.umcg.nl
The Netherlands

Sébastien Parratte, MD, PhD
Service d'Orthopédie et de Traumatologie
Hôpital Sainte Marguerite
270 Bd Sainte Marguerite
BP 29
13274 Marceille Cedex 09
sebparatte@gmail.com
France

Prof. Carlo L. Romano, MD, PhD
Istituto Ortopedico Gaetano Pini
Piazza Cardinal Ferrari, 1
20122 Milan
romano@gpini.it
Italy

Pieter T. J. Spierings, MD, MSc
Spierings Medische Techniek B.V.
Madoerastraat 24
6524 LH Nijmegen
spierings@spieringsmedical.nl
pspierings@spierings.biz
The Netherlands

Prof. Axel W. Stemberger, MD, PhD, MSc
Institut für Experimentelle Onkologie
u. Therapieforschung
TU München, Klinikum r. d. Isar
Ismaninger Str. 22
81675 München
axel.stemberger@lrz.tum.de
Germany

Prof. Eivind Witsø, MD, PhD
Associate Professor
Department of Orthopaedic Surgery
St. Olavs University Hospital Norwegian University
of Science and Technology
7006 Trondheim
eivind.witso@stolav.no
Norway

Contents

NL 1 Infection of Orthopedic Implants –
Bacterial Adhesion and the Role
of Local Antibiotics 1
D. Neut, H. C. van der Mei, S. K. Bulstra,
H. J. Busscher

D 2 New Antibiotic Carriers and Coatings
in Surgery 13
A. W. Stemberger, J. Schwabe, K. Ibrahim,
F. Matl, M. Rößner, S. Vogt, K.-D. Kühn

D 3 Antimicrobial Implant Coating
in Arthroplasty 23
K.-D. Kühn, S. Vogt

NL 4 Bone Cements – Are They Different? . . 31
P. T. J. Spierings

N 5 Cancellous Bone Allograft as an
Antibiotic Carrier – In-Vitro-, In-Vivo-
and Clinical Studies 41
E. Witsø

D 6 Antibiotic-Loaded Bone Cements –
Antibiotic Release and Influence on
Mechanical Properties 47
K.-D. Kühn

D 7 Antibiotic Choices in Bone Surgery –
Local Therapy using Antibiotic-Loaded
Bone Cement 59
L. Frommelt

NL 8 Local Antibiotic-Loaded Carriers
in Orthopedic Surgery –
Pharmacokinetic Aspects 65
G. H. I. M. Walenkamp

FR 9 Vancomycin Bone Cement –
Experimental Data 75
S. Parratte, C. Foucault, M. Drancourt,
J.-N. Argenson

UK 10 Why cement the Total Hip? 87
S. J. Breusch, H. Malchau

UK 11 Diagnosis and Management
of Infected Arthroplasty –
The United Kingdom Experience 95
P. Gaston

GR 12 Management of Septic Joint Arthro-
plasty – The Hellenic Experience 109
K. N. Malizos, N. T. Roidis, T. S. Karachalios,
L. A. Poultsides, K. Bargiotas

I 13 Revision of Infected Hip Prostheses with
Antibiotic-Loaded Preformed Cement
Spacers – The Italian Experience 121
C. L. Romano, E. Meani

NL 14 Treatment of Infected Prostheses –
The Dutch Experience 133
G. H. I. M. Walenkamp

N 15 Revision of Infected Total Hip
Prostheses in Norway and Sweden . . 145
E. Witsø, L. B. Engesæter

N 16 The Norwegian Hip Register –
The Influence of Cement
and Antibiotics on the Clinical
Results of Primary Prostheses 147
L. B. Engesæter

B 17 Girdlestone Resection Arthroplasty
of the Hip – A One-Stage Procedure
to eradicate Infection 155
M. Mulier, J. Stuyck

Infection of Orthopedic Implants – Bacterial Adhesion and the Role of Local Antibiotics

Daniëlle Neut, Henny C. van der Mei, Sjoerd K. Bulstra, Henk J. Busscher

Abstract

Infection is a serious complication following joint replacement surgery that often can only be eradicated by removal of the prosthesis, as the biofilm growth mode on an implant surface protects the infecting bacteria against the host immune system and antibiotic therapy. Over the past decades it has been attempted to prevent and cure joint replacement infections by incorporating antibiotics in polymethylmethacrylate (PMMA) bone cements, both in primary and revision surgery. It has been shown that antibiotic-loaded bone cement has a significant effect on bacterial growth, decreasing the chances of infection and improving the efficacy of infection treatment. However, due to increasing bacterial resistance to antibiotics the current commercially available gentamicin-loaded bone cement has had to be enhanced by incorporating a second antibiotic. In this paper, we review the background of prosthesis-related infections in orthopedics, together with the release mechanisms and properties of antibiotic-loaded bone cements. In addition, the clinical efficacy of antibiotic-loaded bone cements is evaluated analyzing seperatedly the prophylactic and therapeutic use of these products.

Biomaterial-Related Infections

Biomaterials are man-made materials (polymers, metals, alloys or ceramics) designed to interact with living tissue or with a body fluid. Biomaterials are used more and more in modern medicine to replace, support or restore human body function, for example in joint prostheses, prosthetic heart valves or catheters. The application of biomaterials bears one major drawback: the risk of attracting infectious microorganisms (Gristina, 1987). Infecting organisms are able to reach prosthetic devices in two ways.

Firstly, by direct contamination during the surgical procedure, i.e.; from the patient's or surgeon's skin flora or from contaminated air in the operating room (Gristina, 1985). Lidwell (Lidwell et al., 1983) stated that over 95% of prosthetic infections that occur during the first year after implantation, are due to peroperative contamination of the prosthesis. Peroperative contamination studies have been conducted on indirectly involved surgical instruments, like sucker tips, light handles, gloves used for preparation, theater gowns, etc. A total of 63% of the screened operations showed contamination in the field of operation (Davis et al., 1999). However, no studies have been performed on the possible contamination of instruments that are used directly in the planned site for the prosthesis or of tissue samples taken from the planned site of the prosthesis. Maathuis (Maathuis et al., 2005) investigated the possible contamination rate in total hip arthroplasty through instruments used at the direct site of the prosthesis during the primary procedure. Viable microorganisms were cultured from instruments and tissue that had been in direct contact with the actual site of the prosthesis in 30% of all cases, thus potentially constituting a future cause for septic loosening.

Secondly, infections may occur by way of the bloodstream (Gristina, 1985). A hematogenous origin of infection is typically associated with infections that manifest later. In this case, either the bloodstream or the lymphatic vessels transport the pathogens from a distant site of infection (for example from a periodontal or urinary tract infection or a simple scratch or cut) to the prosthesis. However, hematogenous infection only plays a minor role in orthopedic surgery with an incidence of 0.3 – 7% (Ahnfelt et al., 1990; Ainscow and Denham, 1984).

Bacterial adhesion is a complicated process. All biomaterials undergo changes at the surface after

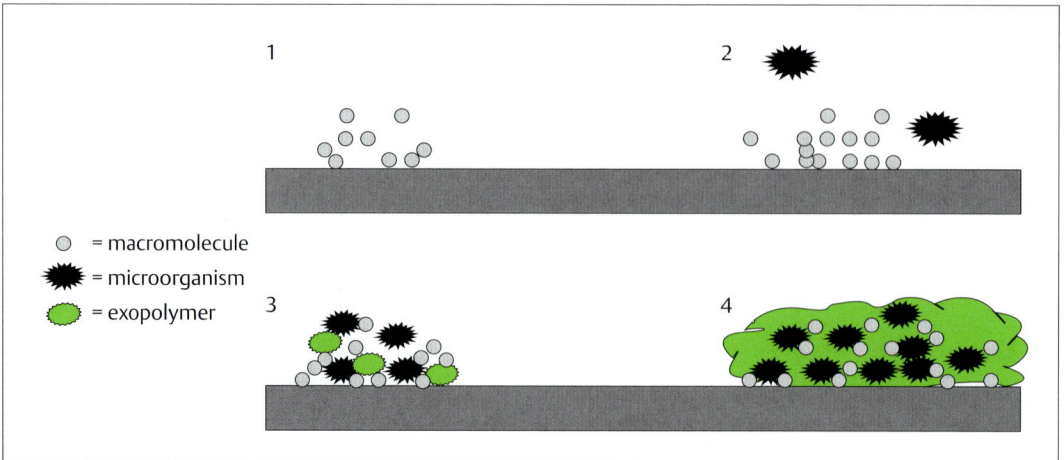

Fig. 1.**1** A schematic representation of the sequential steps in biofilm formation on biomaterials including:
1) formation of a conditioning film,
2) microbial mass transport,
3) initial microbial adhesion and slime (exopolymer) production, and
4) growth of adhering microorganisms embedded in slime to form a multicellular layer – the biofilm.

implantation. The earliest and probably clinically most important phase is the "race for the surface", a contest between tissue cell integration and bacterial adhesion to that same surface (Gristina, 1987). On contact, body fluids immediately coat all surfaces with a layer of host material, primarily serum proteins and platelets. These host proteins promote attachment of bacteria onto the implant by specific receptors and nonspecific interactions that are influenced by the hydrophobicity and charge of the implant and bacterial cell surface. Adhesion progresses to aggregation of bacteria on the surface of the foreign body where they become encased in a hydrated matrix (exopolymer) of polysaccharides and proteins to form a slimy layer known as biofilm (Costerton et al., 1999), (Fig. 1.**1**).

Biomaterial-related infections can cause severe problems, from dysfunctioning of the implanted device (Fig. 1.**2**) to lethal sepsis of the patient. In addition, treatment of these biomaterial-related infections is complicated, as biofilms grow slowly and can resist cellular and humoral immune responses (Costerton et al., 1999). Moreover, microorganisms in a biofilm are much more resistant to antibiotics than their planktonic counterparts (Khoury et al., 1992). Reduced antibiotic susceptibility contributes to the persistence of biofilm infections. The protective mechanisms in biofilms

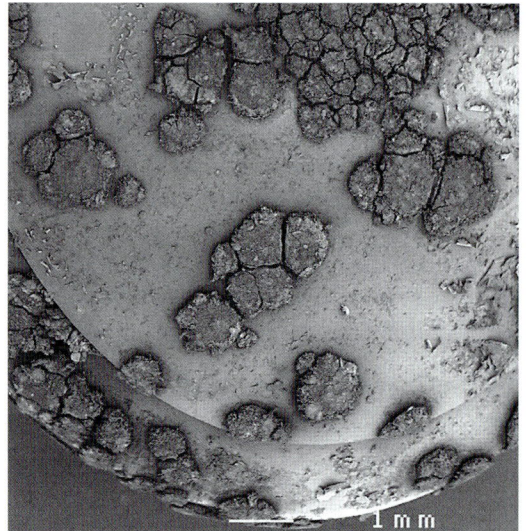

Fig. 1.**2** Biofilm formation is the main cause for the failure of voice prostheses used for speech rehabilitation in patients after total laryngectomy. Bacteria and yeasts easily form a biofilm on the esophageal side of a prosthesis, which leads to dysfunction of the valve and induces leakage of fluids into the trachea and/or increased airflow resistance during speech.

turn out to be distinct from those that are responsible for conventional antibiotic resistance. In biofilms, poor antibiotic penetration and slow growth are hypothesized to constitute a multilayered defence (Costerton et al., 1999). Besides, in the past it was assumed that biofilm bacteria behave much like planktonic bacteria. Now, it is discovered that, while biofilm bacteria have the exact same genetic makeup as their planktonic counterparts, their biochemistry is very different because they switch on a different set of genes. For example, up to 40% of cell wall proteins differ between biofilm and planktonic bacteria. This makes biofilm bacteria difficult to kill because some of the targets for antibiotics are no longer there (Costerton et al., 1995). In addition, some bacteria, such as *Staphylococcus aureus*, form small colony variants, characterized by a reduced growth rate, decreased susceptibility to aminoglycosides, and possible intracellular persistence (Proctor and Peters, 1998).

Biomaterial-related infections will, in general, not clear until the implant is removed and the patient is given antibiotic therapy. This treatment can prolong the patient's hospital stay by several days to weeks and require additional surgery, incuring considerable costs for the health care system and patient's suffering. Therefore, a clear goal is to prevent the development of an infectious biofilm on the biomaterial surface. Over the last four decades, the prophylactic application of antibiotics prior to even minor surgery for biomaterial implantation (Lattimer et al., 1979) and the strict adherence to hygienic rules to prevent contamination of implants during surgery, has reduced the incidence of biomaterial-related infections. Still, a significant number of infections occur. The incidence of biomaterial-related infections varies from about 0.11% for contact lenses (Sharma et al., 2003) to 100% for urinary tract catheters after 3 weeks use (Denstedt, 1998).

Biomaterial-related infections in orthopedic implants

Total joint replacement has been shown to be a highly effective treatment for end-stage osteoarthritis of the major weight-bearing joints. Therefore hip and knee replacements are very common in orthopedic surgery. A current estimate of the rate of hip replacements amounts approximately to one million per year worldwide with over 250000 knee replacements (Sculco, 1995).

This figure is expected to double between 1999 and 2025 as a result of aging populations and growing demands of a higher quality of life. Despite the success of joint arthroplasty, complications persist, including dislocation, osteolysis, aseptic loosening and infection. The infection rate of primary joint arthroplasties is currently estimated between 1 and 3% (Antti-Poika et al., 1990; Harris and Sledge, 1990), despite the use of intraoperative systemic antibiotic prophylaxis, strict hygienic protocols, and special sterile enclosures with laminar flow (Knobben et al., 2006). This may seem a small percentage, but since joint replacement operations are so common, it is a complication that affects a significant number of patients. Moreover, infection remains a devastating complication for both the patient and society. It is associated with a substantial increase in morbidity, which increases hospital admittance time and hence adds significant costs to the health care system. At an average cost of $50000–60000 per treatment, the total costs for the management of infected joint replacements amount $200–250 million in the United States (Sculco, 1995) and approximately triples that amount worldwide.

The infection rate of joint replacements may have been underestimated. A role for bacteria has been suggested in a proportion of the supposed aseptic loosenings of prostheses. It has been noted that peroperative measures against infection not only lead to a decrease in infections, but also in the incidence of aseptic loosening (Josefsson and Kolmert, 1993). This is further supported by evidence from improved methods of infection detection (Neut et al., 2003; Tunney et al., 1998). The reference standard for diagnosing infection is the isolation of responsible pathogens. Peroperative tissue samples provide the most accurate specimens for microbiological cultures, and are frequently used as the standard method in diagnosing infection after joint arthroplasty. Shortcomings of this method are the diagnostic delay and sensitivity of cultures (Hoeffel et al., 1999). Some cultures are easily grown in three days, but especially culturing of anaerobic and slowly growing biofilm organisms can take time. Moreover, the formation of small colony variants may limit the ability of the laboratory to isolate the micro-organism. Also, not infrequently, previous or simultaneous antibiotic treatment in patients with an orthopedic implant may lead to false negative microbiological test results. Therefore, bacteria colonizing the surface of implants, may not be identified by standard culture techniques (Dupont, 1986). If the causative organism cannot be detected, the surgical and/or antibiotic treatment cannot be optimized. There are obvious dangers related to treating an unrecognized infection without adequate antibiotic therapy during revision arthroplasty. The new prosthesis may be implanted into a field contaminated with bacteria. Any organisms colonizing the primary prosthesis, but not identified and eradicated, will likely infect a new implant and put the revision surgery at risk of failure. Improved methods particularly tailored to detect biofilm infections, are required to improve the outcome of prosthetic surgery. Advances in laboratory techniques (Neut et al., 2003) and molecular biological methods, such as PCR techniques (Tunney et al., 1998), provide new diagnostic tools.

Bacteria isolated from orthopedic infections are frequently Staphylococcus species, predominantly coagulase-negative Staphylococci (CNS). Aerobic Gram-negative bacteria cause 10–20% of all deep infections and anerobic bacteria are responsible for another 10–15% (Fitzgerald, 1995; Garvin et al., 1999). With routine hospital culturing, mostly only one causative organism is found on infected implants. However, more extensive culturing techniques reveal that most infections are caused by a mixture of microorganisms (Neut et al., 2003; Tunney et al., 1998).

Biomaterial-Related Infections in Orthopedic Implants

In the field of biomaterials, PMMA bone cement is a material widely used to anchor prostheses during joint replacement surgery. PMMA bone cement was introduced to stabilize metallic hip implants and transfer mechanical loads from the implant to the bone and visa versa (Charnley, 1970). The introduction of antibiotic-loaded bone cement aimed at establishing a decrease of implant infection rates (Buchholz, 1970). The assumption underlying the incorporation of antibiotics in bone cements, is that the antibiotic is gradually released, yielding higher local concentrations than can be achieved by systemic therapy. Furthermore, the local release of antibiotics causes a low rise in serum or urine concentrations, thus minimizing the side effects associated with systemic antibiotics.

Mechanisms of antibiotic release from bone cements

The polymer PMMA, from which bone cements are made, is capable of taking up very small quantities of dissolution fluid into its outermost layers. This dissolution fluid slowly releases the antibiotic molecules contained within the polymer into the surrounding tissue. The sustained release of antibiotics from bone cements is largely influenced by the penetration of dissolution fluids into the polymer matrix, which requires a certain porosity of the cement (Baker and Greenham, 1988; Kuechle et al., 1991). Initially, large amounts of antibiotic are released (Van de Belt et al., 2000), as it is particularly easily available at the surface of bone cement. A point on which all studies have agreed, is that the period of maximum antibiotic release is limited to the first few hours or days after implantation. The maximum effectiveness of the released antibiotic might thus be expected to occur during this period of time (Trippel, 1986). Most if not all of the antibiotic is released from the superficial regions of the cement and fails to be released from the center (Schurman et al., 1978; Wahlig and Dingeldein, 1980). In fact, many in-vitro and in-vivo tests have shown that only small amounts (3–15%) of the antibiotics incorporated in bone cement are actually released (Van de Belt, 2000; Schurmann et al., 1978; Törholm et al., 1983). The release of antibiotics from bone cement is, therefore, largely a surface phenomenon.

The porosity of the polymer matrix depends on air entrapment, while wetting and stirring the cement powder during transfer to the cement gun. It is also influenced by effects of monomer boiling (Wixson et al., 1987). Baker and Greenham (Baker and Greenham, 1988) concluded that bone cement with greater porosity would allow more antibiotic release than cement with less porosity. Therefore, methods of cement preparation designed to improve mechanical properties by decreasing the porosity (such as vacuum mixing or centrifugation) could have adverse effects on elution characteristics. Furthermore, in commercially available antibiotic-loaded bone cement, the antibiotic is evenly dispersed throughout the cement, creating a homogeneous mixture. This uniform antibiotic dispersion cannot be achieved when adding the antibiotic by hand to the bone cement. An uneven dispersion may reduce the mechanical properties of the cement, and cannot always ensure sufficient antibiotic release (Neut et al., 2003).

In-vivo experience with antibiotic-loaded bone cement

Animal studies:

The characteristics of antibiotic release from bone cement applied in rabbits (Rodeheaver et al., 1983) and rats (Wahlig and Buchholz, 1972) correspond largely with the findings of in-vitro experiments. Antibiotic concentrations in serum peak within a few hours at a level that is always below toxicity, and drop to below measurement thresholds within one day (Wahlig and Buchholz, 1972; Bunetel et al., 1994). Local concentrations are much higher than serum concentrations (Rhodeheaver et al., 1983), and have been reported to be measurable up to weeks or months (Wahlig and Buchholz, 1972; Bunetel et al., 1994).

Most in-vitro experiments do not show a complete eradication of bacteria with the application of antibiotic-loaded bone cement (Van de Belt et al., 2001; Konig et al., 2000). However, in animals antibiotic-loaded bone cement appears to prevent infection from peroperative challenge in all (Schurmann et al., 1978; Nijhof et al., 2000), or in most examined cases (Rodeheaver et al., 1983; Welch, 1978; Nijhof et al., 2001). Compared with systemic administration of antibiotics, the application of antibiotic-loaded bone cement has similar (Nijhof et al., 2000; Nijhof et al., 2001) or better results (Petty et al., 1988). However, the protection against hematogenous infection of a joint prosthesis in late postoperative phase is doubtful, as animal experiments have shown (Blomgren and Lindgren, 1981).

Clinical studies:

With the addition of antibiotics to Palacos bone cement in the Endoclinic (Hamburg), a marked decrease of deep infection has been noticed. Between 1972 and 1975 Buchholz (Buchholz et al., 1984) noted an infection frequency of 1.6% for total hip arthroplasties using gentamicin-loaded bone cement. In contrast, the frequency of deep infections for hip prostheses using plain bone cement was 4.9%. Since then, authors have reported similar results. Randomized controlled prospective clinical trials have shown that antibiotic-loaded bone cements provide better protection against deep infection than plain bone cement (Jo-

sefsson and Kolmert, 1993; Josefsson et al., 1990; Chiu et al., 2002). An even greater effect was demonstrated in a retrospective study, when a systemic antibiotic was used in addition to antibiotic-loaded bone cement (Espehaug et al., 1987–1995). Also, with the use of a clean air technique, an additional drop in infection rates after primary procedures was noted if gentamicin-loaded bone cement was used (Persson et al., 1999). As a result, many surgeons now routinely use antibiotic-loaded bone cement in all primary implantations performed. For example, it has been reported that over 90% of orthopedic surgeons in the United States use antibiotic-loaded bone cement for primary arthroplasties. Heck (Heck et al., 1995), and Espehaug (Espehaug et al., 2006) reported that, in Norway, the use of antibiotic-loaded bone cements for the fixation of total hip replacements increased from 40% in 1989 to 94% in 1999.

The prophylactic use of antibiotic-loaded bone cements for the primary fixation of implants must be clearly distinguished from its therapeutic use in revision. The value of using antibiotic-loaded bone cements at re-implantation, if necessary one-stage, of an infected prosthesis has been significantly demonstrated (Lynch et al., 1987). Beads and spacers made of antibiotic-loaded bone cement designed to treat infections prior to re-implantation, constitute another temporary application of these biomaterials.

Clinical aspects of the application of antibiotic-loaded bone cements

Worrisome in the application of antibiotic-loaded bone cements, is the risk of introducing resistant strains by releasing sub-inhibitory antibiotic concentrations for many years. Gentamicin, for instance, has remained detectable in joint fluid aspirations and tissue samples for years after using gentamicin-loaded cement for fixation of a joint prosthesis (Wahlig and Dingeldein, 1980; Törholm et al., 1983). The exact mechanism, by which this antibiotic resistance evolves, is not clear and different options have been reported, including mutation and selection. Thomes (Thomes et al., 2002) stated that gentamicin-loaded bone cement offers an optimal surface for bacterial colonization, and prolonged exposure to gentamicin promotes mutational resistance. Here, it is important to note that antibiotics do not directly cause mutation. They rather provide a situation for selecting the naturally resistant strains, which arise spontaneously: The antibiotic kills the sensitive bacteria, leaving behind those that are resistant. These resistant bacteria then multiply and become predominant. A model, simulating the in-vivo interfacial gap between bone and cement, supports this theory. It was shown that gentamicin-sensitive strains were not able to survive in this gap model, whereas a highly gentamicin-resistant strain was able to survive in the gap environment. This indicates selection as a basis for resistance to gentamicin after using gentamicin-loaded bone cements (Hendriks et al., 2005).

Improvements of commercially available antibiotic-loaded bone cements

Most of the 18 different antibiotic-loaded bone cements, currently available on the European market, contain gentamicin as a sulfate (Kühn, 2000). Gentamicin shows a good release from bone cement, has a broad antimicrobial spectrum, and good water solubility. Several in-vitro and in-vivo studies have, however, indicated bacterial growth on antibiotic-loaded bone cements (Van de Belt et al., 1999; Van de Belt et al., 2001; Oga et al., 1992), with increased occurrence of gentamicin-resistant strains, thus necessitating improvements of the existing gentamicin-loaded bone cements.

The increasing bacterial resistance to gentamicin has prompted renewed interest in the addition of further antibiotics to bone cements, such as tobramycin and cefuroxime (Nijhof et al., 2000; Chiu et al., 2002). From past experience, it is likely, however, that it will only be a matter of time, before the bacteria develop a mechanism of resistance to overcome any new antibiotic which is incorporated in bone cement. Therefore, ongoing research and industrial developments include the use of combinations of antibiotics (multidrug targeting). Multidrug targeting is assumed not only to be more powerful, but also to prevent the emergence of resistant strains through the synergistic action of two antibiotics at the same time (Murray et al., 1998). In Europe, one multidrug-loaded bone cement, containing gentamicin and clindamycin, Copal (a product of Heraeus Medical, Germany), is already commercially available. A combination of gentamicin and clindamycin in bone cement has a theoretical antimicrobial effect on more than 90% of the bacteria common to in-

fected arthroplasties (Kühn, 2000). In addition, the release of gentamicin seems to be enhanced by the release of clindamycin in this cement (Kühn, 2000). This may be an effect of the extra antibiotic, which acts as a soluble additive that leaves a network of voids behind, enhancing further release (Penner et al., 1996). Moreover, bone cements loaded with combinations of gentamicin and clindamycin or fusidic acid are more effective in preventing biofilm formation, than bone cements with gentamicin alone (Neut et al., 2005), (Fig.1.3).

Multidrug targeting may be effective in preventing resistance, but using it is a difficult option in bone cement, as the release of the different antibiotics depends on many factors. For example, vancomycin has a high molecular weight and demonstrates poor release simply because vancomycin is trapped in the matrix of bone cement (Klekamp et al., 1999). Also, combinations of antibiotics must be carefully selected, due to known cross-resistances between different antibiotics. For this reason, the combination of gentamicin and tobramycin is not advizable. And, there is always the possibility of an antagonistic effect in the different ways antibiotics act upon the bacterial life cycle.

Future prevention options for infected joint prosthesis with ultrasound

Low-frequency ultrasound has been implied in new drug delivery systems (Tachibana and Tachibana, 1999). It is a pressure wave that enhances movement of particles in fluid, thus promoting diffusion. Antibiotics are released from bone cement in a biphasic manner, i.e., high elution in the first hours to days post-surgery and slowing down considerably after a few days. Over 80% of the antibiotic remain locked in the bone cement, years after implantation (Van de Belt et al., 2000). It is assumed that the application of low-frequency ultrasound to antibiotic-loaded bone cement will accelerate the release of antibiotics. In addition, there is an effect of low-frequency ultrasound on bacteria, known as the bioacoustic effect (Pitt et al., 1994). This effect refers to the enhanced activity of antibiotics towards biofilm bacteria in an ultrasound field. Electron-spin resonance studies suggest that ultrasound induces uptake of antibiotic by perturbing or stressing the membrane (Rediske et al., 1999).

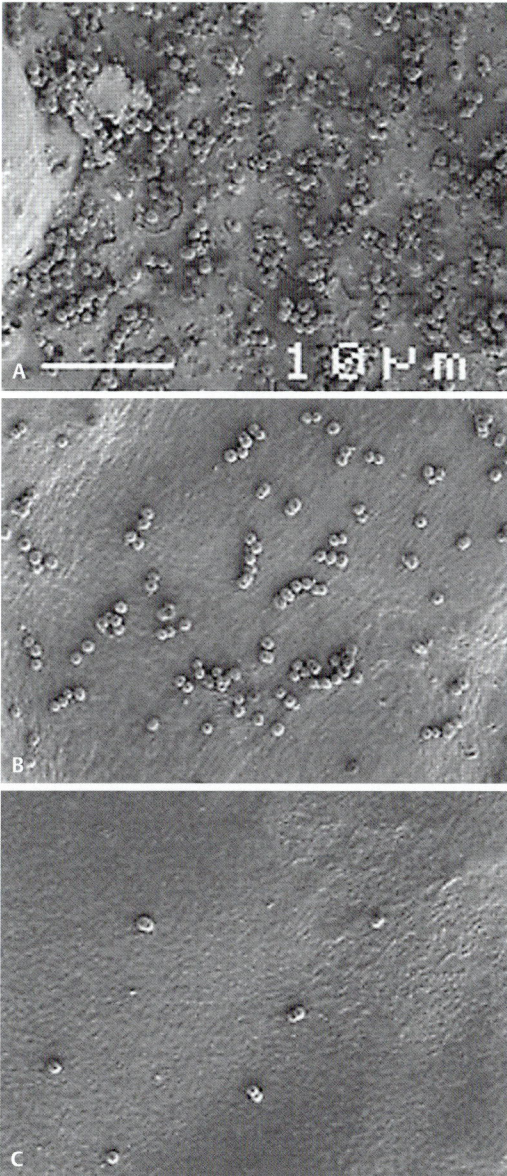

Fig. 1.**3**   SEM pictures of *Staphylococcus aureus* biofilms grown after 24 hours on bone cement discs.
A = plain bone cement,
B = gentamicin-loaded bone cement, and
C = gentamicin / clindamycin-loaded bone cement.

Earlier studies showed a small increase in antibiotic release with the application of ultrasound on antibiotic-loaded cement (Hedriks et al., 2003). Ensing (Ensing et al., 2005) studied rabbits to de-termine whether the bioacoustic effect yielded enhanced bactericidal effects on gentamicin-loaded bone cement. The results demonstrated that ultrasound in combination with gentamicin yields an enhanced killing of bacteria on bone cement, in vivo. However, it is unknown whether this enhanced bactericidal effect is due to the bioacoustic effect, or the increased release of genta-micin from the antibiotic-loaded bone cement, or a combination of both. The clinical value of these observations warrants further evaluation, as it may offer a new treatment option of infected joint prostheses when fixed with antibiotic-loaded bone cement. Moreover, ultrasound can be ap-plied in combination with antibiotics in the early postoperative period to prevent infection, as planktonic bacteria present in the wound and sur-rounding wound tissue, due to inevitable contam-ination during surgery, can then be more effec-tively stopped from forming a biofilm.

Treatment of Chronic Joint Replacement Infections

A prosthesis-related infection is difficult to treat. The immunoincompetent zone around a prosthe-sis (Gristina, 1994), the reduced sensitivity of bac-teria growing in a biofilm (Costerton et al., 1999), and the relatively poor availability of antibiotics from the bloodstream at the site of infection prob-ably all contribute to this fact. Several options for treatment of infected joint replacements have been established depending on multiple factors such as type of infection (acute versus chronic), the isolated pathogen and its susceptibility pat-tern, the fixation of the device, the quality and availability of the bone stock, as well as the train-ing and experience of the orthopedic surgeon and infectious disease physician. For acute infections, long-term therapy involving combinations of anti-biotics have been reported to be successful (Zim-merli et al., 1998). In order to eradicate chronic prosthesis infection, most authors recommend the removal of the device (McDonald et al., 1989; Tattevin et al., 1999) and a two-stage revision ar-throplasty (initial removal and debridement fol-lowed by a period of antibiotic treatment, then re-placement of the implant). Other treatment options are one-stage revision surgery (removal, debridement and reimplantation in one proce-dure) and suppressive antimicrobial therapy for patients unfit for surgery. The one-stage approach includes systemic antibiotics and antibiotic-loaded bone cement. The choice between one-stage or two-stage revision surgery, and type and duration of antibiotic therapy are poorly standardized and, to a great extent, depend on the personal experience of the surgeon.

For successful reimplantation, high local concentrations of antibiotic are needed to cure the infection. These can be achieved by implanting chains of gentamicin-loaded PMMA beads in the compromized tissue. Locally applied gentamicin concentrations by far exceed those achieved by systemic gentamicin treatment. These may be 10–100 times higher than the minimal inhibitory concentration (MIC) of the causative bacteria (Walenkamp, 1997), depending on the local circumstances and the kind of application of the beads. A prospective study of 28 patients with infected total joint arthroplasties showed that the recurrence of infection was not statistically more common in the group treated with conventional systemic antibiotic therapy than in the group treated with gentamicin-loaded beads (Nelson et al., 1993). However, the costs of treatment are considerably lower in patients treated with gentamicin-loaded beads (Blaha et al., 1993). Usually, gentamicin-loaded beads are removed after two weeks, and the absence of viable bacteria in excised soft tissue samples is taken as a sign that the infection is cured and implantation of a new prosthesis can take place.

Up to now, gentamicin-loaded PMMA beads are the only commercially available beads, and therefore are routinely used in prosthesis-related infections, without prior identification of the infecting bacteria and its sensitivity for gentamicin. Neut (Neut et al., 2001) showed bacterial survival on gentamicin-loaded PMMA beads after two-stage revision surgery and most of the bacteria retrieved from the bead surfaces were gentamicin-resistant or had developed resistant sub-populations, raising concern about the efficacy of this treatment option. Increasing emergence of gentamicin-resistant bacteria in joint replacement surgery poses a threat to current clinical practice and new treatment options are being considered. Also, it has been observed that the PMMA beads do not release all of the gentamicin. After 2 weeks in situ, 20–70% of the total amount of gentamicin incorporated in the beads is released into the body and gentamicin concentrations drop significantly (Walenkamp et al., 1986). As a result, incomplete drug release, colonization of beads with bacteria,

and the requirement for surgical bead removal have prompted research into biodegradable materials acting as antibiotic carriers for local drug delivery.

Despite the advantage of achieving high local concentrations of antibiotics with beads, there are more disadvantages to be considered. There is limited joint function requiring bed rest, and the complication of re-implantation surgery due to soft tissue shortening because of scar formation. Also, in two-stage revision, the interval between two operations means impaired mobility and possible stiffening of the joint. Instead of implanting gentamicin-loaded PMMA beads, a more or less functional spacer made of antibiotic-loaded bone cement can be used. The application of various differently shaped temporal spacers has proven to be an effective technique for the treatment of infected hip and knee replacements (Booth and Lotke, 1989; Duncan and Beauchamp, 1993).

References

Ahnfelt L, Herberts P, Malchau H et al. Prognosis of total hip replacement. A Swedish multicenter study of 4664 revisions, Acta Orthop Scand 1990; 238: 1–26.

Ainscow DA, Denham RA. The risk of hematogenous infection in total joint replacements. J Bone Joint Surg Br 1984; 66: 580–582.

Antti-Poika I, Josefsson G, Konttinen Y, Lidgren L, Santavirta S, Sanzen L. Hip arthroplasty infection. Current concepts. Acta Orthop Scand 1990; 61: 163–169.

Baker AS, Greenham LW. Release of gentamicin from acrylic bone cement. J Bone Joint Surg Am 1988; 70: 1551–1557.

Belt van de H, Neut D, Van Horn JR, Van der Mei HC, Schenk W, Busscher HJ. Antibiotic resistance – to treat or not to treat? Nature Med 1999; 5: 358–359.

Belt van de H, Neut D, Van Horn JR et al. Surface roughness, porosity and wettability of gentamicin-loaded bone cements and their antibiotic release. 2000. 21; 1981–1987.

Belt van de H, Neut D, Schenk W, Van Horn JR, Van der Mei HC, Busscher HJ. *Staphylococcus aureus* biofilm formation on different gentamicin-loaded polymethylmethacrylate bone cements. Biomaterials 2001; 22: 1607–1611.

Blaha JD, Calhoun JH, Nelson CL et al. Comparison of the clinical efficacy and tolerance of gentamicin PMMA beads on surgical wire versus combined and systemic therapy for osteomyelitis. Clin Orthop 1993; 295: 8–12.

Blomgren G, Lindgren U. Late hematogenous infection in total joint replacement: studies of gentamicin and bone cement in the rabbit. Clin Orthop 1981; 155: 244–248.

Booth RE, Lotke PA. The results of spacer block technique in revision of infected total knee arthroplasty. Clin Orthop 1989; 248: 57 – 60.

Buchholz HW, Engelbrecht H. Über die Depotwirkung einiger Antibiotika bei Vermischung mit dem Kunstharz Palacos. Chirurg 1970; 40: 511 – 515.

Buchholz HW, Elson RA, Heinert K. Antibiotic-loaded acrylic cement: current concepts. Clin Orthop 1984; 190: 96 – 108.

Bunetel L, Segui A, Langlais F, Cormier M. Osseous concentrations of gentamicin after implantation of acrylic bone cement in sheep femora. Eur J Drug Metab Pharmacokinet 1994; 19: 99 – 105.

Charnley J. The reaction of bone to self-curing acrylic cement. A long-term histological study in man. J Bone Joint Surg Br 1970; 52: 340 – 353.

Chiu FY, Chen CM, Lin CF, Lo WH. Cefuroxime-impregnated cement in primary total knee arthroplasty: a prospective, randomized study of three hundred and forty knees. J Bone Joint Surg Am 2002; 84: 759 – 762.

Costerton JW, Lewandowski Z, Caldwell DE, Korber DR, Lappin-Scott HM. Microbial biofilms. Annu Rev Microbiol 1995; 49: 711 – 745.

Costerton JW, Stewart PS, Greenberg EP. Bacterial biofilms: a common cause of persistent infections. Science 1999; 284: 1318 – 1322.

Davis N, Curry A, Gambhir AK et al. Intraoperative bacterial contamination in operations for joint replacement. J Bone Joint Surg Br 1999; 81: 886 – 889.

Duncan CP, Beauchamp C. A temporary antibiotic-loaded joint replacement system for management of complex infections involving the hip. Orthop Clin North Am 1993; 751 – 759.

Dupont JA. Significance of operative cultures in total hip arthroplasty. Clin Orthop 1986; 211: 122 – 127.

Denstedt JD, Wollin TA, Reid G. Biomaterials used in urology: current issues of biocompatibility, infection, and encrustation. J Endourol 1998; 12: 493 – 500.

Ensing GT, Roeder BL, Nelson JL et al. Effect of pulsed ultrasound in combination with gentamicin on bacterial viability in biofilms on bone cement in vivo. J Appl Microbiol 2005; 99: 443 – 448.

Espehaug B, Engesaeter LB, Vollset SE, Havelin LI, Langeland N. Antibiotic prophylaxis in total hip arthroplasty. Review of 10 905 primary cemented total hip replacements reported to the Norwegian arthroplasty register, 1987 to 1995. J Bone Joint Surg Br 1997; 79: 590 – 595.

Espehaug B, Furnes O, Havelin LI, Engesaeter LB, Vollset SE, Kindseth O. Registration completeness in the Norwegian Arthroplasty Register. Acta Orthop 2006; 77: 49 – 56.

Fitzgerald RH Jr. Infected total hip arthroplasty: diagnosis and treatment. J Am Acad Orthop Surg 1995; 3: 249 – 262.

Garvin KL, Hinrichs SH, Urban JA. Emerging antibiotic-resistant bacteria. Their treatment in total joint arthroplasty. Clin Orthop 1999; 369: 110 – 123.

Gristina AG, Costerton JW. Bacterial adherence to biomaterials and tissue. The significance of its role in clinical sepsis. J Bone Joint Surg Am 1985; 67: 264 – 273.

Gristina AG. Biomaterial-centered infection; microbial adhesion versus tissue integration. Science 1987; 237: 1588 – 1595.

Gristina AG. Implant failure and the immuno-incompetent fibro-inflammatory zone. Clin Orthop 1994; 298: 106 – 118.

Harris WH, Sledge CB. Total hip and total knee replacement (part II). N Engl J Med 1990; 323: 801 – 807.

Heck D, Rosenberg A, Schink-Ascani M, Garbus S, Kiewitt T. Use of antibiotic-impregnated cement during hip and knee arthroplasty in the United States. J Arthrop 1995; 10: 470 – 475.

Hendriks JGE, Ensing GT, van Horn JR et al. Increased release of gentamicin from acrylic bone cements under influence of low-frequency ultrasound. J Control Release 2003; 92: 369 – 374.

Hendriks JGE, Neut D, Van Horn JR, Van der Mei HC, Busscher HJ. Bacterial survival in the interfacial gap in gentamicin-loaded acrylic bone cements. J Bone Joint Surg Br 2005; 87-B: 272 – 276.

Hoeffel DP, Hinrichs SH, Garvin KL. Molecular diagnostics for the detection of musculoskeletal infection. Clin Orthop 1999; 360: 37 – 46.

Josefsson G, Gudmundsson G, Kolmert L, Wijkstrom S. Prophylaxis with systemic antibiotics versus gentamicin bone cement in total hip arthroplasty. A five-year survey of 1688 hips. Clin Orthop 1990; 253: 173 – 178.

Josefsson G, Kolmert L. Prophylaxis with systematic antibiotics versus gentamicin bone cement in total hip arthroplasty. A ten-year survey of 1688 hips. Clin Orthop 1993; 292: 210 – 214.

Khoury AE, Lam K, Ellis B, Costerton JW. Prevention and control of bacterial infections associated with medical devices. ASAIO J 1992; 383: M174 – 178.

Klekamp J, Dawson JM, Haas DW, DeBoer D, Christie M. The use of vancomycin and tobramycin in acrylic bone cement: biomechanical effects and elution kinetics for use in joint arthroplasty. J Arthroplasty 1999; 14: 339 – 346.

Knobben BA, van Horn JR, van der Mei HC, Busscher HJ. Evaluation of measures to decrease intraoperative bacterial contamination in orthopedic implant surgery. J Hosp Infect 2006; 62: 174 – 180.

Konig DP, Schierholz JM, Hilgers RD, Bertram C, Perdreau-Remington F, Rutt J. In-vitro adherence and accumulation of Staphylococcus epidermidis RP 62 A and Staphylococcus epidermidis M7 on four different bone cements. Langenbecks Arch Surg 2001; 386: 328 – 332.

Kuechle DK, Landon GC, Musher DM, Noble PC. Elution of vancomycin, daptomycin and amikacin from acrylic bone cement. Clin Orthop 1991; 264: 302 – 308.

Kühn KD. Bone Cements. Up-to-date comparison of physical and chemical properties of commercial materials. Springer-Verlag Berlin Heidelberg, 2000.

Lattimer GL, Kebish PA, Dickson TB Jr, Vernick CG, Finnegan WJ. Hematogenous infection in total joint replacement. Recommendations for prophylactic antibiotics. JAMA 1979; 242: 2213–2214.

Lidwell OM, Lowbury EJ, Whyte W, Blowers R, Stanley SJ, Lowe D. Airborne contamination of wounds in joint replacement operations: the relationship to sepsis rates. J Hosp Infect 1983; 4: 111–131.

Lynch M, Esser MP, Shelley P, Wroblewski BM. Deep infection in Charnley low-friction arthroplasty, comparison of plain and gentamicin-loaded cement. J Bone Joint Surg Br 1987; 69: 355–360.

Maathuis PGM, Neut D, Busscher HJ, Van der Mei HC, Van Horn JR. Peroperative contamination in primary total hip arthroplasty. Clin Orthop 2005; 433: 136–139.

McDonald DJ, Fitzgerald RH Jr, Ilstrup DM. Two-stage reconstruction of a total hip arthroplasty because of infection. J Bone Joint Surg Am 1989; 71: 828–834.

Murray PR, Pfaller MA, Rosenthal KS, Kobayashi G. Medical Microbiology, Mosby-Year Book, Incorporated, Chapter 20: Antibacterial Agents, 3rd Edition, 1998: 165–168.

Nelson CL, Evans RP, Blaha JD, Calhoun J, Henry SL, Patzakis MJ. A comparison of gentamicin-impregnated polymethylmethacrylate bead implantation to conventional parenteral antibiotic therapy in infected total hip and knee arthroplasty. Clin Orthop 1993; 295: 96–101.

Neut D, Van de Belt H, Stokroos I, van Horn JR, van der Mei HC, Busscher HJ. Biomaterial-associated infection of gentamicin-loaded PMMA beads in orthopedic revision surgery. J Antimicrob Chemother 2001; 47: 885–891.

Neut D, van de Belt H, van Horn JR, van der Mei HC, Busscher HJ. The effect of mixing on gentamicin release from polymethylmethacrylate bone cements. Acta Orthop Scand 2003; 74: 670–676.

Neut D, Van Horn JR, Van Kooten TG, Van der Mei HC, Busscher HJ. Detection of biomaterial-associated infections in orthopedic joint implants. Clin Orthop 2003: 413: 261–268.

Neut D, de Groot EP, Kowalski RS, van Horn JR, van der Mei HC, Busscher HJ. Gentamicin-loaded bone cement with clindamycin or fusidic acid added: biofilm formation and antibiotic release. J Biomed Mater Res A 2005; 73: 165–170.

Nijhof MW, Stallmann HP, Vogely HC et al. Prevention of infection with tobramycin-containing bone cement or systemic cefazolin in an animal model. J Biomed Mater Res 2000; 52: 709–715.

Nijhof MW, Fleer A, Hardus K et al. Tobramycin-containing bone cement and systemic cefazolin in a one-stage revision. Treatment of infection in a rabbit model. J Biomed Mater Res 2001; 58: 747–753.

Oga M, Arizono T, Sugioka Y. Inhibition of bacterial adherence to tobramycin-impregnated PMMA bone cement. Acta Orthop Scand 1992; 63: 301–304.

Penner MJ, Masri BA, Duncan CP. Elution characteristics of vancomycin and tobramycin combined in acrylic bone cement. J Arthroplasty 1996; 11: 939–944.

Persson U, Persson M, Malchau H. The economics of preventing revisions in total hip replacement. Acta Orthop Scand 1999; 70: 163–169.

Petty W, Spanier S, Shuster JJ. Prevention of infection after total joint replacement. Experiments with a canine model. J Bone Joint Surg Am 1988; 70: 536–539.

Pitt WG, McBride MO, Lunceford JK, Roper RJ, Sagers RD. Ultrasonic enhancement of antibiotic action on gram-negative bacteria. Antimicrob Agents Chemother 1994; 38: 2577–2582.

Proctor RA, Peters G. Small colony variants in staphylococcal infections: diagnostic and therapeutic implications. Clin Infect Dis 1998; 27: 419–422.

Rediske AM, Rapoport N, Pitt WG. Reducing bacterial resistance to antibiotics with ultrasound. Lett Appl Microbiol 1999; 28: 81–84.

Rodeheaver GT, Rukstalis D, Bono M, Bellamy W. A new model of bone infection used to evaluate the efficacy of antibiotic-impregnated polymethylmethacrylate cement. Clin Orthop 1983; 178: 303–311.

Schurman DJ, Trindale C, Hirschman HP, Moser K, Kajiyama G, Stevens P. Antibiotic-loaded acrylic bone cement composites. J Bone Joint Surg Am 1978; 60: 978–984.

Sculco TP. The economic impact of infected joint arthroplasty. Orthopedics 1995; 18: 871–873.

Sharma S, Gopalakrishnan S, Aasuri MK, Garg P, Rao GN. Trends in contact lens-associated microbial keratitis in Southern India. Ophthalmology 2003; 110: 138–143.

Tachibana K, Tachibana S. Application of ultrasound energy as a new drug delivery system. Nippon Yakurigaku Zasshi 1999; 114: 138–141.

Tattevin P, Cremieux AC, Pottier P, Huten D, Carbon C. Prosthetic joint infection: when can prosthesis salvage be considered? Clin Infect Dis 1999; 29: 292–295.

Thomes B, Murray P, Bouchier-Hayes D. Development of resistant strains of Staphylococcus epidermidis on gentamicin-loaded bone cement in vivo. J Bone Joint Surg Br 2002; 84: 758–760.

Törholm C, Lidgren L, Lindberg L, Kahlmeter G. Total hip joint arthroplasty with gentamicin-impregnated cement. A clinical study of gentamicin excretion kinetics. Clin Orthop 1983; 181: 99–106.

Trippel SB. Antibiotic-impregnated cement in total joint arthroplasty. J Bone Joint Surg Am 1986; 68: 1297–1302.

Tunney MM, Patrick S, Gorman SP et al. Improved detection of infection in hip replacements. A currently underestimated problem. J Bone Joint Surg Br 1998; 80: 568–572.

Wahlig H, Dingeldein E. Antibiotics and bone cements. Experimental and clinical long-term observations. Acta Orthop Scand. 1980; 51: 49–56.

Walenkamp GH, Vree TB, Van Rens TJ. Gentamicin-PMMA beads. Pharmacokinetic and nephrotoxicological study. Clin Orthop 1986; 205: 171 – 183.

Walenkamp GHIM. Chronic osteomyelitis. Acta Orthop Scand 1997; 68: 497 – 506.

Wahlig H, Buchholz HW. Experimentelle und klinische Untersuchungen zur Freisetzung von Gentamycin aus einem Knochenzement. Chirurg 1972; 43: 441 – 445.

Welch AB. Antibiotics in acrylic bone cement. In-vivo studies. J Biomed Mater Res 1978; 12: 843 – 855.

Wixson RL, Lautenschlager EP, Novak MA. Vacuum mixing of acrylic bone cement. J Arthroplasty 1987; 2: 141 – 149.

Zimmerli W, Widmer AF, Blatter M, Frei R, Ochsner PE. Role of rifampin for treatment of orthopedic implant-related staphylococcal infections: a randomized controled trial. Foreign-Body Infection (FBI) Study Group. JAMA 1998; 279: 1537 – 1541.

D New Antibiotic Carriers and Coatings in Surgery

Axel W. Stemberger, Joachim Schwabe, Karim Ibrahim, Florian Matl,
Michaela Rößner, Sebastian Vogt, Klaus-Dieter Kühn

Introduction

Biomaterials are an undeniable attribute of modern medicine in the Western hemisphere. These materials include contact lenses, dental fillings, resorbable sutures, bone screws, vascular prostheses and artificial joints, and they even offer the possibility of replacing a complete organ such as an artificial heart.

The materials applied at this moment in time have been developed to function for an entire lifetime. Unfortunately, however, it still has not been possible to control interactions with living organisms. Infection and rejection of the implants are reactions which can lead to encapsulation and, as a result, loss of function. This border area between implant and tissue has moved more strongly into the limelight of research into biomaterials (Gristina, 1987).

The infection of biomaterials introduced into the body, such as endoprostheses or vascular prostheses, can prove to be fatal for the patient and presents a major financial burden for the economy. The implant can weaken the body's own immune resistance in the surrounding tissues, and adhering bacteria evade host defense by forming a biofilm. For this reason, the prevention of bacterial colonization is of special interest. The germs colonizing biomaterials mostly are *Staphylococcus epidermidis* and *Staphylococcus aureus* (Christensen et al., 1989).

Injury to the surrounding tissue is unavoidable during implantation, which results in an impaired blood circulation in this area and triggers an inflammatory reaction. Bacteria are more apt to colonize on the surface of the implant, where host defense is weakened, and blood supply is insufficient. When there is a clear manifestation of infection, antibiotics administered systemically unfortunately do not reach a high therapeutic level in the area directly surrounding the implant, so that long-term high doses of antibiotics are usually unsuccessful.

In addition, a reduction in the formation of free radicals within segmental nucleated leucocytes in the framework of the host defense has been described for several materials, such as, e.g., stainless steel, which incurs even more difficulties in eliminating infections associated with (steel) implants (Pascual et al., 1992). The ability of the organism to opsonize and phagocyte bacteria is severely limited.

When examining the relationship between implant, host, and bacteria, a competition for colonization of the implant surface can be observed. If the body's own cells are the first colonists, they form a cell "lawn", made of connective tissue. This makes it difficult for the bacteria to adhere to the surface and thus effectively protects the implant from infection. If, however, the bacteria win the race, they can, like the body's own cells, form a slimy biofilm which in turn protects itself from disintegration through host immune cells. This is called the "race for the surface" (Gristina et al., 1994). Endoprostheses, catheters, heart valves, pacemakers, shunts, etc. are especially susceptible. The biofilm not only protects bacteria from the host immune system, but it also supplies bacteria with a greater resistance against antibiotics due to ionic interactions (Olson et al., 2002; Peters et al., 1982), (Fig. 2.**1**).

High local drug levels can be attained on the implant's surface without systemic side effects through the local application of antibiotics with a "drug delivery system". The combination of gentamicin with a collagen sponge that can be resorbed in the body has been introduced as an additional therapeutic concept for the local control of bone infections (Stemberger et al., 1997).

Resorbable polymers based on polylactic acid (PLA) or polyglycolic acid, have been used in the field of surgical wound closure for a long time.

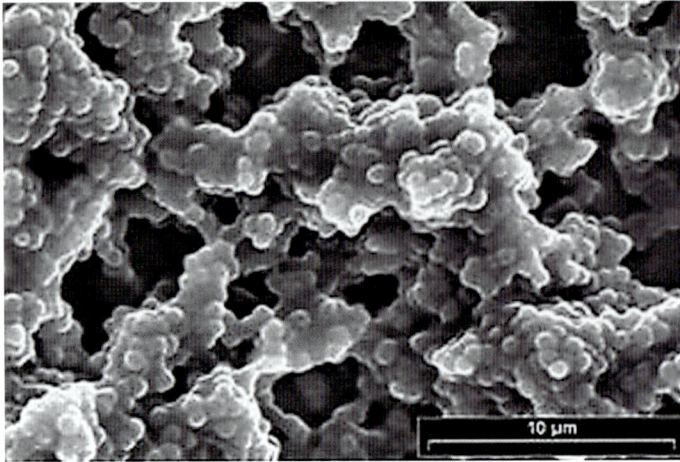

Fig. 2.**1** Biofilm of *Staphylococcus epidermidis*. Scanning electron microscopy (SEM). The scaffoldlike structure of the biofilm creates cavities, through which deeper lying bacteria can easily be supplied with nutrients (With kind permission of the Friedrich-Baur Research Institute for Biomaterials, University of Bayreuth).

The key word here is: resorbable suture materials. The combination of these polymers with drugs for implant coating, the so-called "drug delivery system", is a recently promising area of application for targeted local drug levels. The list of applicable drugs is almost unlimited. According to the indication, they can be applied with antibiotics, anticoagulants, cortisone, growth factors or even for non-viral gene transfer. Through local release, high drug levels can be attained at only the targeted area, and side effects are negligible (Bouma et al., 2002; Gollwitzer et al., 2003; Gollwitzer et al., 2005; Lucke et al., 2003; Lucke et al., 2005).

Schmidmaier showed that local application of growth factors with a PLA-coating of osteosynthesis materials improved fracture healing (Schmidmaier et al., 2001).

After extensive development, a coating with PLA for medullary pins was developed as an infection prophylaxis device for clinical use. No systemic side effects of incorporated gentamicin have been observed.

New developments include the attempt to coat implants directly with hard-to-dissolve drug combinations on the basis of fatty acids or related compounds or to manufacture retarded drug formulations with bioresorbable carriers for targeted local application.

Polytetrafluoroethylene (PTFE) prostheses were coated with various gentamicin salts of lauric acid (laurate compound), palmitic acid (palmitate compound) as well as sodium dodecyl sulfate (SDS compound) using methanol or a mixture of chloroform with methanol. Dental implants were coated exclusively with gentamicin palmitate (Vogt et al. 2003; Vogt et al. 2005).

We conducted examinations to assess PTFE prostheses / dental implants and test tubes (model for thrombogenocity) coated with various gentamicin salts (Figs. 2.**2a** and 2.**2b**) with regard to the following characteristics:

* release of gentamicin in relation to the retarding compound,
* thrombogenicity / antithrombogenicity, and
* antiinfective properties.

Materials and Methods

In order to characterize the release behavior of the retarding gentamicin salts, the coated dental implants as well as the PTFE prosthesis parts were eluted in phosphate-buffered-saline (PBS) at 37 °C. At the points of time t = 15 min, 1 h, 4 h, 8 h and 24 h, samples were taken and the elution medium was replaced completely. The gentamicin released in the eluates in the corresponding time period was examined by means of TDX Assay (Abbott Company, Institut für klinische Chemie und Pathobiochemie, am Klinikum r. d. Isar).

For blood clotting analyses, human blood, that was freshly drawn and not anticoagulated, was carefully filled into coated test tubes, then suctioned off again after a 7-minute incubation period and finally washed three times with PBS. The evaluation of the test tubes with respect to blood

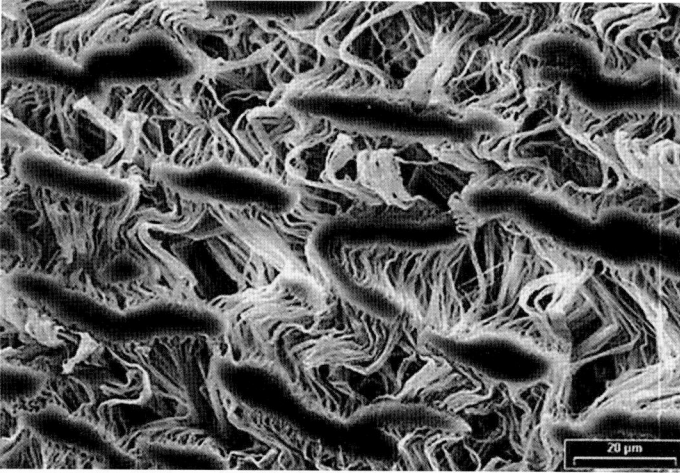

Fig. 2.**2a** SEM characterization of PTFE prosthesis following G palmitate coating.
uncoated

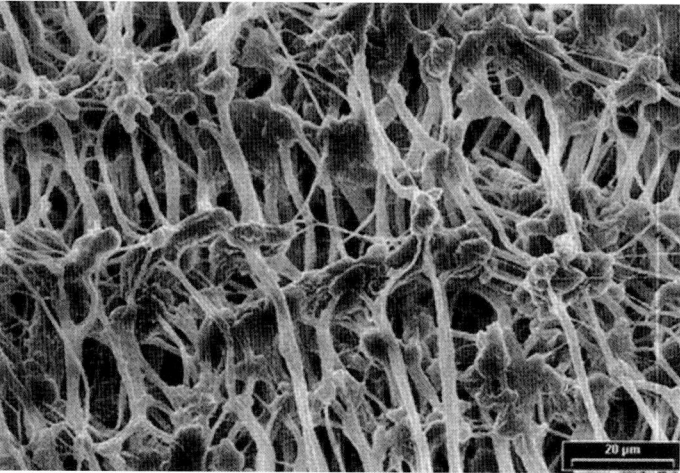

Fig. 2.**2b** coated

clots was carried out macroscopically and documented by photos.

PTFE prostheses with *non*anticoagulated human blood were incubated following the same procedure; after 7 minutes the blood was suctioned off, to be subsequently analyzed for blood deposits.

Investigations to determine the antiinfective characteristics were conducted with a human pathogenic germ (*Staphylococcus epidermidis* ATCC 35984). The bacterial solution consisted of 9/10 PBS and 1/10 tryptic soy broth as nutrient solution. 1 cm-long coated PTFE prosthesis parts with an average coating weight of 1.1 mg were used for incubation. At the beginning of the test,

half of the samples of each type of coating were eluted in 10 mL of PBS for 2 hours. The eluate obtained, was then inoculated with 10 000 colony-forming units (CFU) of *Staphylococcus epidermidis*, and after at least 2 hours of contact time 100 µL of this solution was plated. The further procedure was the same for all eluted/*non*eluted samples. For each, 2 mL of the bacterial solution with increasing germ concentration (1000, 5000, 10 000 CFU/mL) served as incubation solution for the prostheses, which were incubated at 37 °C for 17 hours. For each sample, 50 µL of the incubation solution was analyzed after this time period; the prosthesis parts were removed, washed in PBS three times in order to remove *non*adherent germs and then treated in 1 mL of PBS with ultrasound for 10 minutes. 100 µL of this solution were analyzed for any detached germs to prove the presence of adhering germs.

Release of gentamicin from the different compounds of the coated PTFE prostheses or dental implants was determined by means of TDX assay. Best results were demonstrated for the palmitate compound (Fig. 2.3).

To investigate hemocompatibility after coating with the retarding gentamicin salts, test tubes were coated for orientation tests and then filled with *non*anticoagulated blood from healthy donors. Coated test tubes showed promising hemocompatible results (Fig. 2.4).

PTFE vascular prostheses (Alpha-Research Company, Berlin) were then coated with the different gentamicin compounds and evaluated macroscopically after blood contact with regard to blood deposits and in comparison to the uncoated PTFE vascular prostheses.

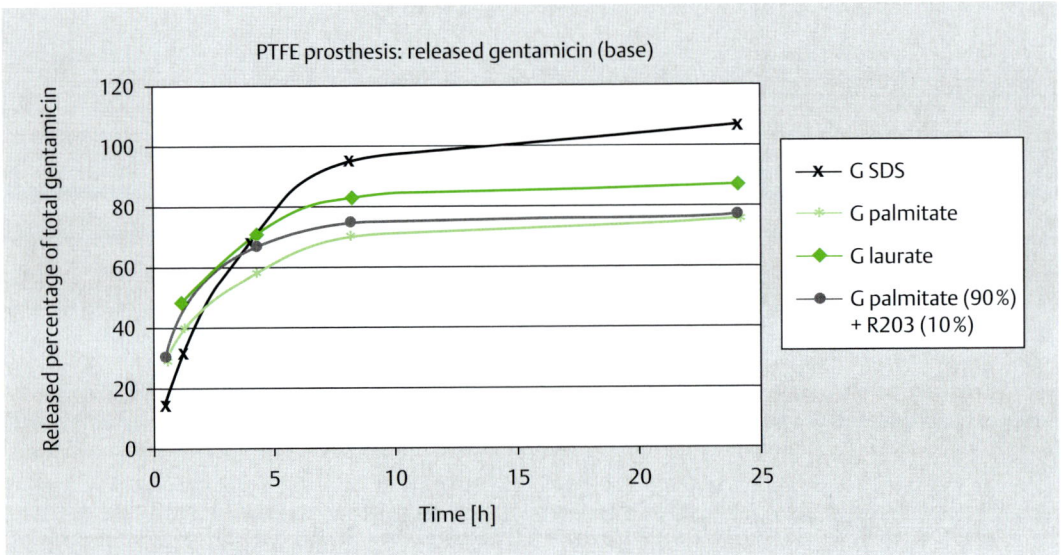

Fig. 2.3   Gentamicin release after coating of PTFE prosthesis with different gentamicin formulations.

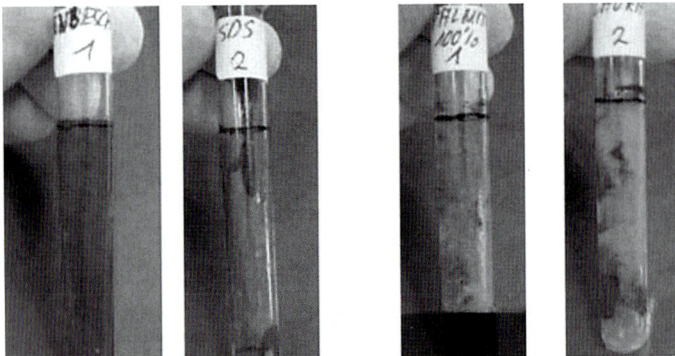

Fig. 2.4   Blood clots adhering on *non*coated test tubes after 7-minute incubation. The applied coating technology reduces thrombus formation.

Results

Coated as well as uncoated PTFE vascular prostheses showed very good hemocompatible characteristics (Figs. 2.**5a** and 2.**5b**).

The data verify that especially coating with gentamicin palmitate can further improve the good hemocompatibility of the PTFE vascular prostheses.

The findings that retarding gentamicin salts on the basis of the palmitate, laurate and SDS compound show evidence of antithrombogenic properties after contact with *non*anticoagulated human blood must be evaluated as unexpectedly positive.

A decisive parameter for the clinical application of PTFE vascular prostheses coated with retarding gentamicin salts, is the resistance against bacterial colonization. As described, uncoated and coated prosthesis parts (length 1 cm) were incubated with *Staphylococcus epidermidis* in rising concentrations of 1000, 5000 and 10 000 CFU/mL and the antiinfective characteristics were tested in relation to the gentamicin salt coating. The resistance of the coated vascular prostheses to colonization was determined after a 2-hour period of elution.

For all the uncoated prostheses, a distinct colonization with *Staphylococcus epidermidis* could be proven, whereas no colonies could be isolated on gentamicin-coated prostheses, independent of the used gentamicin salts (Table 2.**1**).

PTFE prostheses coated with retarding gentamicin palmitate demonstrate a very good protective effect against bacterial colonization. This could also be proven for large amounts of germs (10 000 CFU/mL of *Staphylococcus epidermidis* per cm of prosthesis length). Even after a two-hour elution, the coated prostheses still demonstrated complete protection against bacterial colonization with 10 000 CFU/mL of *Staphylococcus epidermidis*.

With regard to the clinical application, it can be concluded that long-term protection against bacterial colonization can be expected immediately after implantation of the coated prosthesis and after contact of the prosthesis with flowing blood.

Discussion

Infections associated with implants are feared side effects, as many of these complications can lead to implant failure, associated with life-threatening problems. In an attempt to prevent these complications, new techniques and drug compounds have been developed in recent years.

The goal of this study was the development of a locally effective drug delivery system, by coating implants with new antibiotic salts on the basis of fatty acids.

Effective antibacterial levels were determined in vitro, and investigations concerning the adhe-

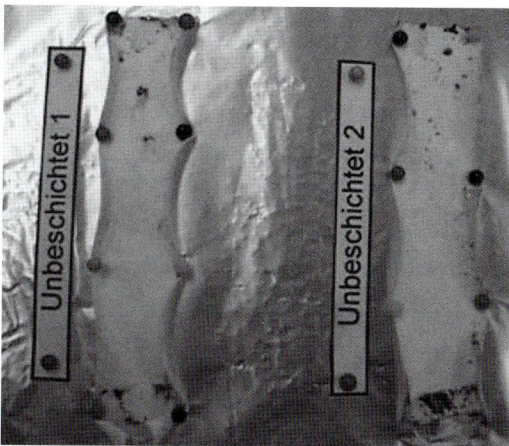

Fig. 2.**5a** Inner surface of PTFE vascular prostheses after blood contact.
Uncoated PTFE vascular prostheses.

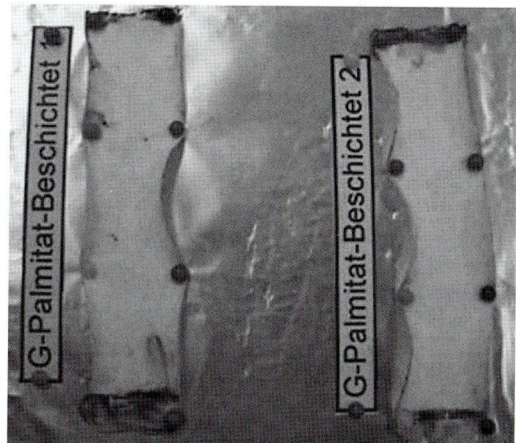

Fig. 2.**5b** PTFE vascular prostheses coated with G palmitate.

Table 2.1 Growth of *Staphylococcus epidermidis* on coated versus uncoated PTFE prostheses

	Elution 2 h	CFU/mL	Supernatant	Prosthesis
Uncoated	No	5 000	+++	+++
Uncoated	No	10 000	+++	+++
G palmitate 7	No	1 000	0	0
G palmitate 9	No	5 000	0	0
G palmitate 11	No	10 000	+	0
G palmitate 1	Yes	1 000	0	0
G palmitate 3	Yes	5 000	96	0
G palmitate 5	Yes	10 000	20	0

sion and ability to prevent colonization of bacteria were carried out.

In addition to their application in vascular prostheses and dental implants, biodegradable materials for bone replacement can also be used as local antibiotic delivery systems. Biodegradable materials for bone replacements are generally intended to fill up bone cavities. Bone cavities resulting from radical debridement during surgical sanitation of osteomyelitis, can also be filled up with suitable materials for bone replacement. In order to effectively protect these implant materials from microbial colonization, replacement materials equipped with broad spectrum antibiotics are advantageous. Palasorb G beads are a recent development. These beads are a composite calci-

um sulfate-dihydrate, calcium carbonate, tripalmitin and gentamicin sulfate (Kühn and Vogt, 2000), (Fig. 2.6).

Palasorb G beads are biocompatible according to ISO10993. During in-vitro conditions, the Palasorb G beads demonstrate delayed release of gentamicin in the serous medium for a time period of several days (Fig. 2.7).

Animal experiments have been started to corroborate the delayed in-vitro release characteristics and the biocompatible cell culture experiments (Fig. 2.8).

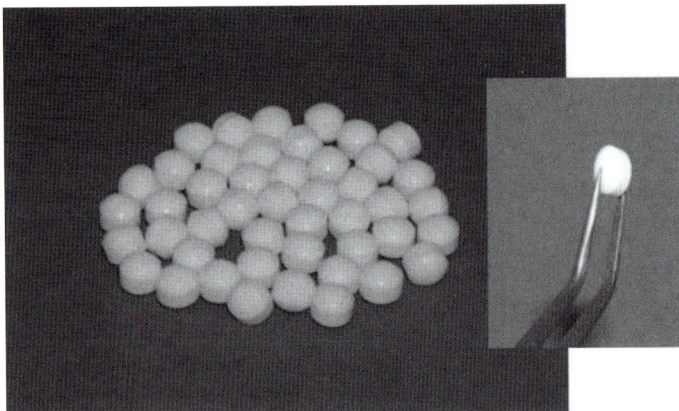

Fig. 2.6 Palasorb G beads (calcium sulfate-dihydrate, calcium carbonate, tripalmitin, gentamicin).

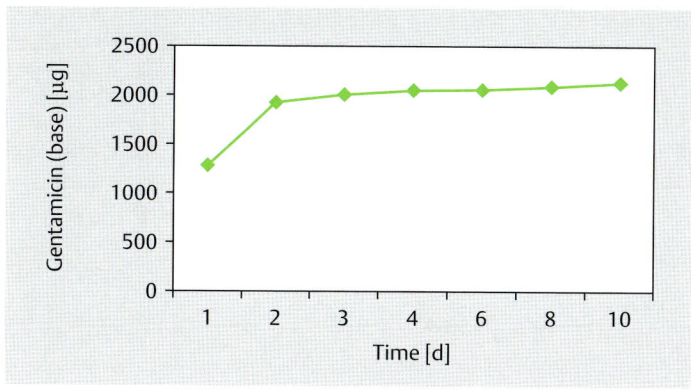

Fig. 2.**7**   In-vitro release of gentamicin from a Palasorb G bead
(37 °C / phosphate buffer pH 7.4).

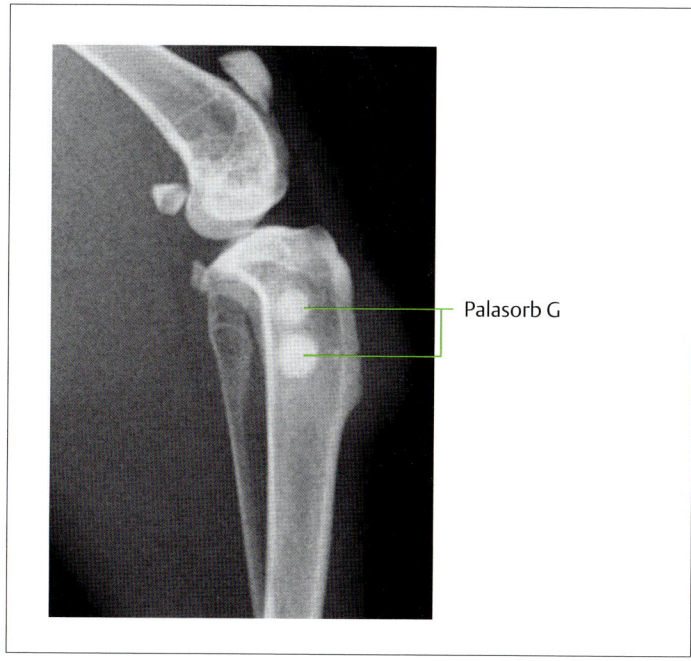

Palasorb G

Fig. 2.**8**   Palasorb G beads following
implantation into a rabbit's femur,
post-operation.

Conclusion

These results confirm both the retarding and the antiinfective characteristics of a gentamicin palmitate. Combinations with known polymers such as poly-d,l-lactide (Resomer, R 203, Boehringer Ingelheim) can lead to improved retarding characteristics of the incorporated antibiotics for heavily strained implants. Promising investigations into new coating technologies are on the way (Fig. 2.**9**).

Acknowledgement: The authors gratefully acknowledge funding from Alpha Research (Berlin, Germany) and Heraeus-Kulzer GmbH (Wehrheim, Germany).

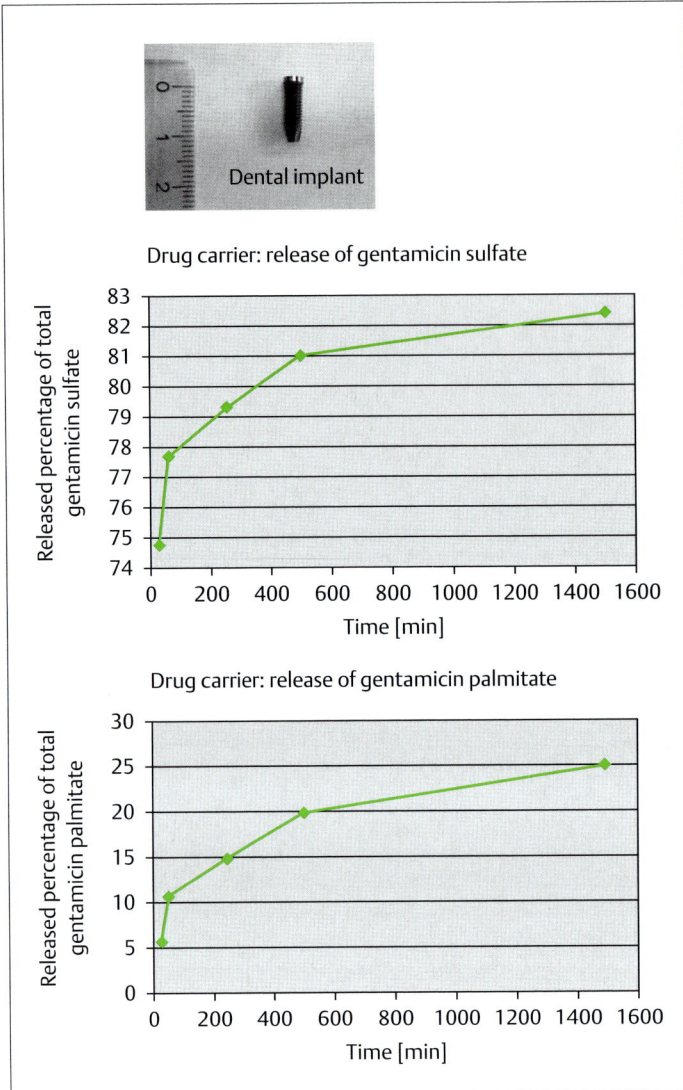

Fig. 2.**9** New coating technology using gentamicin sulfate and palmitate incorporated into a resorbable drug carrier (R 203) for dental implant coating (dental implants provided by Heraeus Kulzer GmbH).

References

Bouma MG, van As HLJJ, Knyer R, Kühn KD, Walenkamp GHIM. In-vitro and in-vivo characteristics of resorbable gentamicin polylactide in the treatment of osteomyelitis. 7th European Symposium on controlled drug delivery. Noordwigk, NL 2002; Proceedings Vol 87: 199–202.

Christensen G, Baddour L, Hasty D, Lowrance J, Simpson W. Microbial and Foreign Body Factors in the Pathogenesis of Medical Device Infections. Edited by A. L. Bisno and F. A. Waldvogel. American Society for Microbiology 1989.

Gollwitzer H, Thomas P, Diehl P et al. Biomechanical and allergological characteristics of a biodegradable poly(D,L-lactic acid) coating for orthopaedic implants. J Orthop Res 2005 Jul; 23 (4): 802–809.

Gollwitzer H, Ibrahim K, Meyer H, Mittelmeier W, Busch R, Stemberger A. Antibacterial poly(D,L-lactic acid) coating of medical implants using a biodegradable drug delivery technology. J Antimicrob Chemother 2003 Mar; 51 (3): 585–591.

Gristina AG. Implantat Failure and the Immuno-Incompetent Fibro-Inflammatory Zone. Clinical Orthopaedics and Related Research 1994; 298: 106–118.

Gristina AG. Biomaterial-Centered Infection. Microbial Adhesion Versus Tissue Integration. Science 1987; 237: 1588–1595.

Kühn KD, Vogt S. Antibiotikum / Antibiotika enthaltendes Knochenersatzmaterial mit retardierter Wirkstofffreisetzung. EP 1671661 A2, 2003.

Lucke M, Wildemann B, Sadoni S et al. Systemic versus local application of gentamicin in prophylaxis of implant-related osteomyelitis in a rat model. Bone 2005 May; 36 (5): 770–778. Epub 2005 Mar 24.

Lucke M, Schmidmaier G, Sadoni S et al. A new model of implant-related osteomyelitis in rats. J Biomed Mater Res B Appl Biomater 2003 Oct 15; 67 (1): 593–602.

Olson ME, Ceri H, Morck DW, Buret AG, Read RR. Biofilm bacteria: formation and comparative susceptibility to antibiotics. Can J Vet Res 2002; 66 (2): 86–92.

Pascual A, Tsukayama D, Wicklund B et al. The Effect of Stainless Steel, Cobalt-Chromium, Titanium Alloy, and Titanium on the Respiratory Burst Activity of Human Polymorphonuclear Leukocytes. Clinical Orthopaedics and Related Research 1992; 280: 281–287.

Peters G, Locci R, Pulverer G. Adherence and growth of coagulase-negative staphylococci on surfaces of intravenous catheters. The Journal of Infectious Diseases 1982; 146: 479–482.

Schmidmaier G, Wildemann B, Bail H et al. Local Application of growth factors (insulin-like growth factor-1 and transforming growth factor-beta 1) from a biodegradable poly(D,L-lactide) coating of osteosynthetic implants accelerates fracture healing in rats. Bone 2001; 28 (4): 341–350.

Stemberger A, Grimm H, Bader F, Rahn HD, Ascherl R. Local treatment of bone and soft tissue infections with the collagen-gentamicin sponge. Eur J Surg Suppl 1997; 578: 17–26. Review.

Vogt S, Kühn KD, Schnabelrauch M. Poröse Implantatkörper mit antibiotischer Beschichtung, ihre Herstellung sowie Verwendung. EP 1364923 A2 2003.

Vogt S, Kühn KD, Gopp U, Schnabelrauch M. Resorbable antibiotic coatings for bone substitutes and implantable devices. Mat.-wiss u. Werkstofftech 2005; 36: 814–819.

(D) Antimicrobial Implant Coating in Arthroplasty

Klaus-Dieter Kühn, Sebastian Vogt

Introduction

Posttraumatic and postoperative osteitis are considered the major complications in traumatic and orthopedic surgery. These infections result in considerable consequences for the patient and substantial medical costs (Darouiche 2001; Schierholz and Beuth, 2001; Safdar and Maki, 2002). In extreme cases, such infections may result in the loss of limbs and life-threatening sepsis. In addition to the compliance with strict hygienic standards and the systemic administration of antibiotics, any method that allows the application of antimicrobial substances directly onto the surface of the implant is highly welcome to prevent the implant surface from being colonized by bacteria and to thus avoid these severe infections.

The posttraumatic and postoperative osteitis is mainly caused by Gram-positive germs, like *Staphylococcus aureus* and *Staphylococcus epidermidis*. These germs are part of the natural skin flora of humans and occur ubiquitously. Recently, also Gram-negative germs have begun to play a more important role.

Nasser (1999) found out that 50–80% of all postoperative infections are associated with the microbial contamination of the operation field. The incubation time for posttraumatic, postoperative infections may amount to several weeks or months. After the microbial colonization on the implant surface, the germs can hardly be destroyed by the natural immune system or systemically administered antibiotics due to the formation of a biofilm. Therefore a local release of antimicrobial substances from the implant surface appears recommendable, in order to effectively prevent a potential colonization (Rushton, 1997; Holtom, 2003). The antimicrobial protection of the implant surface should be provided for several days.

Antimicrobial Protection of Cemented Endoprostheses

Today, two different methods for endoprosthesis fixation are applied: cemented and cementless arthroplasty. For cemented prostheses, the addition of antibiotics, e.g., gentamicin sulfate, to polymethylmethacrylate (PMMA) bone cements has represented a successful method for approximately 30 years (Kühn, 2002). Thermo stability and high water solubility of the antibiotics are fundamental requirements. The antibiotics are added to the cement powder. Following implantation, these PMMA bone cements release antibiotics locally. The occurrence of postoperative infections for total hip and knee replacements has been significantly reduced due to the utilization of antibiotic-containing PMMA bone cements, the strict compliance with hygienic standards, and preoperative systemic antibiotic administration. The antibiotic release from the PMMA bone cements is initiated by secretion and blood. The therein included fluid penetrates the cement surface and provides diffusion into the cement matrix. During this process the antibiotic dissolves into the areas close to the surface and diffuses to the cement surface. This means the release of the antibiotic from the cement matrix depends on the surface properties and follows the rules of diffusion. This process is also closely related to the hydrophilic properties of the bone cement. Therefore, the release of active agents proceeds proportionally to the water absorption on the one hand and to the available cement surface on the other hand. The composition of the polymers in the bone cement and thus the water absorption of the cement significantly influence the release of the active agent (Fig. 3.**1**).

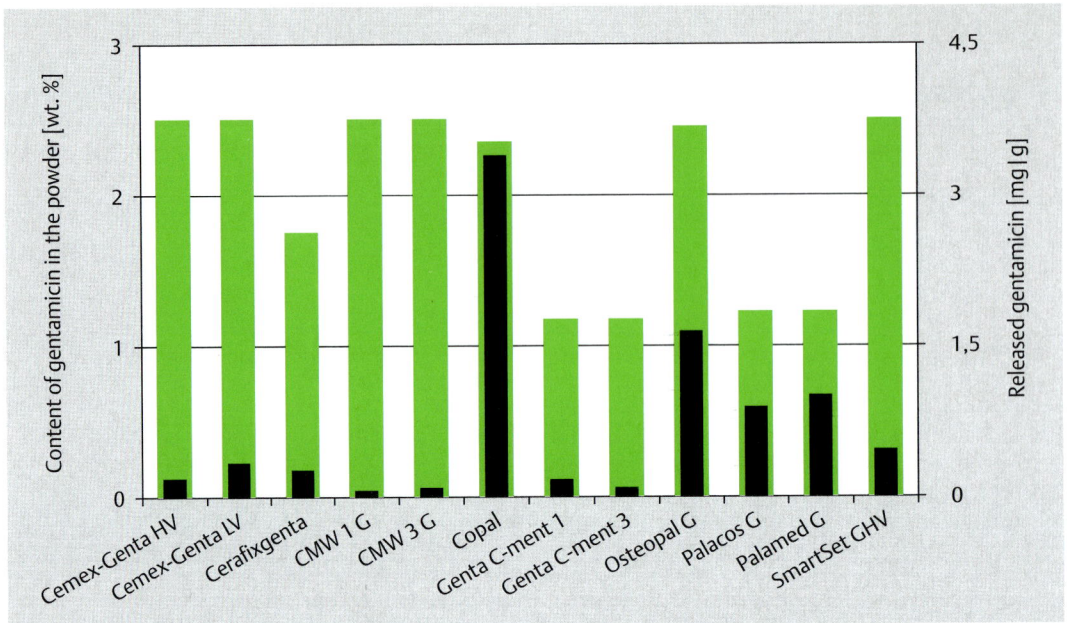

Fig. 3.1   Release of gentamicin from PMMA bone cements – A comparison of various bone cements (Kühn et al., 2005).

Antimicrobial Protection of Cementless Endoprostheses

The local antimicrobial protection of the surface of cementless endoprostheses has more or less been disregarded until today. The following methods for the local protection of the implant surface are known: One option is the integration of antibiotics/antiseptics into a polymer layer-forming carrier system (Kanellakopoulou and Giamarellos-Bourboulis, 2000; Anderson, 2003; Price et al., 1996; Gollwitzer et al., 2003; Lucke et al., 2003). A further method is to include antibiotics/antiseptics into porous hydroxylapatite coatings (Alt et al., 2006). Another alternative is to coat implant devices with heavy metal/heavy metal salts (Illingworth et al., 2000; Darouiche, 1999; Trerotola et al., 1998; Grzybowski and Trafny, 1999; Ziegler et al., 2003). A relatively new and until today more or less neglected method, is the coating with self-adhesive, low-soluble antibiotic salts (Kühn et al, 2003; Vogt et al., 2005). Four local coating methods are listed in Table 3.1.

Polymer layer-forming carrier system with incorporated antibiotics/antiseptics

The development of polymer layer-forming carrier systems with incorporated antibiotics can be attributed in particular to Gollwitzer et al., (2003). These coatings are composed of biodegradable polyesters, e.g., polylactide, including gentamicin sulfate as antibiotic. They offer the benefit that different soluble antibiotics/antiseptics may be included without requiring chemical modifications of the active substance, and that registered polymers like polylactide can be applied as layer-forming material. Thus, the registration process is less extensive compared to novel carrier systems and novel active agents, respectively. However, these coatings also reveal drawbacks. In general, active substance suspensions are used for the coating process. These active substance suspensions have to provide homogeneity during the coating process in order to achieve reproducible loading concentrations. In principle, active substance release does not proceed synchronously to the degradation rate of the polymer layers. For the application of polymer layer-forming carriers, based on hydroxycarboxylic acid, the formation of

Table 3.**1**   Advantages and disadvantages of 4 local coating methods

Approach	Advantages	Disadvantages
Polymer layer-forming carrier with incorporated antibiotics	▪ Antibiotics may be highly soluble in water ▪ Different antibiotics may be used without modification ▪ Use of approved layer-forming material	▪ Coating technology with suspensions complex ▪ Release of antibiotics not synchronic with layer degradation ▪ Polymer layer-forming materials (PLLA) degrade slowly, releasing degradation products (acid release) ▪ Layer as additional barrier to bone growth
Antibiotics in porous hydroxyl apatite coatings	▪ Use of easily soluble antibiotics ▪ No modification required ▪ No polymer layer-forming material ▪ No degradation products ▪ Use of typical HA-coated implants	▪ Limited protraction of antibiotic release ▪ Easily soluble antibiotics are quickly dissolved from the surface ▪ Limited to HA-coated implants
Coating with heavy metals or heavy metal salts	▪ Silver or copper (ions) with broad antimicrobial effect ▪ Relatively cost-saving	▪ Silver and copper ions are potentially cytotoxic ▪ Unspecific effect ▪ Silver ions react with human proteins ▪ Silver ions form hardly soluble salts ▪ Silver ions are easy to reduce
Coating with self-adhesive low-soluble antibiotic salts	▪ No polymeric layer ▪ No acidic degradation products ▪ Antibiotic release synchronic with layer degradation ▪ Simple coating technology	▪ Sparingly soluble salts of antibiotics accessible by ion exchange ▪ Problem of registration / approval

acid degradation products has to be taken into consideration.

Antibiotics / antiseptics included in porous hydroxyl apatite coatings

In 2006 Alt (Alt et al., 2006) reported first experiences with implants in animals that were furnished with a porous hydroxyl apatite coating, including gentamicin sulfate and gentamicin crobefat in their cavities. This option offers the benefit that polymer layers are not necessary and, therefore, the imponderabilities of degradation products can be avoided. In addition, ordinary commercially available hydroxyl apatite-coated prostheses and implant devices can be used. This method, however, reveals the drawback that a delayed active substance release can only be achieved by the application of active substances with low solubility. The adhesion of commercially registered antibiotics in the hydroxylapatite layer is relatively low. The loading capacity is mainly determined by the pore volume of the hydroxyl apatite coating.

Coating with heavy metal / heavy metal salts

During the last years, the application of heavy metals and heavy metal salts as microbiocides have received considerable attention (Illingworth et al., 2000; Darouiche, 1999; Ambrosius et al., 1998; Grzybowski and Trafny, 1999; Ziegler et al.,

2003). Particularly silver in form of nano particles and low soluble silver salts have been of special interest. The applicability of copper also has been extensively investigated. Heavy metals and heavy metal salts offer a beneficially broad antimicrobial efficacy at relatively low costs. Furthermore, heavy metals and heavy metal salts can be applied to a variety of surfaces and can be integrated into implants so that effectual metal concentrations at the implant surface are provided. However, the low selectivity of heavy metals is disadvantageous. Heavy metal ions, like silver ions, do not specifically react with microbial structures, but are likely to react with human or animal cells and cell components. Thus, the antimicrobial depth effect of silver ions in the bone tissue is limited because silver ions may react with components of the bone tissue, forming low soluble salts. Furthermore, heavy metal ions can be easily reduced. In general, for the use of heavy metals / heavy metal salts as a component of antimicrobial coatings the considerable potential of cytotoxicity should be taken into consideration. Currently, the company Implantcast GmbH manufactures and sells custom-made products in Germany.

Coating with self-adhesive, low-soluble antibiotic salts

Antibiotics based on aminoglycosides feature a broad range of efficacy. The bactericidal antibiotics gentamicin and tobramycin are aminoglycoside antibiotics, and have been used successfully for PMMA bone cements for years. Gentamicin and tobramycin are employed in the sulfate form.

Gentamicin sulfate is the substance most often used in PMMA bone cements for local antimicrobial protection. Gentamicin sulfate consists of a mixture of gentamicin C1, C1a and C2a+b. It is highly water soluble and does not reveal extensive adhesion on metal surfaces. Being a cationic antibiotic, it possesses five proton amino groups. Gentamicin adds itself to bacterial ribosomes and disrupts or inhibits the bacterial protein synthesis. As a result, nonsense proteins that damage bacterial membranes are formed.

By transferring the water soluble gentamicin sulfate into a low-soluble gentamicin fatty acid salt, it can be used as coating material (Kühn et al., 2003; Vogt et al., 2005).

Gentamicin sulfate can be converted into a gentamicin fatty acid salt by ion exchange, whereby sulfate ions are replaced by fatty acid anions (Fig. 3.**2**). Suitable fatty acid anions are laurate, myristate and palmitate. The protonic gentamicin base remains unchanged during the ion exchange process. The antimicrobially active gentamicin base is not chemically modified. Also, the proportion between gentamicin C1 and C1a and C2a+b is not modified. The gentamicin fatty acid salts are waxy solids featuring an extensive adhesion property on a variety of surfaces in thin layers. The fatty acid anions are *non*toxic and can be metabolized in the human organism by β-oxidation, which generates carbon dioxide and water.

The antimicrobial active substance of the gentamicin sulfate and the gentamicin palmitate is the protonic gentamicin base.

Gentamicin palmitate is of special interest for antimicrobial coating. This salt is a colourless to yellowish waxy solid that dissolves in organic solvents. Gentamicin palmitate can be applied to the surface of cementless endoprostheses by spray coat method (Figs. 3.**3** and 3.**4**). The loading capacity can be largely varied (up to 300 µg gentamicin base / cm^2). Depending on the test conditions, the gentamicin release takes place within a period of 10 – 14 days under in-vitro conditions. The coated endoprostheses can be sterilized by gamma radiation.

In a study, we compared the gentamicin base release of gentamicin palmitate-coated, sandblasted titanium plates with the gentamicin release of Palacos R+G (Fig. 3.**5**).

The results demonstrate a continuous gentamicin release from the gentamicin palmitate coating, similar to Palacos R+G. Therefore, it can be assumed that the local protective ability of the gentamicin palmitate coating on the implant surface is similar to the antimicrobial protection of the cement surface of Palacos R+G.

First trials on an animal test model investigating the osteointegration of gentamicin palmitate-coated, sand-blasted titanium bars, did not reveal any undesired side effects. The osteointegration of the coated titanium bars was comparable to the osteointegration of *non*coated titanium bars.

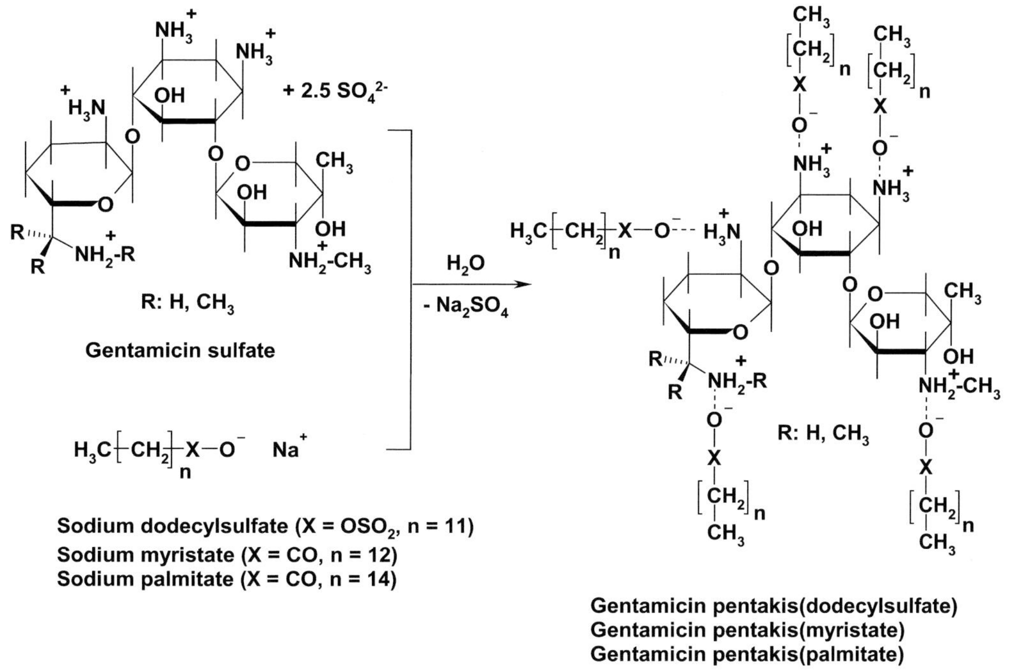

Fig. 3.**2** Synthesis of sparingly soluble fatty acid salts of gentamicin by ion exchange (Vogt et al., 2005).

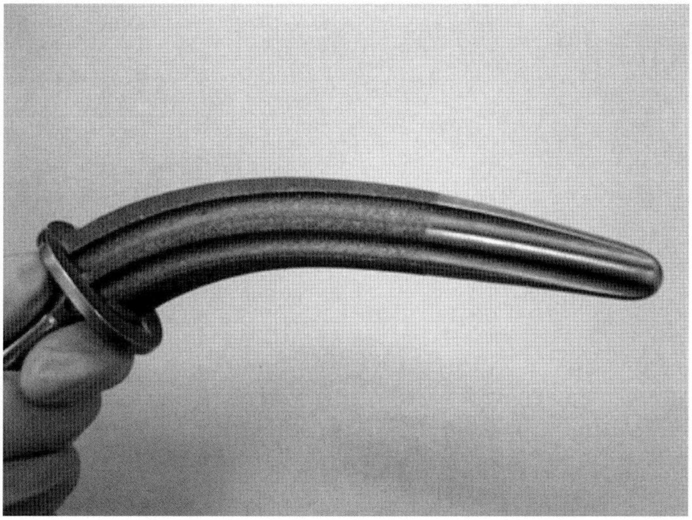

Fig. 3.**3** Uncoated hip endoprosthesis.

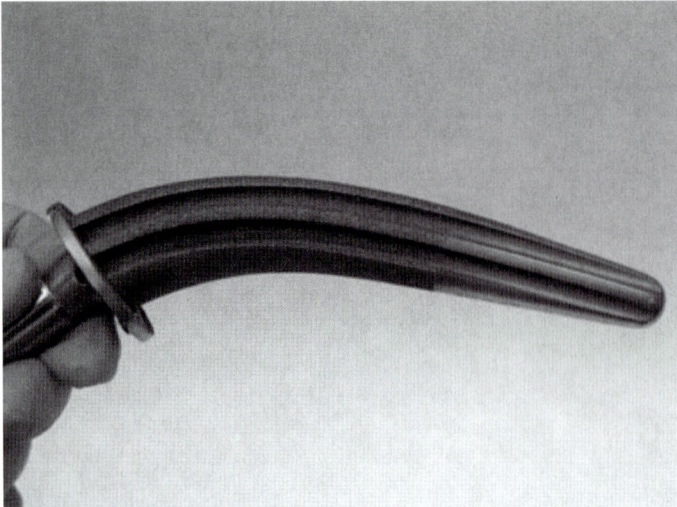

Fig. 3.**4** Gentamicin palmitate-coated hip endoprosthesis.

Summary and Preview

A variety of methods for antimicrobial coating of endoprostheses have been discussed:
1. Polymer layer-forming carrier systems with incorporated antibiotics,
2. Antibiotics included in porous hydroxyl apatite coating,
3. Coating with heavy metal / heavy metal salts, and
4. Coating with self-adhesive, low-soluble antibiotic salts.

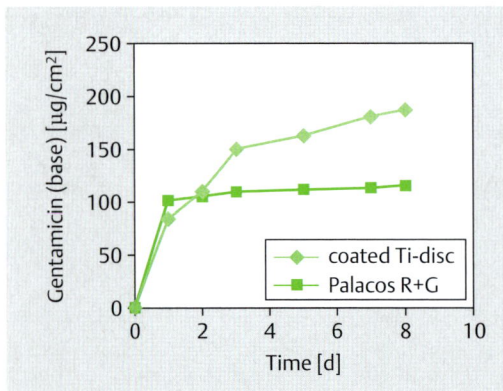

Fig. 3.**5** Release results of a coated titanium plate (loading capacity 853 µg gentamicin palmitate / cm², 221 µg gentamicin base / cm²) compared to the gentamicin release from Palacos R + G.

Gentamicin palmitate was used as an example to illustrate coating with low-soluble antibiotic salts in detail. The active substance release with this coating is comparable to the active substance release from antibiotic-containing PMMA bone cements.

Antimicrobial-coated endoprostheses are designed to provide a sustainable benefit for the patient in the future, and to profoundly contribute to substantial cost reductions by a decline of septic revisions. It can be assumed that antimicrobial-coated endoprostheses will gain the same recognition in the future as antibiotic-loaded PMMA bone cements.

References

Alt V, Bitschnau A, Osterling J et al. The effects of combined gentamicin-hydroxyapatite coating for cementless joint prostheses on the reduction of infection rates in a rabbit infection prophylaxis model. Biomaterials. 2006; 26: 4627 – 4634.

Anderson AB. Combining local drug delivery and implantable medical devices. Med Device Technol 2003; 14 (7): 16 – 19.

Darouiche RO. Anti-infective efficacy of silver-coated medical protheses. Clin Infect Dis 1999; 29 (6): 1371 – 1377.

Darouiche RO. Device-associated infections: a macroproblem that starts with microadherence. Clinic Infect Dis 2001; 33 (9): 1567 – 1572.

Gollwitzer H, Ibrahim K, Meyer H, Mittelmeier W, Busch R, Stemberger A. Antibacterial poly (D,L-lactic acid) coating of medical implants using a bio-degradable drug delivery technology. Antimicrob Chemother 2003; 51 (3): 585–591.

Grzybowski J, Trafny EA. Antimicrobial properties of copper-coated electroconductive polyester fibers. Polim Med 1999; 29 (1–2): 27–33.

Holtom PD. Newer methods of antimicrobial delivery for bone and joint infections. Instr Course Lect 2003; 52: 745–749.

Ilingworth B, Bianco RW, Weisberg S. In vivo efficacy of silver-coated fabric against staphylococcus epidermidis. J Heart Valve Dis 2000; 9 (1): 135–141.

Kanellakopoulou EJ, Giamarellos-Bourboulis EJ. Carrier systems for the local delivery of antibiotics in bone infections. Drugs 2000; 59 (6): 1223–1232.

Kühn KD. Bone Cements. Up-to-date comparison of physical and chemical properties of commercial materials. Springer-Verlag, Berlin Heidelberg, 2000.

Kühn KD, Vogt S, Schnabelrauch M. Porous implants with antibiotic coating, their preparation and use EP 1374923 B1, 2003.

Lucke M, Schmidmaier G, Sadoni S et al. Gentamicin coating of metallic implants reduces implant-related osteomyelitis in rats. Bone 2003; 32 (5): 521.

Nasser S. The incidence of sepsis after total hip replacement arthroplasty. Semin Arthroplasty 1999; 5 (4): 153–159.

Price JS, Tencer FA, Arm DM, Bohach GA. Controlled release of antibiotics from coated orthopaedic implants. Biomed Mater Res 1996; 30: 281.

Rushton N. Applications of local antibiotic therapy. Eur. J Surg 1997; 578: 27–30.

Safdar N, Maki DG. The commonality of risk factors for nosocomial colonization and infection with antimicrobial-resistant staphylococcus aureus, enterococcus, gram-negative bacilli, clostridium difficile, and candida. Ann Intern Med 2002; 136 (11): 834–844.

Schierholz JM, Beuth J. Implant infections: a haven for opportunistic bacteria. J Hosp Infect 2001; 49 (2): 87–93.

Trerotola SO, Johnson MS, Shah H et al. Tunneled hemodialysis catheters: use of a silver-coated catheter for prevention of infection – a randomized study. Radiology 1998; 207 (2): 491–496.

Vogt S, Kühn KD, Gopp U, Schnabelrauch M. Mat.-wiss. u. Werkstofftechn. Resorbable antibiotic coatings for bone substitutes and implantable devices 2005; 36: 814–819.

Ziegler G, Gollwitzer H, Heidenau F, Mittelmeier W, Stenzel F. Anti-infectious, biocompatible titanium oxide coatings for implants, and method for the production thereof WO2004/026346 A2, 2003.

(NL) Bone Cements – Are They Different?

Pieter T. J. Spierings

Introduction

Bone cement is the common name for fast-curing resins, which are used for fixation of artificial joint prostheses. Any material that is biocompatible, is able to fill the space between implant and bone, cures at room temperature, and is set in approximately 10 minutes can be called bone cement. Contrarily to what the name "cement" suggests, bone cement bonds neither to a prosthesis nor to bone. Despite the fact that most bone cements show adhesive properties during the curing process, this adhesive property is lost immediately after curing. Cements are used purely as filler materials. This specific ability to fill even the smallest crevices secures a strong mechanical interlock with any nonsmooth surface, like trabecular bone or a rough or structured metal surface. Hence cements stabilize the implant by mechanical interlock only. By filling the gap between implant and bone, cements transfer the joint load and because their modulus of elasticity is much less than that of bone and metal, they are capable of smoothing interface stresses.

Various types of bone cements have been applied commercially. The most commonly used types are acrylic cements based on methylmethacrylate (MMA) polymers. Other types of cements have been used clinically in the past, but they soon were abandoned. Glass ionomer cements, resorbable CaP-cements and bioactive cements were assumed to bond better to bone, to be more biocompatible and to enhance bone ingrowth. None of them were successful. Several types of fibers have been tested to reinforce cements such as glass, carbon and Kevlar fibers. These types failed because of granulomatous reactions on wear particles. So far, only acrylic cements have stood the test of time.

In the following chapters various differences of properties of commercially available acrylic cements will be discussed.

Chemistry

The basic material polymethylmethacrylate (PMMA) has been used for more than a century. It is well-known under the trade names Plexiglas and Perspex. In 1902, Otto Rhöm wrote a thesis on the synthesis of this artificial material. Today, Rhöm GmbH is still one of the leading manufacturers of acrylic monomers and polymers used in industry and in bone cements. The breakthrough to apply PMMA for orthopedic surgery was in 1943, when a patent was filed on a method to polymerize PMMA at room temperature by means of tertiary amines. Shortly afterwards, various researchers and clinicians started experiments with this material as an anchorage medium for implants. In 1952, Haboush was the first to publish on the application of cold curing PMMA for the fixation of a hip prosthesis (Haboush, 1952). The first commercial cements were released in the beginning of the seventies. Little has changed since then. Most original cements like Palacos, CMW, Surgical Simplex and Zimmer bone cements, are still on the market with an unchanged chemical composition. One major modification was the addition of antibiotics in the eighties.

All acrylic cements are composed of a powder and a liquid component. A typical composition is shown in Table 4.1.

The powder component mainly contains PMMA. If all monomer molecules of the powder polymer are identical, we call it a homopolymer. If a polymer is composed of different types of monomer molecules, we call it a copolymer. Bone cements may contain up to 10% w/w copolymers. Often manufacturers use a combination of two different powders. By slightly adjusting the ratio between the two powders they are able to compensate for any batch differences in the base materials and to keep the handling characteristics of the cement constant. The liquid component

Table 4.1 Traditional chemical composition of cold curing PMMA bone cement

Powder	polymethylmethacrylate	90 % w/w
40 g	radiopacifier	9 % w/w
	benzoyl peroxide	1 % w/w
Liquid	methylmethacrylate	98 % w/w
20 m/L	N-N dimethyl-p-toluidine	2 % w/w
	hydroquinone	25 – 100 ppm

mainly contains MMA, but also up to 5 % butyl-methacrylate (BMA) can be used. In exceptional cases like Boneloc cement, 50 % high molecular weight monomers are used. Methylacrylate (MA) monomer cannot be used because of it's bad smell.

There are many variables beyond the chemical description on the package insert, which determine the properties of a cement (Table 4.2).

Probably the most determining factor to characterize a type of cement is the type of molecule used for the powder component. Table 4.3 shows the types of polymer molecules used for various well-known cements.

Mechanical properties

Acrylic cement is a fairly brittle material and much stronger under compression than in tension (Kühn, 2000). Maximum tensile strain-to-failure is 2 %. This makes it vulnerable for enclosures like air voids and clusters of radiopacifier beads, which act as stress risers. The static tensile strength is in the order of 30 – 50 Mpa. In cyclic loading up to 10^7 cycles, the tensile strength is reduced to ± 10 Mpa. In static compression loading cement will not fracture but deform. Maximum compression strain is ± 7 %. Static compressive strength after polymerization of the residual monomer at 4 weeks after mixing is in the order of 90 – 120 Mpa. Cyclic compression loading at a physiological stress level of 5 –

Table 4.2 Additional parameters affecting cement properties

Powder/liquid ratio
Types of copolymer powder
Mixture ratio of polymers
Shape, mean size and size distribution of the powder beads
Molecular mean weight distribution
Moisture concentration
Particle size of BPO
Ratio of free and residual BPO
Type and particle size of radiopacifier
Reactor size, temperature and catalyst
Types of monomer
Mixture ratio of monomers
Filling weight accuracy

Table 4.3 Cement brands classified by type of powder copolymer

Type of copolymer	Brand
MMA homopolymer	CMW1
	CMW3
MMA/MA copolymer	Palacos R
	Palamed
	Osteopal
	Bone cement R
	SmartSet HV
MMA/BMA copolymer	Sulfix/Duracem
	Biolos1
	Biolos3
	Boneloc
MMA/Styrene copolymer	Surgical Simplex Ro
	CMW Endurance
	Zimmer Osteobond

Table 4.**4**   Effect of type of copolymer on mechanical properties

Elasticity	Molecule	Tglass [°C]
Ductile ↑	Methylacrylate	6
	Butylmethacrylate	20
	Ethylmethacrylate	65
↓	Methylmethacrylate	105
Brittle	Styrene	120

10 Mpa will not lead to failure. In-vivo failure is always associated with fatigue tensile fractures which are propagated through air enclosures (Topoleski, 1995).

Differences in the mechanical properties mainly depend on the type of copolymer. Small molecules like MA in the powder, will give the cement a more ductile behavior, while styrene will make the cement brittle. This effect of the type of molecule runs parallel with the glass transition temperature of these polymers (Table 4.**4**).

The failure strain in a static tensile test will express the effect of the type of copolymer, as can be seen in Table 4.**5**.

An MMA-MA copolymer cement like Palacos will have a high tensile strength and-strain because of its forgiveness for air inclusions due to its ductility. It will also exhibit a larger creep rate than a styrene cement. A styrene copolymer cement like Simplex, on the other hand, will exhibit a low failure strain in tensile testing, but also a low creep rate (Lee, 2005). Palacos shows a compression/tensile strength ratio of 2:1 in static testing while Surgical Simplex has a ratio of 3:1, see Table 4.**5**. A homopolymer cement like CMW 1 yields intermediate results.

Next to the chemical composition, the preparation method will have great effect on the strength of the reconstruction. Avoiding laminations, blood entrapment and a minimal cement layer thickness are important factors that are in the hands of the surgeon. Vacuum mixing can contribute significantly to the strength of the cement. A 30 % increase in static strength and fracture strain can be achieved, and the longevity in a fatigue test can be increased up to 10 times by vacuum mixing (Lewis, 1997).

Thermal properties

All acrylic cements produce heat during polymerization. The heat is released by opening of the double bond of the monomer molecule, while it forms a polymer chain. The amount of heat generation purely depends on the number of monomer molecules. The adiabatic temperature rise of a number of cements representing the amount of heat generated is listed in Table 4.**6**.

The temperature rise of the polymerizing cement resulting from this heat generation also depends on other factors like the powder/liquid (P/L) ratio and the speed of polymerization. The traditional cements with a P/L ratio of 40 g/20 mL all exhibit a similar adiabatic temperature rise of ±105° C. The so-called low temperature cements are in the range of 70–90 °C (Spierings, 2005).

In vivo, the temperature rise is much less because the cement cures in a thin layer and the surrounding bone and prosthesis act as a heat sink. In a test according to ISO5833:2002, the cement temperature rise is measured in the centre of a 6 mm thick plate surrounded by a plastic mold, see Figure 4.**1**.

The temperature rise is recorded as a function of time and the peak temperature and tempera-

Table 4.**5**   Mechanical properties as a function of type of copolymer (manual mixing, tensile test). MA-copolymer cements are relatively flexible with good tensile strength. Styrene-copolymer cements are relatively brittle with good compression strength.

Cement	Powder	Static tensile fracture strain	Tensile strength [MPa] at 28 days	Compression strength [MPa] at 28 days
Palacos R	MMA/MA copolymer	2.1 %	50	93
CMW 1	MMMA homopolymer	1.4 %	36	107
Surgical Simplex	MMA/Styrene copolymer	1.2 %	34	110

Table 4.6 Temperature rise of polymerizing bone cement in an adiabatic mold. Traditional cements, beneath the dotted line, with a powder/liquid ratio of 40 g/20 mL show a temperature rise of ± 105 °C. Low-temperature cements, above the dotted line, show an adiabatic rise of 70 to 90 °C.

Cement type	Temperature rise in adiabatic mold [°C]
Boneloc	71
Implast	76
Cemex RX	90
Sulfix-6	90
Zimmer LVC	104
Palacos R Genta	104
Palacos E flow	104
Palacos R	104
CMW3	105
Surgical Simplex RO	106

ture gradient can be derived from the graph in Figure 4.2.

The maximum ISO temperature rise of a number of bone cements is listed in Table 4.7.

A large difference in temperature rise is to be seen, and not all low-temperature cements perform much better than traditional cements.

Theoretically, the heat generation threatens the viability of the endosteal bone surrounding cemented implants. The thermal bone necrosis will lead to bone remodeling, and it is during this stage that the cemented reconstruction may be prone to aseptic loosening. For this reason, low-temperature cements were developed. Various methods are in use to reduce the amount of heat generation (Table 4.8).

Unfortunately, these methods will have a drawback. Adding water to the liquid, functions as a heat sink, but leads to a porous cement with reduced mechanical strength. A high P/L ratio reduces the number of monomers per weight unit of the powder, but leads to less comfortable mixing and the risk of an inhomogeneous mixture. High-molecular weight monomers, like in Boneloc cement, reduce the number of monomers per weight unit of the monomer, but bear the risk of difference in reactivity, polymer-incompatibility and segregation resulting in a weak matrix and weak matrix-powder bond. In general, all methods designed to reduce heat generation, will result in reduced mechanical strength. A reduced temperature at the cement-bone interface can also be obtained by method 4 in Table 4.8. A more gradual release of the polymerization heat will result in a decreased heat load of the bone, thereby reducing thermal bone tissue injury. The maximum temperature rise in an ISO 5833 test of 2 cements with a similar amount of heat generation is listed in Table 4.9.

Surgical Simplex cures more exponentially and has a 4 times higher maximum temperature gradient than Palacos R. This results in a 20 °C higher peak temperature than in Palacos R. The peak temperature rise is 46 °C for Palacos R and 66 °C for Surgical Simplex RO.

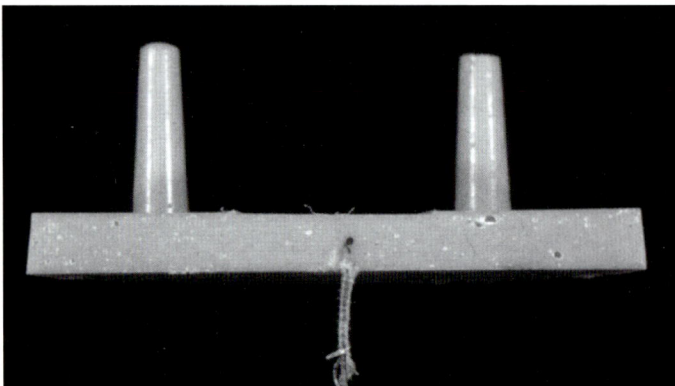

Fig. 4.1 Temperature test specimen according to ISO5833:2002.

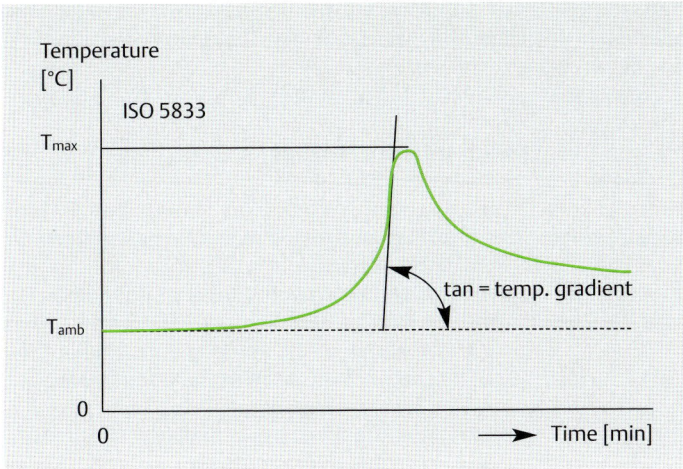

Fig. 4.**2** Temperature development as function of time according to ISO5833:2002.

Table 4.**7** Temperature rise in the center of a 6 mm thick cement specimen according to ISO 5833. Traditional cements, beneath the dotted line, all with the same amount of heat generation, show a large difference in temperature rise. Note that low temperature cements, above the dotted line, with less heat generation are not necessarily lower in peak temperature than traditional cements.

Cement type	Temperature rise in ISO 5833 mold [°C]
Boneloc	36
Cemex RX	44
Sulfix-6	47
Palacos R	46
Zimmer LVC	52
Palacos E flow	58
CMW3	60
Surgical Simplex RO	66

Table 4.**8** Various methods to reduce the temperature rise of curing cements. Methods 1 to 3 reduce the amount of heat generation. Method 4 reduces temperature rise by less exponential polymerization.

1. High molecular weight monomers (Boneloc)

2. High powder / liquid ratio (Cemex RX)

3. Addition of water to the liquid (Implast)

4. Gradual polymerization rate (Palacos)

Table 4.**9** Equal heat generation but different temperature rise of Surgical Simplex and Palacos R

	Adiabatic test	ISO 5833 / 1 test	
Type of cement	Temp. rise	Max. temp. gradient	Temp. rise
Surgical Simplex	106 °C	179 °C / min	66 °C
Palacos R	104 °C	42 °C / min	46 °C

The question arises, however, whether there is a clinical benefit from reducing the endosteal heat load. Cemented implants do not tend to fail during the remodeling period, which occurs during the first postoperative year. There are no clinical studies showing a benefit from low temperature cements for the survival of cemented implants. On the other hand, early animal studies already demonstrated that the thermally induced damage of the endosteal cortex is by far exceeded by the damage resulting from surgical disruption of the vascularisation, and the toxic effect of the cement's monomer (Feith, 1975).

Viscosity

Manufacturers often characterize and name their cement in terms of viscosity. Viscosity is a major parameter to describe the cement's handling characteristics. We will discuss high-, medium- and low-viscosity cements. In Figure 4.3 the viscosity

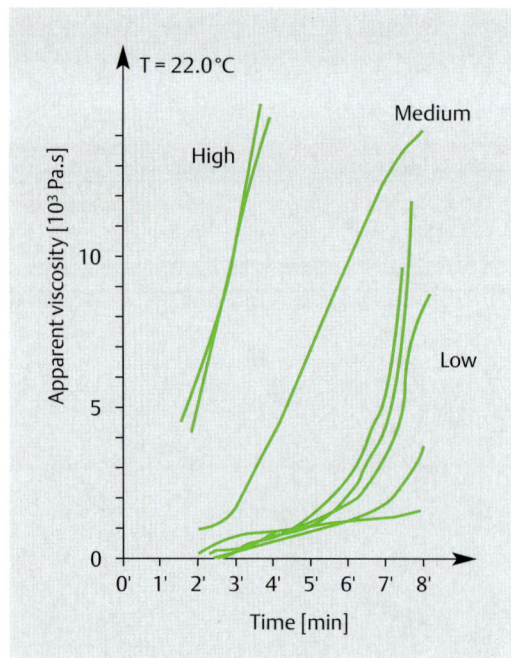

Fig. 4.3 High-, medium- and low-viscosity cements. Note the different viscosity gradients. Low-viscous cements initially take longer, but then polymerize much faster during the working period.

as a function of time is shown for a series of commercially available high-, medium- and low-viscosity cements.

High-viscosity cements

High-viscosity cements are those, which have such a high viscosity after mixing that they can only be handled manualy. This automaticaly implies that these cements are more difficult to use in a mechanical mixing system. Therefore, it is common use to cool these cements. Cooling decreases the viscosity, thereby enabling mixing in a bowl or cartridge vacuum system and easing extrusion through a nozzle. It also increases the setting time, which makes cooled cement suitable for more time-consuming modern cementing techniques like vacuum mixing and pressurizing (Table 4.10).

Reducing viscosity by cooling does not alter the shape of the viscosity development curve, but shifts it in time. The gradual viscosity development remains unchanged after cooling. Cooled high-viscosity cement will behave like uncooled medium-viscosity cement (Fig. 4.4).

The best known high-viscosity cements on the market are Palacos R and CMW1. Palacos R shows superior performance in both the Swedish and Norwegian register. The superior performance of Palacos R is not related to its high-viscosity behavior. In Sweden, 99 % of all cemented procedures are performed with cooled cement.

Table 4.10 Effect of cement cooling on the setting time and handling of Palacos R

Tcement [°C]	Setting time [min:sec.]	Extrusion comfort
4	13:00	very good
10	10:45	good
14	10:30	reasonably / good
18	10:15	reasonably
22	9:20	difficult

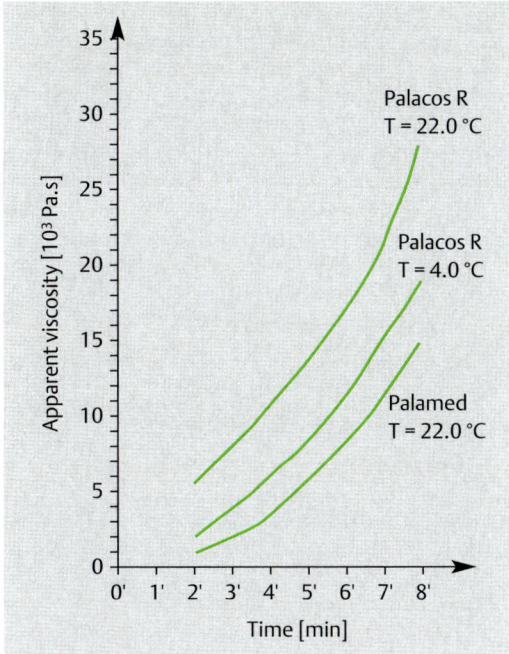

Fig. 4.**4** Cooling of Palacos R reduces the viscosity. The viscosity curve is shifted in time. Cooled Palacos R and uncooled medium-viscous Palamed cement will behave alike.

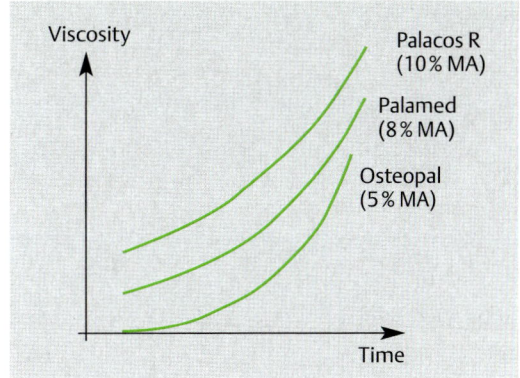

Fig. 4.**5** Effect of MA copolymer percentage on viscosity development. MA is a hydrophylic polymer and will absorb the monomer faster than PMMA. This results in a higher viscosity.

A low initial viscosity in combination with a normal setting time implies that the viscosity develops more exponentially than with traditional cements. Since there is a specific viscosity window, in which cement can be handled, the working time for low-viscosity cements is much shorter (Fig. 4.**6**).

Medium-viscosity cements

Medium-viscosity cements have an intermediate viscosity development, which makes them suitable for both manual and uncooled syringe application. Only few medium-viscosity cements exist. Surgical Simplex RO has the longest history. In the nineties Palamed was developed. It is a medium viscosity variant of Palacos R. It contains slightly less hydrophilic MA and has a slightly lower P/L ratio (Fig. 4.**5**). The idea was to create a cement with similar mechanical properties as Palacos R, but with no need for cooling, when applied in a syringe vacuum mixing system.

Low-viscosity cements

In the eighties, new cements were introduced with a very low initial viscosity. These cements were developed to ease retrograde extrusion of cement through the nozzle of a cement gun. Table 4.**11** lists a number of low viscosity cements.

Table 4.**11** Cement brands classified in terms of viscosity

Viscosity	Brand
Low	Osteopal
	CMW3
	Cerafix
	Zimmer regular
	Zimmer LVC
	Sulfix / Duracem
Medium	Surgical Simplex Ro
	Palamed
High	Palacos R
	Bone Cement R
	CMW1
	SmartSet HV

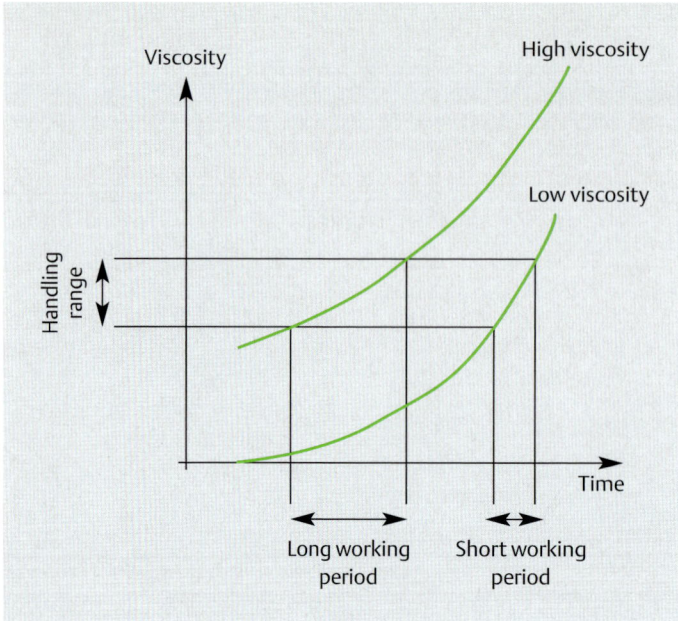

Fig. 4.**6** Effect of viscosity on the working period. The more exponential viscosity development of a low-viscosity cement reduces the working period.

Timing is, therefore, more critical, and deviations from the ideal time frame may lead to less favorable results. Early extrusion is technically a mess. The cement will leak easily, and will be difficult to contain for pressurization. Late extrusion will make it more difficult to operate the gun, and to insert the implant smoothly.

The initial viscosity can be decreased by various methods, like reducing the P/L ratio, decreasing the amount of BPO and/or DMPT, using larger powder beads, or using less hydrophylic polymers (Table 4.**12**).

Table 4.**12** Variables that affect the viscosity of cement

1. Powder/liquid ratio
2. Concentration of initiator and catalyst
3. Size and shape of polymer beads (CMW)
4. Type and amount of copolymer (Palacos)

Discussion

The choice for a particular type of bone cement is often made on historical grounds. In Europe, Palacos R cement has been the leading manufacturer on the market for decades. The same applies for Surgical Simplex RO on the American market. It is probably not by chance that both market leaders also supply the best long-term clinical results in the Scandinavian registers. However, these two cements are opposites in terms of chemistry and mechanical behavior. Palacos is a ductile cement with a large fracture strain, high tensile strength, and large creep rate. Surgical Simplex RO is a brittle cement, with a small fracture strain, less tensile strength, and a low creep rate. What they have in common, are the handling characteristics. In Scandinavia, Palacos R is predominantly applied when cooled. This increases the working and setting time, and it will behave as a medium-viscosity cement. Surgical Simplex RO, prepared at room temperature, already has a medium-viscosity development and a long setting time without cooling. They are both also normal temperature cements. It is unclear, why a homopolymer PMMA cement like CMW1, which is more or less in between Palacos and Simplex in terms of mechanical properties, performs less well clinically. Unfortunately, no direct comparative fatigue tests comparing these cements are published. A bone cement fatigue standard only exists since 2001 and comparative testing is very expensive and time-consuming (ASTM, 2001).

Other cement manufacturers recognized the success of Palacos R and Surgical Simplex RO and copied the formulations. Bone Cement R (Biomet) and SmartSet HV (DePuyCMW) have a similar chemistry as Palacos R. Bone Cement R shows fully equivalent properties in chemical testing, static and dynamic mechanical testing, handling, and antibiotics release. SmartSet HV deviates from the original. It has a higher viscosity, shorter setting time, and higher static strength. Also, Surgical Simplex RO was copied by Osteobond (Zimmer) and Endurance (DePuyCMW). Their chemistry and properties are alike, but not equivalent.

Conclusion

Users should be careful when selecting a type of bone cement. Low-temperature cements not only have no proven benefit, but also bear the risk of less mechanical performance. Low-viscosity cements are not required for the application of modern cementing techniques, but do have more difficult handling characteristics than medium or high viscosity cements. Their viscosity development is exponential and the working time is shorter. The best results are obtained with normal-temperature, medium- and high-viscosity cements. Palacos R and Surgical Simplex RO show the best clinical performance in large-scale registers.

References

ASTM F2118 – 2001. Test method for constant amplitude of force controlled fatigue testing of acrylic bone cements materials. ASTM International, USA 2001.

Feith R. Side-Effects of Acrylic Cement Implanted into Bone. Ph.D. Thesis, University of Nijmegen 1975.

Haboush EJ. A new operation for arthroplasty of the hip based on biomechanics, photoelasticity, fast-setting dental acrylic and other considerations. Scientific Exhibit, AAOS, Chicago, January 1952.

ISO 5833:2002, Implants for surgery-Acrylic resin cements. International Standardization Organisation, Switzerland 2002.

Kühn K-D. Bone Cements. Up-to-date comparison of physical and chemical properties of commercial materials. Springer-Verlag, Berlin Heidelberg, 2000.

Lee C. The Mechanical Properties of PMMA Bone Cement. In: Breusch SJ, Malchau H. editors, The Well-Cemented Total Hip Arthroplasty, Heidelberg. Springer Medizin Verlag 2005; 60 – 66.

Lewis G. Properties of Acrylic Bone Cement: State of Art Review. JBMR 1997; 38: 155 – 182.

Norwegian Arthroplasty Register 1987 – 2004. Scientific Exhibition 72nd Annual Meeting AAOS, Washington, February 2005.

Spierings PTJ. Testing and Performance of Bone Cements. In: Breusch SJ, Malchau H. editors, The Well-Cemented Total Hip Arthroplasty, Heidelberg. Springer Medizin Verlag 2005; 67 – 78.

Swedish National Hip Arthroplasty Registry 1979 – 1998. Scientific Exhibition 67th Annual Meeting AAOS, Orlando, March 2000.

Topoleski LDT, Ducheyne P, Cuckler JM. A fractographic analysis of in vivo poly(methylmethacrylate) bone cement failure mechanisms. JBMR 1990; 24: 135 – 154.

(N) Cancellous Bone Allograft as an Antibiotic Carrier – In-Vitro-, In-Vivo- and Clinical Studies

Eivind Witsø

Introduction

Loosened hip and knee prostheses are usually associated with loss of bone stock. To restore the skeleton morcelized cancellous bone can be impacted or transplanted when these prostheses are revised. At our department, this technique has been used since the early 1990s. In 2000, cancellous bone impaction was performed in approximately one quarter of all revisions of total hip prostheses in Norway (Norwegian Arthroplasty Register, 2003). In many cases, bone cement is not used when loosened hip prostheses are revised. Although the patients receive systemic antibiotic prophylaxis, and are operated in theaters with laminar air flow, cancellous bone impaction in uncemented revisions without applying antibiotic-containing bone cement, might expose the patient to an increased risk of postoperative infection. Therefore, in one- and two-stage revision procedures, the possibility of using bone grafts as a vehicle for antibiotic delivery is of special interest. In 1947, De Grood (De Grood, 1947) was the first to report on mixing penicillin with cancellous bone when filling bone defects. Two patients were successfully treated for residual cavities after osteomyelitis. Since then, several in-vitro- and in-vivo studies, as well as clinical studies on cancellous bone have been published (Miclau et al., 1993; Witsø et al., 1999; Winkler et al., 2000; Witsø et al., 2000; Witsø et al., 2002; Buttaro, 2003; Witsø et al., 2004; Buttaro et al., 2005a; Buttaro et al., 2005b; Buttaro et al., 2005c).

In-Vitro- and In-Vivo Studies

Different techniques have been used to impregnate cancellous bone allograft with antibiotics. Antibiotic powder was mixed with the bone graft (Buttaro et al., 2003, Buttaro et al., 2005) or bone grafts were impregnated in an antibiotic solution (Winkler et al., 2000; Witsø et al., 2004). The in-vitro elution of antibiotics in broth or albumin shows high early release with an exponential decay (Witsø et al., 1999; Winkler et al., 2000). The exponential decay indicates that the amount of antibiotic released each day, is proportional to the residual amount. The slope of the curve is antibiotic-specific (Fig. 5.1). After an initial phase of exponential decay, the aminoglycoside shows a period of slow release for several days, or even weeks.

Approximately 99.9% of the total amount of aminoglycoside adsorbed to bone is eluted during 6 weeks (Witsø et al., 2002). The release of vancomycin increases proportionally with the time used for antibiotic impregnation of bone, and the amount of vancomycin released decreases when aminoglycoside and vancomycin are combined in the impregnation fluid. The release of aminoglycoside and vancomycin from antibiotic-impregnated cancellous bone also depends on factors such as the pH of the impregnating fluid, the concentration of antibiotics in the impregnating fluid, and the degree of bone morcelization (Witsø et al., 2002). Generally, the amount of vancomycin released from cancellous allograft is not lower than that of an aminoglycoside. This is contrary to other studies on the release of aminoglycosides and glycopeptides from bone cement and poly-methylmethacrylate (PMMA) beads (Adams et al., 1992; Mader et al., 1997; Klekamp et al., 1999). We observed a more rapid release of aminoglycoside compared to vancomycin. The fraction of the total amount eluted during the first 24 hours of aminoglycoside and vancomycin was 80% and 30%, respectively (Witsø et al., 2002). In conclusion, by optimizing the conditions for antibiotic impregnation of bone, more than 70 mg of aminoglycoside (netilmicin) and more than 100 mg of vancomycin is released from 1 g of cancellous bone in vitro (Witsø et al., 2002).

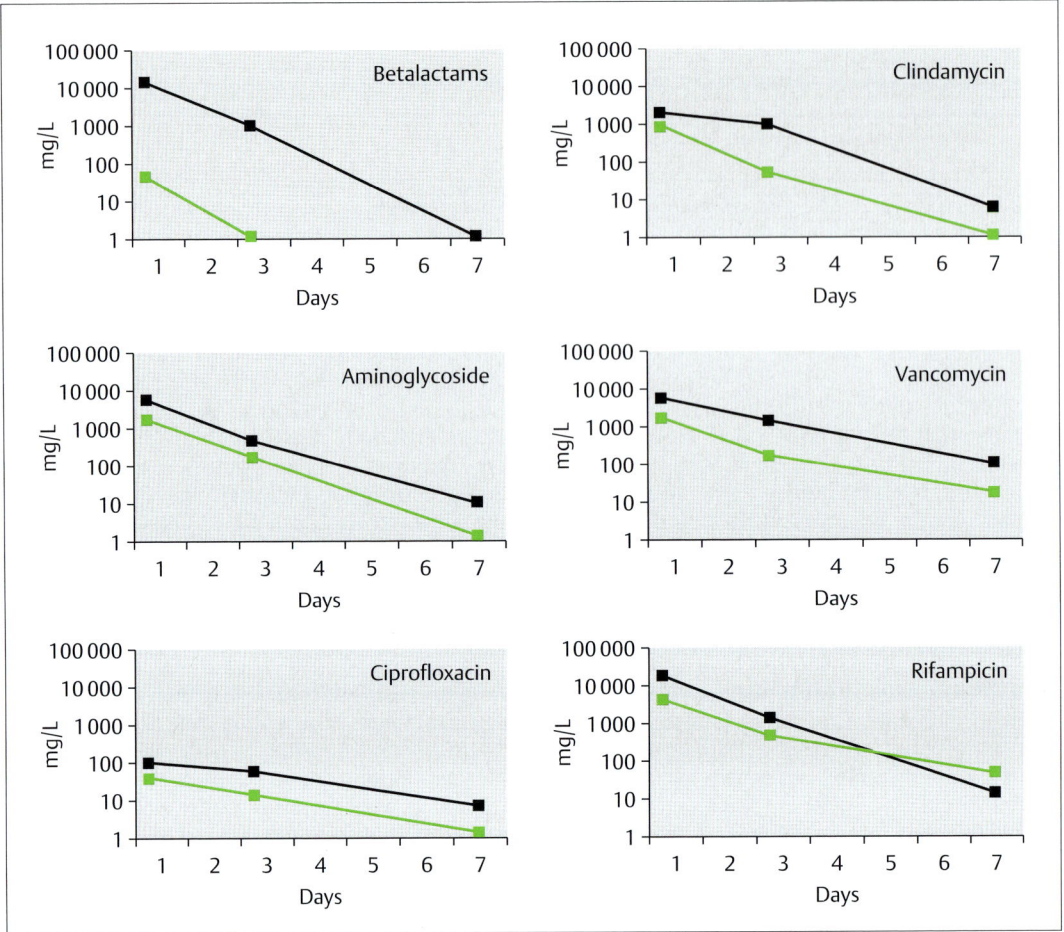

Fig. 5.1 Antibiotics have a similar elution profile when released from cancellous bone in vivo (green) and in vitro (black).

Antibiotic impregnation of bone graft could have a detrimental effect on osteogenesis. Ciprofloxacin reduces fracture healing when injected subcutaneously in rats, and topically applied chloramphenicol and methicillin powder diminishes the osteogenesis in corticocancellous grafts (Huddleston, 2000; Gray and Elves, 1981). Miclau (Miclau et al., 1995) showed that tobramycin concentrations <200 mg/L had no effect on osteoblast replication, while concentrations >400 mg/L impaired osteoblast replication. The effect of vancomycin on osteogenesis has been thoroughly studied. Vancomycin-supplemented bone allografts in pigs have the same osteogenic activity as nonsupplemented bone (Petri, 1984). In an excellent study (Acta Orthopedica Scandinavica Award article, 2002) comparing the healing processes in vancomycin-supplemented bone allografts used for the treatment of tibia defects in pigs, and nonsupplemented allografts, no radiographic, histological or immunohistochemical differences were shown (Buttaro et al., 2003). Similar results have been presented in a case report involving two patients (Buttaro, 2005).

Clinical Studies

Few studies have been published on clinical pharmacokinetics and the possible adverse effects of antibiotic release from cancellous bone impregnated with antibiotics (Witsø et al., 2004; Buttaro et al., 2005). Bone grafts impregnated with an aminoglycoside or vancomycin, show extremely high local concentrations when impacted in the femur canal or acetabulum (Fig. 5.2).

The local antibiotic concentration exceeded the MIC of vancomycin against most strains of *Staphylococcus aureus* and *Staphylococcus epidermidis* for at least 48 hours (Buttaro et al., 2005). The antibiotic concentration in the wound drainage fluid in patients receiving cancellous bone impregnated with aminoglycoside, is considerably higher than concentrations recorded when using gentamicin-containing bone cement (Wahlig and Dingeldein, 1980; Wahlig et al., 1984; Salvati et al., 1986; Bunetel et al., 1989; Bunetel et al., 1990; Lindberg et al., 1991).

No studies have answered the question, over which period of time high local antibiotic concentrations are needed to obtain an effective infection prophylaxis. The prolonged release of antibiotics from antibiotic-containing bone cement offered no protection against late hematogenous infections (Elson et al., 1977; Blomgren and Lindgren, 1981). From an ecological and pharmacokinetic point of view, a high initial release with rapid decay and complete release of aminoglycoside from cancellous bone should be superior to the sustained release of the antibiotic from bone cement. It can be speculated that the high initial release of antibiotics from cancellous bone might reduce the need for systemic antibiotic prophylaxis. However, only a randomized clinical study can address this issue adequately. In vivo, bone impregnated with betalactams showed an almost complete release within one to two days. Generally, in clean, elective orthopedic surgery the trend is moving towards a very short-time use of systemic antibiotics for prophylaxis (Walenkamp, 2001). Hence, cancellous bone impregnated with beta-lactamase-stable penicillins and cephalosporins could be a prophylactic option when performing revision arthroplasties in cases of aseptic loosening. However, due to the risk of hypersensitivity, the beta-lactams have been avoided as local antibacterial agents (Wininger et al., 1996).

There are two reports on toxic serum levels of gentamicin when using gentamicin-containing PMMA spacers and beads or gentamicin-containing sponges (Van Raaij et al., 2002; Swieringa and Tulp, 2005). On the other hand, impaction of 50 g of cancellous bone impregnated in 100 mg/mL aminoglycoside solution (netilmicin) did not result in toxic serum levels, and renal or otovestibular toxicity was not reported (Witsø et al., 2004). Also, no nephrotoxicity was reported when an average of three morcelized femoral heads, mixed with 3 g of vancomycin, was impacted in the femur and/or the acetabulum (Buttaro et al., 2005).

Conclusion

In conclusion, the use of antibiotic-impregnated cancellous bone might be an alternative or a supplement to the use of antibiotic-containing bone cement in revisions of aseptic and septic loosened hip and knee prostheses. In a clinical study on two-stage revisions of 30 total hip arthroplasties, the reinfection rate was 3% when using vancomy-

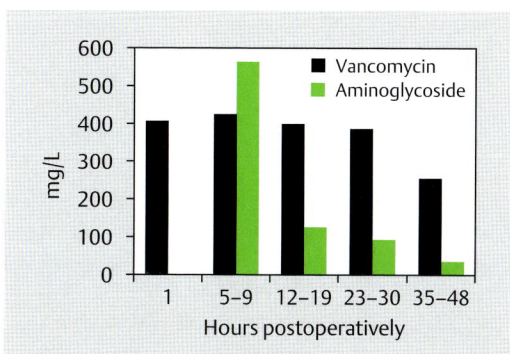

Fig. 5.2 The impaction of cancellous bone impregnated with antibiotics results in very high local concentrations of antibiotics in the hip joint.

cin-supplemeted impacted bone allograft (Buttaro et al., 2005). In addition to revision prosthetic surgery, antibiotic-containing allografts could be used when grafting *non*healed fractures, in particular infected pseudarthroses. By preference, randomized clinical studies comparing the use of antibiotic-impregnated bone graft with other local antibiotic carriers, should be conducted.

References

Adams K, Couch L, Cierny G, Calhoun J, Mader JT. In-vitro and in-vivo evaluation of antibiotic diffusion from antibiotic-impregnated polymethylmethacrylate beads. Clin Orthop1992; 278: 244–252.

Blomgren G, Lindgren U. Late hematogenous infection in total joint replacement: Studies of gentamicin and bone cement in the rabbit. Clin Orthop 1981; 155: 244–248.

Bunetel L, Segui A, Cormier M, Langlais F. Comparative study of gentamicin release from normal and low viscosity acrylic bone cement. Clin Pharamcokinet 1990; 19 (4): 333–340.

Buttaro M, Pusso R, Piccaluga F. Vancomycin-supplemented impacted bone allografts in infected hip arthroplasty. Two-stage revision results. J Bone Joint Surg Br 2005; 87: 314–319.

Buttaro M, Morandi A, Garcia Rivello H, Piccaluga F. Histology of vancomycin-supplemented impacted bone allografts in revision total hip arthroplasty. Case report. J Bone Joint Surg Br 2005; 87: 1684–1687.

Buttaro M, Gimenez MI, Greco G, Barcan L, Piccaluga F. High local levels of vancomycin without nephrotoxicity released from impacted bone allograft in 20 revision hip arthroplasties. Acta Orthopaedica 2005; 76 (3): 336–340.

Buttaro M, Della Valle AMG, Piñeiro L, Mocetti E, Morandi AA, Piccaluga F. Incorporation of vancomycin-supplemented bone allografts. Radiographical, histopathological and immunohistochemical study in pigs. Acta Orthop Scand 2003; 74 (5): 505–513.

Gray JC, Elves MW. Osteogenesis in bone grafts after short-term storage and topical antibiotic treatment. An experimental study in rats. J Bone Joint Surg Br 1981; 63 (3): 441–445.

Grood de DM. Het plomeren van restholten na osteomyelitis met "bone-chips". Ned Tijdschr V Gen 1947; 91.III.32: 2192–2196 (In Dutch).

Elson RA, Jephcott AE, McGechie DB, Verettas D. Bacterial infection and acrylic cement in the rat. J Bone Joint Surg Br 1977; 59 (4): 452–457.

Huddleston PM, Steckelberg JM, Hanssen AD, Rouse MS, Bolander ME, Patel R. Ciprofloxacin inhibition of experimental fracture-healing. J Bone Joint Surg Am 2000; 82 (2): 161–173.

Klekamp J, Dawson JM, Haas DW, DeBoer D, Christie M. The use of vancomycin and tobramycin in acrylic bone cement. Biomechanical effects and elution kinetics for use in joint arthroplasty. J Arthroplasty 1999; 14 (3): 339–346.

Lindberg L, Önnerfält R, Dingeldein E, Wahlig H. The release of gentamicin after total hip replacement using low or high viscosity bone cement. Int Orthop 1991; 15: 305–309.

The Norwegian Arthroplasty Register 2003. ISBN: 82-91847–06–1 (In Norwegian).

Mader JT, Calhoun J, Cobos J. In vitro evaluation of antibiotic diffusion from antibiotic-impregnated biodegradable beads and polymethylmethacrylate beads. Antimicrob Agents Chemother 1997; 41 (2): 415–418.

Miclau T, Edin ML, Lester GE, Lindesy RW, Dahners LE. Bone toxicity of local applied aminoglycosides. J Orthop Trauma 1995; 9 (5): 401–406.

Miclau T, Dahners LE, Lindsey RW. In-vitro pharmacokinetics of antibiotic release from locally implantable materials. J Orthop Res 1993; 11 (5): 627–632.

Petri WH. Osteogenic activity of antibiotic-supplemented bone allografts in the guinea pig. J Oral Maxillofac Surg 1984; 42: 631–636.

Raaij van TM, Visser LE, Vulto AG, Verhaar JA. Acute renal failure after local gentamicin treatment in an infected total knee arthroplasty. J Arthroplasty 2002; 17 (7): 948–50.

Salvati EA, Callaghan JJ, Brause BD, Klein RF, Small RD. Reimplantation in infection. Elution of gentamicin from cement and beads. Clin Orthop 1986; 207: 83–93.

Swieringa AJ, Tulp NJ. Toxic serum gentamicin levels after use of gentamicin-loaded sponges in infected total hip arthroplasty. Acta Orthop 2005; 76 (1): 75–77.

Wahlig H, Dingeldein E. Antibiotics and bone cements. Acta Orthop Scand 1980; 51: 49–56.

Wahlig H, Dingeldein E, Buchholz HW, Buchholz M, Bachmann F. Pharmacokinetic study of gentamicin-loaded cement in total hip replacements. Comparative effects of varying dosage. J Bone Joint Surg Br 1984; 66 (2): 175–179.

Walenkamp GHIM. Prevention of infection in orthopedic surgery. European Instructional Course Lectures. 2001 EFORT (ISBN: 0–9525921–3–4) 2001; 5: 8–17.

Winkler H, Janata O, Berger C, Wein W, Georgopoulos A. In-vitro release of vancomycin and tobramycin from impregnated human and bovine bone grafts. J Antimicrob Chemot 2000; 46: 423–428.

Wininger DA, Fass RJ. Minireview. Antibiotic-impregnated cement and beads for orthopedic infections. Antimicrob Agents Chemother 1996; 40 (12): 2675–2679.

Witsø E, Persen L, Løseth K, Bergh K. Adsorption and release of antibiotics from morcelized cancellous bone. Acta Orthop Scand 1999; 70 (3): 298–304.

Witsø E, Persen L, Løseth K, Benum P, Bergh K. Cancellous bone as an antibiotic carrier. Acta Orthop Scand 2000; 71 (1): 80–84.

Witsø E, Persen L, Benum P, Bergh K. Release of netilmicin and vancomycin from cancellous bone. Acta Orthop Scand 2002; 73 (2): 199–205.

Witsø E, Persen L, Benum P, Aamodt A, Schnell Husby O, Bergh K. High local concentration without systemic adverse effects after impaction of netilmicin-impregnated bone. Acta Orthop Scand 2004; 75 (3): 339–346.

(D) Antibiotic-Loaded Bone Cements – Antibiotic Release and Influence on Mechanical Properties

Klaus-Dieter Kühn

Introduction

One of the major applications of polymers in medicine, particularly in arthroplasty, is the anchorage of artificial joints. Clinical tests have proven that bone cements on PMMA basis are suitable for this indication. Every surgical intervention involves an infection risk for the patient. This applies in particular to elderly and weak persons who are subject to an endoprosthetic revision operation. Such an operation is often associated with extensive soft tissue injuries. Also, the implantation of foreign body materials favors the occurrence and aggravation of an infection, due to the weakened immune system of the human body. No matter, whether an initial or a late-onset infection, this type of complication always stands for a medical disaster. The particular susceptibility of the artificial joint to germ colonization on its surface cannot be avoided by systemic antibiotic administration only, as the regular blood stream does not transport sufficient active substances to the source of infection, which again is a result of the impaired blood supply around the infected tissue. Already at an early stage, local antibiotic therapy was considered the key to success for the prevention of serious infections. In this context, antibiotic containing bone cements, used for the fixation of artificial joints, were introduced as local drug carriers.

History

The first investigations were conducted by Buchholz, Hamburg, at the end of the sixties. He added various antibiotics to the bone cement Palacos R from Kulzer GmbH & Co. KG, a 100 % affiliate of today's Heraeus Kulzer GmbH. He chose Palacos R bone cement because its properties seemed ideal to him. Moreover, Palacos R, developed by Kulzer

and introduced to the market in 1958, was the bone cement used for almost all joint replacement operations in Germany at that time.

Further tests carried out by Buchholz in the laboratories of his bacteriologist, Dr. Lodenkämper, showed an antibiotic effect of antiobiotic-containing Palacos R over a period of 14 days. The effect of the antibiotic on the mechanical stability of the bone cement – which was reason for concern – was investigated by a variety of mechanical and physical tests at Heraeus Kulzer (Table 6.1).

Further joint investigations were arranged by adding various antibiotics in different quantities to Palacos R bone cement. Gentamicin was supplied by E. Merck, Darmstadt. It was supplied directly to Buchholz in a lyophilized form that had initially been intended for analysis purposes. The typical green color of Palacos R cement powder provided a visible control for the uniform distribution of the gentamicin in the cement powder. The results collected in 1969 / 1970 were published by Buchholz and Engelbrecht (Buchholz and Engelbrecht, 1970).

By that time, Buchholz required a sterile, industrially manufactured gentamicin-containing Palacos R to avoid any difficulties that could result from manual adding of gentamicin to the cement powder. Therefore, he established a first direct contact between Heraeus Kulzer and E. Merck. It was Heraeus Kulzer's intention to buy the gentamicin from E. Merck and implement the industrial adding and mixing of gentamicin to the Palacos R powder. When Heraeus Kulzer approached E. Merck with these plans, they had to realize that Schering Plough, United States, was the patent owner of gentamicin. E. Merck, on the other hand, owned a licence for Germany and Austria. Schering delivered the same antibiotic, amongst others, to Germany using a different brand as E. Merck.

Before antibiotic-containing Palacos R was launched Ruckdeschel and Hessert (Ruckdeschel et

Table 6.1 Admixture of antibiotics to bone cement: Influence on mechanical properties

	Bending strength [kg/cm²]	Impact strength [kg/cm³]	Young's Modulus [kg/cm²]
Palacos R plain	960 ± 69	12.9 ± 1.9	16550
With 1 ampoule erycin	852 ± 51	10.8 ± 0.7	15600
With 2 ampoules erycin	823 ± 9	9.0 ± 0.6	16100
With 1 ampoule megacillin	883 ± 14	10.2 ± 0.4	16000
With 2 ampoules megacillin	827 ± 6	9.8 ± 0.6	17350
With 0.5 g gentamicin	814 ± 18	10.3 ± 0.3	16500
With 1.0 g gentamicin	807 ± 18	8.5 ± 0.6	16700

(Modified: Buchholz and Engelbrecht, 1970)

al., 1973) published that 80% of the gentamicin admixed to the cement powder had been detected in the body within the first 24 hours. These results required further investigations. In order to exclude any ototoxic damages, E. Merck initiated extensive in-house pharmacokinetic investigations on gentamicin-containing Palacos R. The results have been described in detail in numerous publications.

During the launch of antibiotic-containing Palacos R, the so-called drug law was implemented in Germany in the early seventies. This new law implied that a manufacturer of drug-containing products needed a manufacturing licence in accordance with the new drug law. Unfortunately, Heraeus Kulzer did not possess such a manufacturing licence at that time, and, therefore, depended on a cooperation partner with a manufacturing licence that permitted to place pharmaceuticals on the market.

Negotiations between Heraeus Kulzer and E. Merck quickly revealed that, due to the licence contracts with Schering Plough, E. Merck had to market the gentamicin-containing Palacos R as a Merck and not as a Heraeus Kulzer product, because Merck was not allowed to assign sublicences to Heraeus Kulzer.

In the end, Heraeus Kulzer had to manufacture their gentamicin-containing Palacos R under the brand name Refobacin Palacos R for E. Merck exclusively in Germany and Austria. For all other European countries Heraeus Kulzer sold the product exclusively to Schering Plough under the brand name Palacos R with Gentamicin. Heraeus Kulzer remained the holder of all property rights

on the gentamicin-containing Palacos R products (Fig. 6.1).

Antibiotic Requirements for the Usage in Acrylic Bone Cement

Foreign implants, e.g., acrylics, are especially sensitive to bacterial surface contamination as the germs may spread there almost unhampered by the immune defence of the body. Bacteria rapidly generate a protective mucus layer and go into a nonoperative state with low sensitivity to antibiotics. Therefore, local antibiotic treatment is important. The pharmacokinetics of antibiotic release from the matrix is of clinical importance. The local antibiotic concentrations achieved, must be clearly above the minimal inhibitory concentration (MIC) and the minimal bactericidal concentration of the germs.

Several antibiotics were tested for usage as an additive to PMMA bone cement to ensure infection prophylaxis and to protect the cement from bacterial colonization. However, a number of known antibiotics are inadequate for addition to PMMA bone cements. Suitable antibiotics require several physico-chemical properties to allow admixture to bone cement as an efficient microbiological additive. They should be:
- highly soluble in water,
- sterilizable by γ-irradiation or by gassing with ethylene oxide,
- heat stable and chemically inert during polymerization,

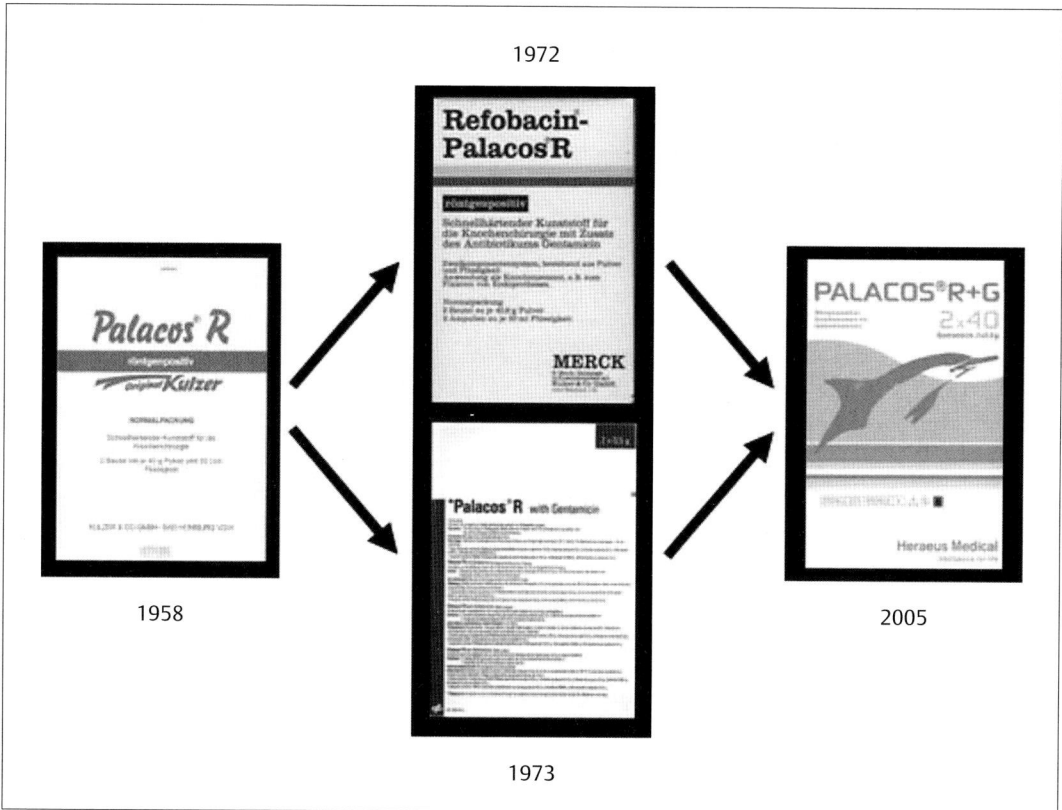

Fig. 6.**1**   The different package sizes of Palacos bone cement:
left: Palacos R from Kulzer in the sixties
mid up: Refobacin Palacos R distributed by E. Merck
mid down: Palacos R with gentamicin distributed by Schering Plough
right: Palacos R +G from Heraeus Kulzer.

* without or with low influence on the mechanical strength of the bone cement,
* easily released from cured bone cement, and
* stable during storage of the finished cement powder before usage.

The following biological factors should be provided:

* broad antibacterial spectrum including gram-positive and gram-negative germs,
* good bactericidal effect in low concentrations,
* low rate of primary resistant germs,
* low rate of development of resistances,
* low protein bonding, and
* low allergic potential.

Gentamicin meets these requirements almost completely. Gentamicin has an ototoxic and nephrotoxic potential. However, when using gentamicin-containing bone cement in total joint replacements, the serum gentamicin levels remain low during the postoperative time period. So the risk of ototoxic and nephrotoxic effects seems to be negligible. Based on these requirements and release tests, gentamicin was the favorite antibiotic for bone cements from the early seventies onwards (Wahlig and Buchholz, 1972; Frommelt and Kühn, 2005).

Methods for Detection of Gentamicin

Gentamicin sulfate is an aminoglycoside antibiotic consisting of a mixture of several structurally very similar aminoglycosides, which do not have a chromophore or fluorophore. The major components of gentamicin are gentamicin C_1, C_{1a}, C_2 and C_{2a}. Several methods can be used to determine the antibiotic content in the polymer powder, as well as the antibiotic release from the acrylic bone cement. To measure gentamicin in the cement powder, the powder is suspended in water and subsequently filtered and analyzed. To determine its release, specimens of gentamicin-loaded bone cement are prepared and stored in aqueous buffer solution for a given time. Of course, each method requires calibration with a gentamicin standard.

High performance liquid chromatography (HPLC) is often used for the detection of antibiotics. HPLC is a form of column chromatography and is sometimes referred to as high pressure liquid chromatography. For gentamicin, the reversed-phase technique with a post-column derivatization is used. The gentamicin-containing buffer solution is forced through a nonpolar column of the stationary phase at high pressure. Having left the column, the separated gentamicin molecules are derivatized with o-phthaldialdehyde to form a fluorophore, which is subsequently analyzed by a fluorescence detector. HPLC results show great accuracy and chromatograms even display the distribution of the isomers of gentamicin (Fig. 6.2).

Another method for antibiotic detection is the agar diffusion test. For this test, plates prepared with agar as cell-culture medium are inoculated with gentamicin-sensitive bacteria. The agar plates are then prepared with the elutions and incubated at elevated temperatures for a given time. The concentration of the eluted gentamicin is determined with an optical analysis system by measuring the inhibition zones on the agar plates. This test measures the actual microbiological activity of the gentamicin solution. Specific immunological methods for the determination of gentamicin can be used, like fluorescent polarization immunoassays (FPIA), radioimmunoassays (RIA) or enzyme immunoassays (EIA). These assays make use of the principle of competitive binding. For FPIA the assays are supplied in kit form containing the reagents and the gentamicin standard. Tracers, samples, and diluted antisera are combined, and the polarization of tracer fluorescence is determined in a specially designed fluorometer. Immunoassays are reliable methods for detection of gentamicin in serum, as well as in aqueous solutions. A rarely applied method for detection of gentamicin is the capillary electrophoresis.

Release Characteristics

The release of antibiotics is a surface and diffusion process. Release kinetics of gentamicin from bone cements are mainly controlled by a combination of surface roughness and porosity (Van de Belt et

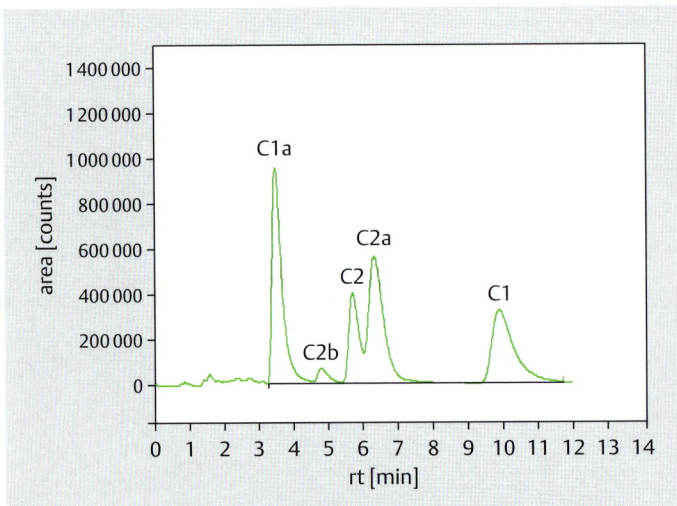

Fig. 6.2 A HPLC chromatogram of gentamicin with C 1a, C 2b, C 2, C 2a and C 1 peaks.

al., 2000), whereby the release through pores in the bone cement matrix influences the total release rate. Another important property affecting gentamicin release, is the water uptake of the cement because water is needed to dissolve antibiotics out of the surface area (Fig. 6.3).

Different antibiotic-loaded cements on the market show different release rates, mainly due to hydrophilic properties of the polymer components (Kühn et al., 2005a; Frommelt and Kühn, 2005). It is also important to note that antibiotics are released from a thin surface layer. Therefore, size and roughness of the surface area also are relevant factors influencing the overall release of an antibiotic out of the bone cement. After all, most of the antibiotic will not be eluted during the lifetime of the implant.

Release of gentamicin is related to the surface area of the bone cement. The larger the specific surface (i.e., the surface per weight), the higher the release of gentamicin (Walenkamp et al., 1986). This occurs, because larger surfaces mean a greater amount of gentamicin particles directly on the surface. Test specimens with a specific surface area of 8.0 cm² per g cured cement have a definitely higher release of gentamicin than specimens with a specific surface area of 3.1 cm² per g cured cement (Fig. 6.4).

The release rate of gentamicin depends on the quality of the gentamicin. The word quality, in this context, however, is not used in terms of chemical purity. Gentamicin used for bone cements, e.g., in Europe has to comply with the European pharmacopeia (Ph. Eur.) where chemical purity is strictly defined. All manufacturers of gentamicin-loaded bone cement have to adhere to these legal requirements. Optimized particle size distribution of the gentamicin particles results in

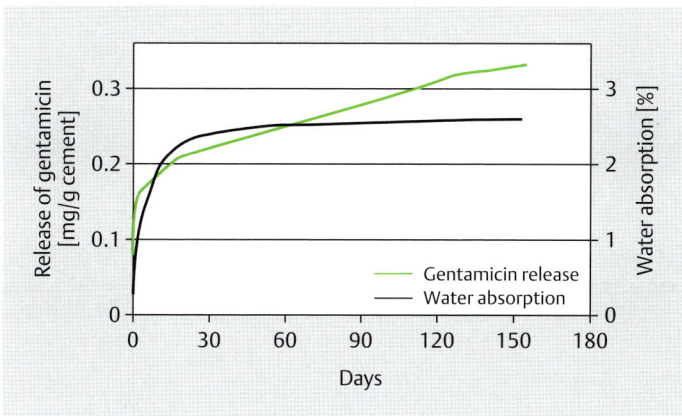

Fig. 6.**3** Release of gentamicin from a high-viscous bone cement manually mixed. Mixing ratio: 40 g cement powder with added 0.5 g gentamicin and 20 mL liquid. Incubation at 37 °C in phosphate buffer solution; detection by agardiffusion test (Wahlig and Buchholz, 1972). Test specimens: cylinder with diameter 25 mm and height 10 mm. Water uptake of the same high-viscous bone cement. Incubation at 37 °C in phosphate buffer solution; gravimetrical detection.

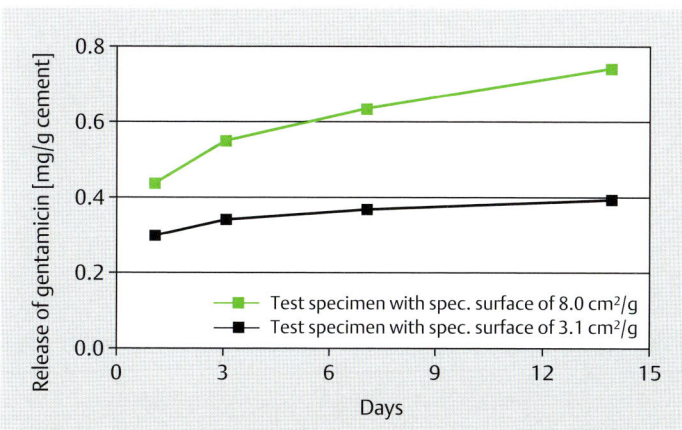

Fig. 6.**4** Release of gentamicin from a high-viscous bone cement manually mixed. Mixing ratio: 40 g cement powder with added 0.5 g gentamicin and 20 mL liquid. Incubation at 37 °C in phosphate buffer solution; detection by HPLC. Dimensions of test specimens: 8.0 cm² per g: blocks with 15 mm × 10 mm × 3.3 mm. 3.1 cm² per g: cylinder with diameter 25 mm and height 10 mm.

optimal release of gentamicin and, therefore, in a more efficient prophylaxis against colonization of the bone cement surface.

In Fig. 6.**5** results are shown for the release of gentamicin from specimens prepared using the same high-viscous bone cement matrix and the same mixing technique. Also, the same amount of gentamicin was applied. The samples, which all comply with Ph. Eur., differ in the morphology of the added gentamicin. It is clearly visible that dif-

ferent morphologies and particle sizes result in different release rates. In-vitro trials also showed that a high load of gentamicin in the cement increases the release rate (Fig. 6.**6**).

This occurs, because the more highly loaded cement contains more gentamicin particles right on the surface, which are released into the human body directly after application of the cement. As already stated, release through pores in the matrix of the cement is to be assumed. Vacuum mix-

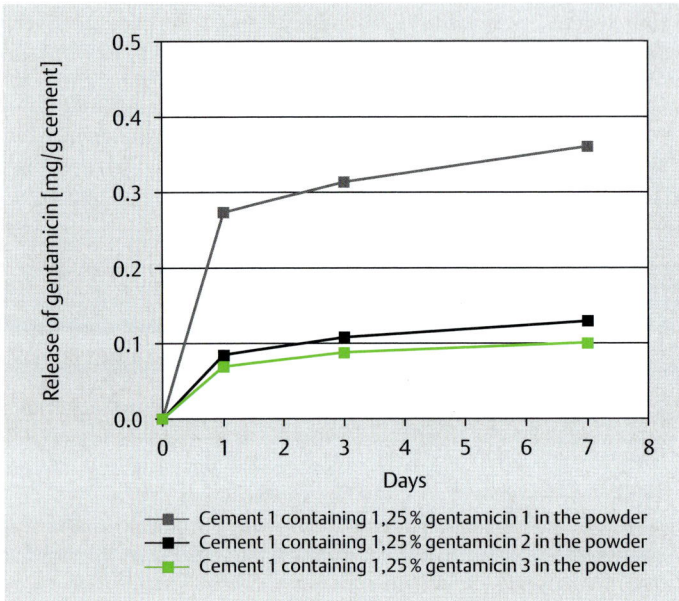

Fig. 6.**5** Release of gentamicin from a high-viscous bone cement manually mixed. Mixing ratio: 40 g cement powder with added 0.5 g gentamicin and 20 mL liquid. Incubation at 37 °C in phosphate buffer solution; detection by FPIA. Test specimens: cylinder with diameter 25 mm and height 10 mm. Gentamicin sulfate with three different morphologies were added.

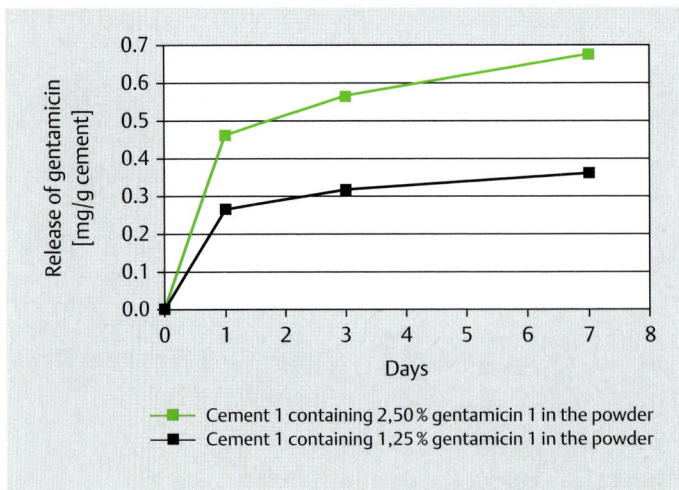

Fig. 6.**6** Release of gentamicin from a high-viscous bone cement manually mixed. Mixing ratio: 40 g cement powder with added 0.5 g or 1.0 g gentamicin and 20 mL liquid. Incubation at 37 °C in phosphate buffer solution; detection by FPIA. Test specimens: cylinder with diameter 25 mm and height 10 mm.

ing of bone cement results in cement with low porosity, i.e., there are almost no voids in the cement matrix. As these voids accelerate the diffusion of gentamicin from the inner matrix to the surface of the cement, the release of gentamicin decreases if voids are missing. Therefore, vacuum mixing slightly lowers the release of gentamicin (Fig.6.**7**).

All of the test results show a high initial release of gentamicin with a subsequently low release within the following days. The high initial release during the first 24 hours provides a high local antibiotic level near to the surface of the cement in the adjacent tissue. High local postoperative concentrations of antibiotics result in a rapid eradication of sensitive germs at the operation site without adverse toxic drug effects. Antibiotic levels far above the MIC might even kill resistent germs, which may be sensitive to high levels. The subsequent release of gentamicin during the following days is of clinical importance, because biofilms that protect bacteria against the immune defense might form on bone cements. Gentamicin-loaded bone cements reduce biofilm formation up to 72 hours after inoculation (Van de Belt et al., 2001). In addition, the antibiotic release protects the surface against colonization by hematogenic germs that cause infections. Currently, a variety of antibiotic-loaded bone cements are available on the market. Usually, gentamicin sulfate is added to the cement powder. Other commercial models may include tobramycin, clindamycin, colistin and erythromycin. In surgical practice, further antibiotics are added to the cement powder prior to the mixing process in order to combat individually isolated germs. For problem germs such as methicillin-resistant *Staphylococcus aureus* (MRSA), the use of vancomycin is advisable.

Mechanical Influence of Antibiotics on PMMA Bone Cement

The addition of antibiotics to bone cement powder influences the mechanical properties of bone cement (Kühn et al., 2005b). As the antibiotic particles are not incorporated in the polymer matrix, they act as a foreign body in the cured cement. However, the antibiotic content in industrially manufactured bone cements is low and varies from 1.25–2.5 wt%. Only one industrially manufactured bone cement has a content of 5 wt%. Here, it has to be mentioned that the antibiotic is not added as a pure substance, but in form of an antibiotic salt, i.e., gentamicin is added as gentamicin sulfate, tobramycin is added as tobramycin sulfate, and clindamycin is added as clindamycin hydrochloride. Therefore, the real content of antibiotic substance is slightly higher. This is, however, a small amount and the influence on mechanical properties is negligible.

In-vitro studies in the seventies (Lee et al., 1978) demonstrated the effect of several variables on the mechanical strength of bone cement. Variables like kind and quantity of used radiopaque fillers, kind and quantity of used antibiotics, mixing techniques, and insertion techniques were investigated. The addition of antibiotics weakens the cement. Weakening depends on the kind and quantity of antibiotic added. Lautenschlager (Lau-

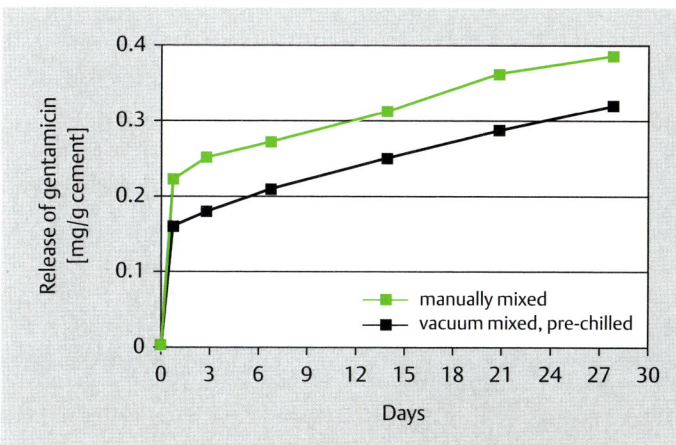

Fig.6.**7** Release of gentamicin from a high-viscous bone cement manually mixed and mixed with a vacuum mixing system. Mixing ratio: 40 g powder cement powder with added 0.5 g gentamicin and 20 mL liquid. Incubation at 37 °C in phosphate buffer solution; detection by FPIA. Test specimens: cylinder with diameter 25 mm and height 10 mm.

53

tenschlager et al., 1976a; Lautenschlager et al., 1976b; Soltesz et al., 1998) showed that the addition of gentamicin sulfate antibiotic powder to acrylic bone cement caused gradual, parallel decreases in the mechanical properties of compressive strengths (Table 6.2).

On the other hand, the influence on mechanical properties remains small. This was also stated by Davies (Davies et al., 1989) and Kühn (Kühn, 2000). Davies found that the addition of 0.5 g of gentamicin to Palacos R did not significantly alter its fatigue properties and the addition of 0.5 g of erythromycin and 0.24 g of colistin did not decrease the fatigue life of Simplex P, respectively. Kühn showed that the difference in fatigue strength between antibiotic and plain bone cement is small (Table 6.3).

Today, it is accepted that the addition of antibiotics lowers the mechanical strength of bone cement. However, the weakening is not clinically

Table 6.**2** Compressive strength of PMMA bone cement with addition of antibiotic powder; used bone cement: Simplex P

	Added antibiotic: (gentamicin) [g / 40 g powder]	Compressive strength [MPa]
Plain cement	0	80.7
Cement with added antibiotic	2	77.7
	5	68.5
	10	51.3

(Modified: Lautenschlager and Jacobs, 1976)

Table 6.**3** Bending strength of PMMA bone cement test specimens after 10 000 000 cycles of dynamic testing. The tests were performed in 4-point-bending mode at 37 °C in Ringer's solution. The static bending strength, i.e., the bending strength before the start of dynamic testing, is shown in the right column.

Cement	Viscosity during mixing	Bending strength after 107 cycles (MPa)	Quasi-static bending strength (MPa)
Palacos R	high	17.8	67.6
CMW1	high	12.3	57.1
Refobacin-Palacos R	high	17.0	60.4
CMW1 G	high	14.1	61.5
Palamed	medium	17.6	62.0
Simplex P	medium	14.2	60.1
Palamed G	medium	17.4	58.6
AKZ	medium	11.5	61.0
Osteopal	low	26.0	65.6
CMW3	low	10.4	59.7
Osteopal G	low	20.0	58.6
CMW3 G	low	6.2	60.0

(Kühn, 2000)

relevant and all industrially manufactured bone cements meet the mechanical requirements of the worldwide ISO standard for acrylic bone cements. Therefore, the use of industrially manufactured bone cements is safe and with regard to its benefits, the use of antibiotic-containing bone cements is preferable.

The addition of antibiotics to bone cements by the surgeon himself has to be seen critically, as the admixture might be inhomogeneous. Furthermore, the quality of the antibiotic is questionable, as several antibiotics are lyophilized and present as a lumpy powder. Manual mixing of antibiotics might result in inhomogeneous bone cement with poor mechanical properties, so that industrially manufactured bone cements, if available, should be preferred. Antibiotics should not be added as aqueous solutions to acrylic bone cements because water interferes with the polymerization process and weakens the cement considerably (Marks et al., 1976).

Infections with Resistant Organisms – a Challenge to Drug-Carrying Bone Cements

For several years, an increase of infections caused by resistant and multiresistant organisms (e.g., MRSA/MRSE), was observed in Europe as well as worldwide. This development also impacts on bone surgery. Increasingly, joint endoprostheses are subjected to septic revisions provoked by problem germs and in particular by multiresistant germs. This process is an extreme challenge to surgeons and manufacturers of bone cements, alike.

For infected joint endoprostheses, single-stage revisions as well as two-stage revisions are performed today. In both cases, careful surgical debridement of the affected area is mandatory. The application of bone cements in septic revisions is usually performed in two ways:

1. Customized addition of antibiotics to the bone cement by the surgeon

Here, the choice of the added antibiotic is based on the patient's antibiogram. Currently, this procedure is widely applied, as no commercially-manufactured bone cements are available containing antibiotics that are capable of dealing adequately with multiresistant problem organisms.

Customized addition of antibiotics offers the benefit that exactly those antibiotics are selected that fit the individually established antibiogram. There are however some drawbacks:

The distribution of the antibiotic particles in the cement might not be uniform, resulting in *non*reproducible release kinetics. The effect of the added antibiotic/antibiotics on the working properties are often unknown and the mechanical long-term behavior cannot be predicted.

As a legal consequence of customized addition of antibiotics, the surgeon becomes responsible manufacturer and thus assumes liability for the product quality.

It is crucial that the quantity of 4 g antibiotics per 40 g cement powder is not exceeded. Moreover, antibiotics must not be mixed with the monomer liquid. The addition of 2 g antibiotics to 40 g cement powder generally offers a satisfactory release of antibiotics and acceptable mechanical properties. The thermal stability of the intended antibiotic should be proven prior to the incorporation into the cement powder. Moreover, it has to be identified whether the antibiotic may lead to undesired side effects during the polymerization process of the bone cement, which may affect or impede antimicrobial efficacy. As a guideline for daily practice Hendrich and Frommelt (Hendrich and Frommelt, 2004) recommended the following antibiotic dosage for PMMA bone cements (Table 6.4).

The applied antibiotics are categorized with respect to their structure, type and kind of efficacy (Table 6.**5**).

2. Industrially manufactured bone cements loaded with appropriate antibiotics

Industrially manufactured bone cements loaded with appropriate antibiotics present an alternative to the customized addition of antibiotics. This type of bone cement offers the following benefits:

- reproducible, uniform distribution of the antibiotics in the cement powder,
- reproducible release kinetics of the active agents, and
- reproducible mechanical properties.

A significant drawback of industrially manufactured bone cements is, however, that the incorporated antibiotic combinations may not yield the desired efficacy for the entire spectrum of septic revisions, due to the large variety of infective or-

Table 6.4 Recommended admixture of antibiotics to PMMA bone cements for the treatment of infections caused by different bacteria

Antibiotic Dosage per 40 g PMMA bone cement powder	Bacteria
1.0 g Clindamycin + 1.0 g Gentamicin	*Staphylococcus aureus / epidermidis* *Streptococcus / Propioni bacteria*
3.0 g Cefuroxim + 1.0 g Gentamicin	*Staphylococcus aureus / epidermidis* *Streptococcus / Propioni bacteria*
2.0 g Vancomycin + 1.0 g Ofloxacin + 1.0 g Gentamicin	Methicllin- / Oxacillin resistent Staphylococci (MRSA / MRSE)
2.0 g Vancomycin + 1.0 g Ampicillin + 1.0 g Gentamicin	Enterococci
2.0 g Ceperazon + 2.0 g Amikazin	*Pseudomonas aeruginosa*
2.0 g Ofloxacin + 1.0 g Gentamicin	*Pseudomonas aeruginosa*

(Modified: Hendrich and Frommelt, 2004)

ganisms. Thus, the application of one type of bone cement for all septic revisions is not possible. In conclusion, industrially manufactured bone cements intended for revisions need to supply an antibiotic combination that covers the broad germ spectrum common for septic revisions. At present, the combination of gentamicin and clindamycin is often used successfully in septic revisions. The bone cement Copal from Heraeus Kulzer GmbH was the first bone cement on the market for revisions to provide the combination of gentamicin and clindamycin.

References

Belt van de H, Neut D, Schen W, van Horna JR, van der Mei HC, Busscher HJ. Surface roughness, porosity and wettability of gentamicin-loaded bone cements and their antibiotic release. Biomaterials 2000; 21: 1981 – 1987.

Belt van de H, Neut D, Schenk W, van Horn JR, van der Mei HC, Busscher HJ. Infection of orthopedic implants and the use of antibiotic-loaded bone cements. A review. Acta Orthop Scand 2001; 72: 557 – 571.

Buchholz HW, Engelbrecht H. Über die Depotwirkung einiger Antibiotika bei Vermischung mit dem Kunstharz Palacos. Chirurg 1970; 40: 511 – 515.

Davies JP, O'Connor DO, Burke DW, J Biomed Materials Research 1989; 23: 379 – 397.

Frommelt L, Kühn KD. Antibiotic-loaded Cement. In: Breusch S, Malchau H (eds.): The well-cemented total hip arthroplasty, Springer 2005.

Hendrich C, Frommelt L. Keim-orientierte Antibiotikatherapie bei Protheseninfektionen. In: Hendrich C,

Table 6.5 Recommended antibiotics according to their structure, type and efficacy

Antibiotic	Type of Antibiotic	Efficacy
Clindamycin	Lincosamide antibiotic	Bacteriostatic to bactericidal / perturbance inhibition of the bacterial protein synthesis
Gentamicin / Amikacin	Aminoglycoside antibiotic	Bactericidal / perturbance inhibition of the bacterial protein synthesis, formation of nonsense proteins
Vancomycin	Glycopeptide antibiotic	Bactericidal / inhibition of the bacterial cell wall crosslink
Ofloxacin	Chinolone antibiotic	Bactericidal / inhibition of the DNA torque
Cefuroxim / Cefperazon / Ampicillin	β-Lactame antibiotic	Bactericidal / inhibition of the bacterial cell wall crosslink

(Modified: Kayser et al., 1998)

Frommelt L, Eulert J (eds.) Septische Knochen- und Gelenkchirurgie. Berlin; Springer Verlag 2004.

Kayser FH, Bienz KA, Eckert J, Zinkernagel RM. Medizinische Mikrobiologie. Georg Thieme Verlag Stuttgart 1998; 181 – 200.

Kühn KD. Bone cements. Up-to-date comparison of physical and chemical properties of commercial materials. Springer-Verlag Berlin Heidelberg, 2000.

Kühn KD, Ege W, Gopp U. Acrylic bone cements: composition and properties. Orthop Clin North Am 2005a; 36: 17 – 28.

Kühn KD, Ege W, Gopp U. Acrylic bone cements: Mechanical and physical properties. Orthop Clin North Am 36, 2005b; 29: 20 – 39.

Lautenschlager EP, Marshall GW, Marks KE, Schwartz J, Nelson CL. Mechanical strength of acrylic bone cements impregnated with antibiotics. J Biomed Materials Research 1976; 10: 837 – 845.

Lautenschlager EP, Jacobs JJ, Marshall GW, Meyer PR. Mechanical properties of bone cements containing large doses of antibiotic powders. J Biomed Materials Research 1976; 10: 929 – 938.

Lee AJC, Ling RSM, Vangala SS. Some clinicaly relevant variables affecting the mechanical behaviour of bone cement. Arch Orthop Traumat Surg 1978; 92: 1 – 18.

Marks KE, Nelson CL, Lautenschlager EP. Antibiotic-Impregnated Acrylic Bone Cement. J Bone and Joint Surgery 1976; 58-A: 358 – 364.

Ruckdeschel G, Hessert GR, Schoellhammer T. Quantitative in vitro-Untersuchungen zur Frage der Gentamycinabgabe aus Polymethylmethacrylat-Polymerisatblöcken. Arch Orthop Unfallchir 1973; 74: 291 – 300.

Soltesz U, Schäfer R, Kühn KD. Einfluss von Mischbedingungen und Beimengungen auf das Ermüdungsverhalten von Knochenzementen. DVM. 1. Tagung das DVM-Arbeitskreises "Biowerkstoffe". Mechanische Eigenschaften von Implantatwerkstoffen 1998; 89 – 94.

Walenkamp GHIM, Vree TB, van Rens Th IG. Gentamicin-PMMA beads. Pharmacokinetic and nephrotoxicological study. Clin Orthop 1986; 205: 171 – 183.

Wahlig H, Buchholz HW: Experimentelle und klinische Untersuchungen zur Freisetzung von Gentamicin aus einem Knochenzement. Chirurg 1972; 43: 441 – 445.

(D) Antibiotic Choices in Bone Surgery – Local Therapy using Antibiotic-Loaded Bone Cement

Lars Frommelt

Summary

Osteomyelitis and periprosthetic infections are difficult to treat, because of the localized nature of the infection in bone tissue. Systemic administration of antibiotics yields only low concentrations at the site of infection, and often sessile bacteria in biofilm, characterized by an elevated resistance to antibiotics, are the pathogenic organisms underlying these infections. In the presence of foreign material a local immune defect of granulocytes reduces phagocytosis of bacterial pathogens. Bone infections are treated by surgical debridement and extraction of any foreign material. This procedure offers the possibility to place antibiotic-loaded carriers at the site of infection, so that extremely high local drug concentrations can be achieved.

Antibiotic-loaded acrylic cement (ALAC) is a carrier system amongst others that is widely applied, and its antibiotic elution properties are well studied in vivo and in vitro. Unfortunately, not all antibiotics can be used in polymethylmethacrylate (PMMA) bone cement and only few are available in standardized commercial preparations. Often, supplementary antimicrobial agents are necessary, which can only be added to the bone cement by hand-mixing in the operating theater. This is done by preparing a mixture of PMMA powder with antibiotic powder before polymerization of the bone cement. For the mechanical properties of ALAC, as well as the elution properties, the homogeneity of this mixture is crucial. Instructions for hand-mixing and choosing suitable antimicrobial agents are available.

Studies in animals and humans theoretically support the advantages of this therapy. Adverse effects are reported infrequently. Drawbacks of local therapy with ALAC are the limited availability of appropriate antibiotics and the increasing emergence of multiresistant pathogens.

Introduction

Antibiotic-loaded PMMA bone cement is frequently used in prophylaxis and therapy of bone infections – especially in periprosthetic infections of artificial joint replacements. These infections are difficult to treat, and the pathogens cannot be eradicated in the presence of all foreign material or sequesters by systemic antimicrobial treatment alone. Surgical removal of all foreign material, as well as infected bone and soft tissue, respectively is necessary to gain control of this condition. Supplementary antimicrobial therapy ensures the success of the surgical procedure. From a pharmacokinetical point of view bone tissue is functionally a lower compartment, so that systemic antibiotics (and other drugs) are unable to penetrate bone tissue in sufficient amounts if there is an infection.

However, effective concentrations of antimicrobial agents can be achieved at the site of the infection if the antibiotics are applied locally.

Pharmacokinetics of Antibiotics, Bacterial Susceptibility and Alteration of Cellular Host Defense

Mader and co-workers (Mader and Adams 1988) studied tissue concentrations of systemically administered antibiotics in bone infection. The results showed that most antimicrobial agents are available in bone tissue only in low concentrations that rarely exceed 10 % of the levels available in the serum compartment. This concentration often proves insufficient in eradicating bacterial pathogens.

Periprosthetic infection and osteomyelitis are chronic infections determined by sessile bacteria. Sessile bacteria are characterized by a prolonged generation time, the formation of biofilm (Costerton et al., 1999), and an elevated minimal inhibitory concentration (MIC), which may be a thousand-fold, compared with their free-living planktonic counterparts (Stewart and Costerton, 2001). In addition, biofilm is able to protect sessile bacteria from host-defence mechanisms. Biofilm interferes directly with phagocytosis and a local immunodefect of cellular defense is induced in the presence of foreign material and sequesters (Zimmerli et al., 1984).

The combination of reduced availability of antibiotics, reduced susceptibility of sessile bacterial pathogens, inhibited phagocytosis of bacteria in biofilm, and local immunodefect in the presence of foreign material, results in a condition that is difficult to treat.

PMMA Bone Cement as Carrier for Local Therapy

The local application of antibiotics is held responsible for inducing bacterial resistance to antimicrobial agents. Nowadays, this approach remains justified for only very few conditions. One of these is the infection of bone tissue.

In local antibiotic therapy, a carrier for the application of antimicrobial agents has to meet two requirements: It should guarantee sufficient concentration at the site of infection, as well as a "controlled" delivery of the drugs, so that possible adverse drug effects like deafness or renal failure can be prevented.

As early as 1970, Buchholz and Engelbrecht (Buchholz and Engelbrecht, 1979) showed that antimicrobial agents can be eluted from PMMA bone cement if crystalline antibiotics are mixed with polymer powder before polymerization of the bone cement. Buchholz successfully performed one-stage revisions in patients suffering from periprosthetic infection using ALAC (Buchholz et al., 1979).

The elution of antibiotics from PMMA bone cement is characterized by an extremely high peak concentration at the very beginning, which tails down very soon to a low level elution for a certain period of time. Adams and co-workers (Adams et al., 1992) demonstrated different elution profiles in in-vivo animal experiments, but all antibiotics investigated showed concentrations exceeding $30 \mu g/mL$ in wound discharge for at least 28 days. In conclusion, PMMA bone cement is suitable as delivery system for antibiotics in local therapy

and the elution characteristics are proven both in vitro and in vivo.

Characteristics of Bone Cement for Delivery of Antibiotics

Currently available bone cements are based on methylmethacrylate (MMA). Different co-components for polymerization and various methods of preparation determine the wide ranged variety of PMMA, e.g., plexiglas and bone cement are both PMMA. For the preparation of bone cements, a dough is made of liquid MMA and prepolymerized PMMA powder. Curing results from polymerization of MMA with the PMMA particles (Kühn, 2000). Antibiotics can be incorporated and released by diffusion in this meshwork of "new" polymer chains (Low et al., 1986), both in an aqueous environment as in the human body. The elution properties relate directly to the ability of water uptake of the type of bone cement (Van de Belt et al., 2001). Absorption of water by bone cements is determined by the hydrophobicity of the components, as well as the physical configuration of the bone cement, resulting in porosity and roughness.

The amount of antibiotics released from PMMA depends on the surface available for diffusion. This is why extremely high concentrations are obtained from the surface of ALAC directly after implantation. Elution from areas beneath the surface depends on the porosity, rendering a "capillary" approach for water. This allows aqueous body fluids to "wash out" antibiotics by diffusion.

Particle size of incorporated substances influences the elution properties. Large, well soluble particles that are washed out, enlarge the area for diffusion by leaving void spaces behind, which again allow diffusion from lower areas. Thus, for a short period of time, a dynamic enlargement of the surface takes place.

Unfortunately, the addition of antibiotics (and other substances) alters the mechanical properties of the bone cement. There is a direct correlation between the decrease of mechanical properties of ALAC, the amount of antibiotics added, and the reduced homogeneity of the preparation of antibiotic powder plus PMMA particles. The latter influences not only mechanical properties, but also the elution properties. Commercially available preparations of ALAC are standardized, with respect to homogeneity of the mixture of particles and particle size of the substances added. Thus, the properties of these preparations are known and reliable. This kind of standardization cannot be obtained in hand-mixed preparations in the operating theater. Therefore, if industrial preparations are available, they should be preferred.

Characteristics of Antibiotics for ALAC Preparations

The intention when adding antibiotics to PMMA bone cement is to gain control of an established bone infection or to protect medical devices from bacterial colonization. Antimicrobial agents used in ALAC have to meet the following physico-chemical requirements to be effective in elution:

❖ high solubility in water,
❖ heat resistance (polymerization),
❖ no chemical interaction with the components of bone cement, and
❖ low effect on the mechanical properties of bone cement.

Antimicrobial agents used in ALAC should be highly effective, eluted in sufficient concentrations, and must not be inactivated at the site of application. The frequency of adverse drug effects should be low. The "biological" profile should include the following properties:

❖ bactericidal effect on bacteria in low concentrations (except clindamycin),
❖ low rate of primarily resistant germs,
❖ low frequency of emerging resistances,
❖ low frequency of allergic adverse reactions,
❖ low toxic properties, and
❖ low protein-bonding.

In the individual case, it is often impossible to meet all these criteria. When treating infection, the benefit to the patient must be balanced against possible risks.

Unfortunately, the behavior of antibiotics in ALAC is not predictable by theoretical issues alone: For each antimicrobial agent and each type of bone cement the elution properties must be proven in experiments. This also applies to combinations.

The choice of an antimicrobial agent should be done in the knowledge of the experimental elution data and the susceptibility pattern of the pathogen in each patient. Local and systemic antimicrobial therapy in bone infections – especially if a foreign body is involved – must be tailored to the individual patient. Empirical therapy is not appropriate in these chronic infections – with the exception of life-threatening septicemia.

Due to multiresistant pathogens emerging worldwide, often no industrial preparations of ALAC with incorporated suitable antibiotics are available. In these cases, hand-mixing in the operation theater is necessary if a specific local therapy with ALAC is to be performed.

Appropriate antibiotics for the preparation of ALAC matched with possible pathogens are listed in Table 7.**1**.

How to Prepare ALAC by Hand-Mixing

In order to obtain good antibiotic elution and fair mechanical properties by hand-mixing in the operation room, the preparation of the mixture of powders has to be performed just as a pharmacist would (Frommelt and Kühn, 2005). Because the bone cement is directly incorporated in the human bone, this must be done under sterile conditions. All equipment and the antibiotic powder have to be free of microbial contamination.

An appropriate sterile container and a sterile spatula are required. In a first step, the whole amount of sterile antibiotic powder is transferred into the container under aseptic conditions. Then the same amount oft PMMA powder is added to the antibiotics in the container. Both quantities must be mixed well. In a second step, the same proportion of PMMA powder as in the container is added and both quantities are mixed well again. These last two procedures are repeated until no PMMA powder is left. After antibiotic/PMMA mixing is completed, MMA monomer liquid is added, according to the manufacturer's instructions. This procedure warrants a maximum of homogeneity (Fig. 7.**1**).

Antibiotic powders used should be commercial preparations designed for intravenous use. If antibiotics are not available as powders, the preparation should be prepared by pharmacists in their laboratories.

The addition of dissolved antibiotics to bone cement interferes with the polymerization of PMMA, leads to a dramatic loss of mechanical properties of the bone cement, and alters the elution properties of antibiotics unpredictably. Therefore, liquid antimicrobial agents must never be mixed with PMMA bone cement.

Table 7.1 Options for appropriate antimicrobial agents for preparation of ALAC in the operating theater after assessment of susceptibility patterns of pathogens in the individual case

Antimicrobial agent	Pathogen	Note
Amikacin	■ *Pseudomonas aeruginosa*	In combination with a second antibiotic like cefoperazon or ofloxacin
Ampicillin	■ *Enterococcus fecalis* ■ Streptococci ■ Anerobes	
Cefuroxim	■ Staphylococci (MSSA, CNS – methicillin susceptible) ■ Streptococci	
Cefotaxim	■ Enterobacteriaceae	Combination with gentamicin necessary
Cefoperazon	■ *Pseudomonas aeruginosa*	Combination with amikacin or genta-micin or tobramycin
Clindamycin	■ Staphylococci ■ Streptococci ■ Propionibacteriae ■ Anerobes	Commercially available (in combination with gentamicin)
Gentamicin	■ Diverse	Preferred for prophylaxis and combina-tion Several brands available
Ofloxacin	■ Enterobacteriaceae ■ *Pseudomonas aeruginosa*	
Vancomycin	■ Staphylococci (MRSA, CNS – methicillin resistant) ■ *Corynebacterium amycolatum* ■ Enterococcus spp	■ Poor elution properties, ■ Poor bacteriostatic character, and ■ Use in combination, if possible.
General rules		

MSSA = methicillin-susceptible *Staphylococcus aureus*; CNS = coagulase-negative staphylococci; MRSA = methicillin-resistant *Staphylococcus aureus*

Conclusions and Clinical Impact

ALAC may be used for both prophylaxis and therapy. If bone cement is used for fixation of permanently indwelling devices, it substitutes the surface of artificial joint replacements and protects the surface from being colonized by bacteria that originate from the human flora or, as in the case of infection, from remaining bacteria in the operation field. ALAC may also be used as a carrier for antibiotics in cavity management after debridement of infected bone tissue. For this type of application beads should be used, because their spherical shape offers the largest surface area and thus an optimum of antibiotic elution.

In periprosthetic infection, ALAC is of benefit in one- or multiple-staged revision arthroplasty with exchange of the joint prosthesis (Robbins et al., 2001). In revision arthroplasty, local antibiotic therapy has to be supplemented by an appropriate systemic antibiotic regimen.

Instructions for adding and mixing antibiotics to bone cement

Most prosthesis infections can be effectively treated with industrially manufactured bone cements containing antibiotics. However, due to increasing levels of resistance, extra antibiotics have to be added to the bone cement in more and more cases. The following abridge instructions will guide you throught the process of mixing addittional antibiotics to bone cement.

1. Pour in the components

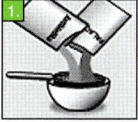

The antibiotics to be used are added to the stirring vessel and mixed with the same quantity of PMMA polymer powder.

2. Homogenise

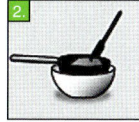

For homogenisation the mixture is passed through a stainless steel sleve using a spatula.

3. Add more

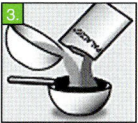

Double the volume by adding same quantity of PMMA as is in the bowl and the compound is mixed homogeneously with the spatula and stainless steel sleve. The procedure is repeated until the PMMA polymere powder has been completely mixed.

4. Add powder to liquid

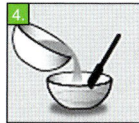

Finally, the PMMA polymer powder is added to the monomer liquid and the mixture is processed in accordance with the user information for the bone cement being used.

Instructions for Mixing Bone Cements Containing Antibiotics

Important:

Generally you should never add more than 4 g antibiotic to 40 g PMMA-bone-cement.
For optimum results the antibiotics being used must meet the following requirements:

• Heat-resistant
• Chemically resistant to monomers
• Water-soluble
• Low microbe count

If medical products are modified, it is the doctor who holds liability!

By adding an antibiotic the doctor assumes liability for the bone cement they have modified. If there are industrially manufactured bone cements which contain antibiotics, they are preferable because of their controlled production process and the liability being assumed by the manufacturer responsible.

Fig. 7.1 Instructions for adding and mixing antibiotics to bone cement.

Numerous empirical data are available on the treatment with ALAC of bone and foreign body-associated infections in bone tissue. The concepts reported are developed empirically, and are sometimes based on personal beliefs, so that a variety of approaches result in outcomes that are at least comparable. There is, however, little exact knowledge of which specific measures lead to success in the individual cases. The theoretical advantages of ALAC in controlling bone infection are supported by the results of investigations in animals and clinical studies in humans. The studies report a low frequency of adverse reactions to local antibiotic therapy (Wininger and Fass, 1996). Controlled studies – especially in comparison with systemic antibiotic therapy – are needed.

In conclusion, local therapy using antibiotic-loaded acrylic cement is a well-established method for the local application of antibiotics in the therapy of bone infections. Nowadays, emerging multiresistant pathogens like methicillin-resistant *Staphylococcus aureus*, vancomycin-resistant enterococci and others limit this therapy, as only a small choice of antibiotics is suitable for application in bone cement.

References

Adams K, Couch L, Cierny G, Calhoun J, Mader JT. In vitro and in vivo evaluation of antibiotic diffusion from antibiotic-impregnated polymethylmethacrylate beads. Clin Orthop Relat Res 1992; 278: 244–252.
Belt van de H, Neut D, Schenk W, van Horn JR, van der Mei HC, Busscher HJ. Infection of orthopedic implants and the use of antibiotic-loaded bone cements: A review. Acta Orthop Scand 2001; 72: 557–571.

Buchholz HW, Elson RA, Lodenkämper H. The Infected Joint implant. In: McKibbin B (ed) Recent Advances in Orthopaedics 3. Curchhill Livingston New York 1979; 139–161.

Buchholz HW, Engelbrecht H. Über die Depotwirkung einiger Antibiotika bei Vermischung mit dem Kunstharz Palacos. Chirurg 1970; 41: 511–515.

Costerton JW, Stewart PS, Greenberg EP. Bacterial biofilm: a common cause of persistent infections. Science 1999; 284: 1318–1322.

Frommelt L, Kühn KD. Antibiotic-Loaded Cement. In: Breusch S, Malchau H. (eds.) The Well-Cemented Total Hip Arthroplasty. Springer Berlin-Heidelberg-New York 2005; 86–92.

Hendrich C, Frommelt L. Keimorientierte Antibiotikatherapie bei Protheseninfektionen. Septische Knochen- und Gelenkchirurgie. Springer Berlin Heidelberg 2004.

Kühn KD, Bone Cements. Up-to-date comparison of physical and chemical properties of commercial materials. Springer-Verlag Berlin Heidelberg, 2000.

Low HAT, Fleming RH, Gilmore MFX, McCarthy ID, Hughes SPF. In vitro measurement and computer modeling of the diffusion of antibiotic in bone cement. J Biomed Eng 1986; 8: 149–155.

Mader JT, Adams KR. Experimental osteomyelitis. In: Schlossberg D (ed) Orthopedic Infection. Springer New York 1988; 39–48.

Robbins GM, Masri BA, Garbuz DS, Duncan CP. Primary Total hip arthroplasty after infection. J Bone Joint Surg Am 2001; 83: 601–614.

Stewart PS, Costerton JW. Antibiotic resistance of bacteria in biofilms. Lancet 2001; 358: 135–138.

Winninger DA, Fass RJ. Antibiotic-impregnated cement and beads for orthopedic infections. Antimicrob Agents Chemotherap 1996; 40: 2675–2679.

Zimmerli W, Lew PD, Waldvogel FA. Pathogenesis of foreign body infection. Evidence for a local granulocyte defect. J Clin Invest 1984; 73: 1191–1200.

Local Antibiotic-Loaded Carriers in Orthopedic Surgery – Pharmacokinetic Aspects

Geert H. I. M. Walenkamp

History

Since the discovery of bacteria by Pasteur in 1864, a more causal therapy of osteomyelitis has been possible. In 1880, he identified the same bacterium in an osteomyelitic abscess as in a furuncle and stated: "Osteomyelitis is the furuncle of the bone." Lister applied these findings, and tried to prevent postoperative infections by disinfection. He treated open fractures locally with carbolic acid tampons and plaster to prevent osteomyelitis, but this combination was later also used to treat established infections. Also, other authors implanted alloplastic materials with closure of the skin, such as plaster with 5% carbolic acid (Dreesman, 1896) and plaster with cod liver oil (Löhr, 1934).

Another approach since 1889 was to fill the cavity with patients' own blood instead of packing it with gauzes. The coagulum was left intact and had to be organized. The results, however, were not favorable, and did not improve with addition of antiseptics. When antibiotics became available, they were mixed with the blood coagulum, forming the so-called antibiotic plug (Winter, 1951).

Antiseptics were applied as irrigation of infected cavities. In 1915, Carrel described irrigation with hypochlorite (Dakin's fluid: NaClO) (Carrel et al., 1915; Dakin, 1915). When antibiotics became available, most advocates of irrigation or suction-drainage systems admixed antibiotics with the instillation fluid (Grace and Bryson, 1950; Willenegger, 1963; Boda, 1979).

Prigge was the first to describe the use of bone grafts in osteomyelitis in cases where no muscle flaps were feasible (Prigge, 1946). After debridement and saucerisation he packed the cavity temporarily with penicillin-instilled gauzes. In a second stage, he performed a bone graft with cancellous bone. Coleman performed the debridement of osteomyelitis and the implantation of cancellous bone graft in one stage, admixing antibiotics to the graft (Coleman et al., 1946). In 1973, Papineau described a similar method (Papineau, 1973). He debrided in several stages, and packed the open wound with antibiotic-containing gauzes. During a second stage, a massive bone graft was applied, and the bone was eventually stabilized with an intramedullary nail.

So, ever since antibiotics were available, local application was frequently practiced. They were, however, also increasingly used for prevention of wound infection. Buchholz used antibiotic-containing solutions for regular lavage during operation, and he sutured cloths soaked in antibiotics to the fascia (Buchholz and Gartenmann, 1972). In his search for a more effective reduction of the postoperative deep infections of hip prostheses (3%), he demonstrated that bone cement was capable of a sustained release of various substances, such as the residual monomer and CuS. So, in a pilot study, he admixed four heat stable antibiotic powders with bone cement and found that, except tetracycline, the antibiotics indeed were released by a diffusion process for at least 2 weeks in a bactericidal concentration.

In June 1969, he wrote a letter to the producer of Palacos, Kulzer GmbH (Wehrheim, Germany) asking to investigate, whether antibiotics could indeed be effectively admixed without decreasing the physical properties of the bone cement. They started a study with the Merck Company (Darmstadt, Germany). Helmut Wahlig and Elvira Dingeldein tested a combination with gentamicin as the most effective. Subsequently, many combinations of antibiotics and bone cements were tested, mainly in the years 1970–1978 (Fig. 8.1).

Like other authors, they found that when gentamicin was chosen, the combination with Palacos resulted in the best release (Wahlig et al., 1972; Kühn, 2000).

Controlled delivery: 3996 patents and 8392 articles (Modified: Bruinewoud, thesis 2005)

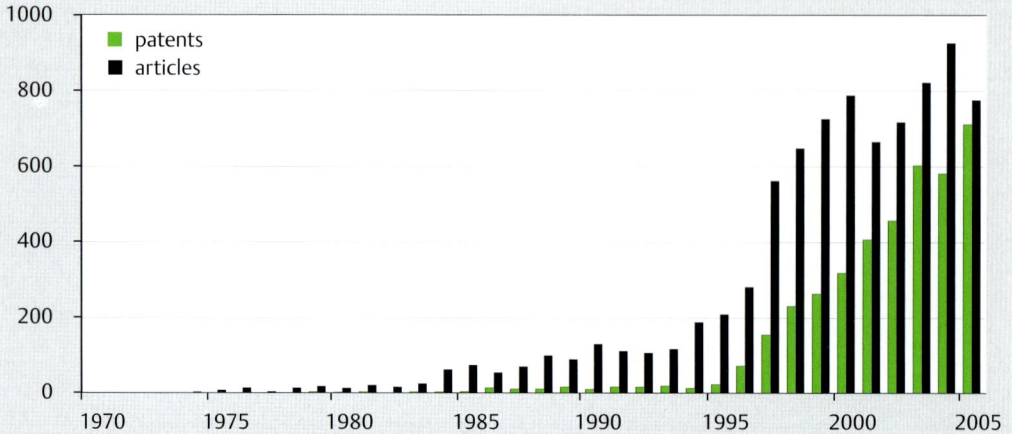

Fig. 8.**1**   Publications and patents on drug delivery since 1970 (Modified: Bruinewoud, 2005).

Antibiotic-Loaded Carriers: Pharmacokinetic Properties

Bone cement is based on methylmethacrylate and is made by mixing the liquid monomer with the polymer powder (PMMA). During the curing process, a network of newly formed PMMA chains is formed. Various substances such as antibiotics can be mixed and will incorporate in between these PMMA chains. They can be released by diffusion when the PMMA absorbs water, which is a process determined by the hydrophobicity of the cement (Kühn, 2000). The antibiotic release is influenced by the porosity and roughness of the cement. The release of antibiotics is limited to a depth of 100 μm (Schurman et al., 1978). The initial high release is a surface phenomenon that lasts for some hours. This is followed by a period of sustained release – a bulk phenomenon – which depends on the penetration of fluid through interconnected pores in the cement (Van de Belt et al., 2000).

Once the antibiotic-loaded cement was on the market, it was also used to treat osteomyelitis. Filling bone cavities after debridement, however, appeared to be ineffective in clinical practice (Voorhoeve and Stöhr, 1973; Jenny et al., 1977; Klemm, 1977), which was confirmed later on in animal experiments (Fitzgerald, 1983). Therefore,

in 1972, Klaus Klemm started to knead small beads of bone cement mixed with antibiotics, to treat osteomyelitis (Klemm, 1993). Since 1976 they have been manufactured at the Kulzer Company and distributed by Merck (Darmstadt).

Many antibiotics and many bone cements have been tested, and still new combinations are being produced. In-vitro and in-vivo studies of the combinations are not standardized, so it is difficult to ascertain what product could be the best choice.

In-vitro studies measure the release of the diffused antibiotic out of the carrier. This can be done in several ways.

Static measurements:

An antibiotic (AB)-loaded cement block with a certain volume and surface is put in a bottle filled with a watery fluid. The release can be measured by two different methods:

1. The bath fluid is exchanged every time unit (first hours, later days) and replaced by fresh fluid. In every exchanged fluid the AB concentration is measured. In this method the fluid has a small volume, e.g., 10 mL with a block of 5 mL (method 1a).
2. A large bath fluid (e.g., 500 mL or 1 L) remains around the cement all the time, but a very

small amount is taken every time unit for cumulative measurements of the AB concentration and replaced by the same amount of fresh fluid (method 1b) a cumulative measurement.

Dynamic measurements:

The release is studied while some kind of continuous stream of bath fluid around the carrier is maintained, and the AB concentration in that fluid is measured.

These methods try to simulate in-vivo conditions in patients where a hematoma around the carrier is formed, resorbed and replaced. Antibiotics are transported in the surrounding tissues by diffusion, so the diffusion characteristics of the AB carrier combination are decisive. The objective in local treatment with antibiotics, is to achieve the highest possible local concentration, since most of the antibiotics used are more effective when applied in higher concentrations.

Because the release is a diffusion process, the maximum release takes place in the very beginning when the gradient between the carrier and its surrounding is highest. The release will diminish in time, at the same rate as the gradient – the "motor" for diffusion – decreases. The diffusion process also governs the distribution of the antibiotic in the surrounding tissues. Thus, the antibiotic concentration will diminish in time and distance.

When the fluid is replaced at regular intervals (method 1a) or as described in cumulative measurements (method 1b), the diffusion process shows a characteristic release curve (Figs. 8.**2a** and 8.**2b**). In effect, the in-vivo results will be somewhere in between the two, because no such a continuous replacement of the hematoma occurs, nor is there a zero diffusion of the antibiotic into the surrounding.

In-vivo results can only be measured in animal experiments and in treated patients.

Wahlig and Dingeldein studied tissue concentrations in dog osteomyelitis. They proved that the concentration in the hematoma and in the tissue decreases in the weeks following implantation. They also demonstrated that concentrations decreased proportionally to an increase of tissue density: fibrous tissue, cancellous bone, cortical bone (Wahlig et al., 1978), (Fig. 8.**3**). It appeared not to be necessary that the bone was alive. Elson proved that also dead bone is well-penetrated and diffused by antibiotics that are released from bone cement (Elson et al., 1977).

We were able to confirm the above mentioned relation of concentration to time and distance to the carrier in animal experiments with sheep (Kaarsemaker et al., 1997) and rabbits (Walenkamp et al., 2007).

When using collagen with gentamicin, attention must be paid to the different properties of different products. First, gentamicin collagen was compared with gentamicin PMMA beads. In an in-vitro study the gentamicin was immediately released within a few hours (Sandberg et al., 1990), resulting in a very high local concentration in the exsudate, but for only a short time period. In order to extend the time period of release, another product was developed with a protracted release. This was achieved by replacing the gentamicin sulfate partly by the inactive gentamicin crobophat. This is transformed to the active sulfate form over a period of some weeks, which results in a longer period of high release and high local concentrations.

How to use Local Antibiotic Carriers in Patients – Practical Guidelines

In general, antibiotic-loaded carriers may be used for prevention as well as for therapy of infection. For prevention, a high local antibiotic concentration will be effective, even if this is only for a short time. One or two days, maybe even a few hours can be sufficient. For therapeutic use, the carrier may be more effective if the antibiotic concentration is high for a long period, preferably for 2 – 4 weeks. The diffusion of the antibiotic into the infected tissues takes time, as well as the killing process of the bacteria. In osteomyelitis, there is some evidence that a long-term treatment of even months with systemic antibiotics is more effective than short treatment periods (Hedström, 1974). So, resorbable carriers with a short half-life such as some gentamicin collagen products or hand-mixed combinations with autologous bonegrafts, may be indicated as preventive local antibiotics. Whereas products that are able to maintain a high concentration for weeks, are preferable for therapeutic applications.

When gentamicin PMMA beads are used for cavity management, the highest gentamicin concentration can be achieved, if the cavity is filled with as much beads as possible, creating a maxi-

In-vitro gentamicin release in exchange bath fluid

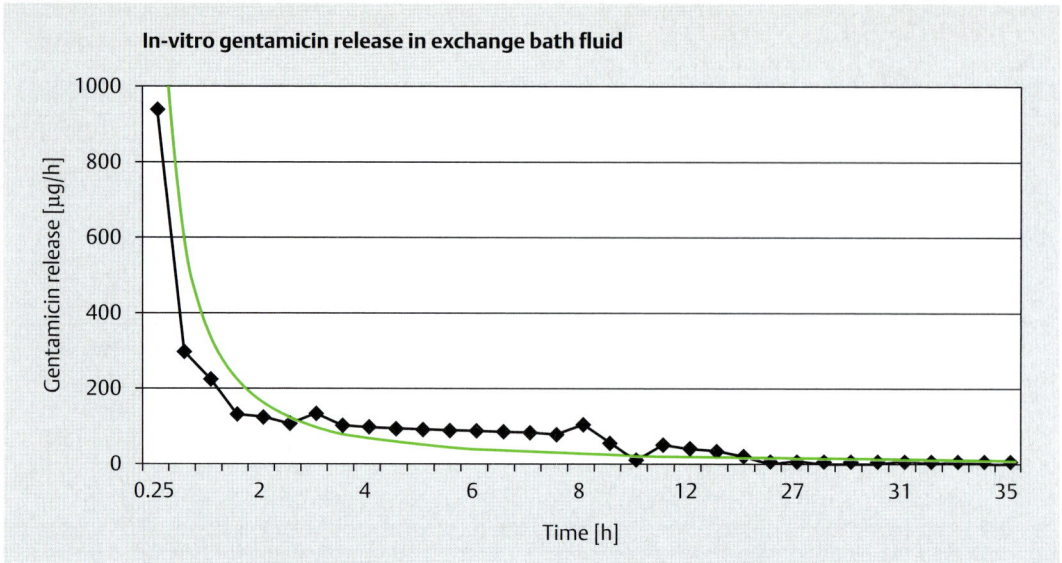

Fig. 8.**2a**   In-vitro release studies with polylactide-gentamicin pellets, method 1a (Walenkamp et al., 2007).

In-vitro cumulative gentamicin release

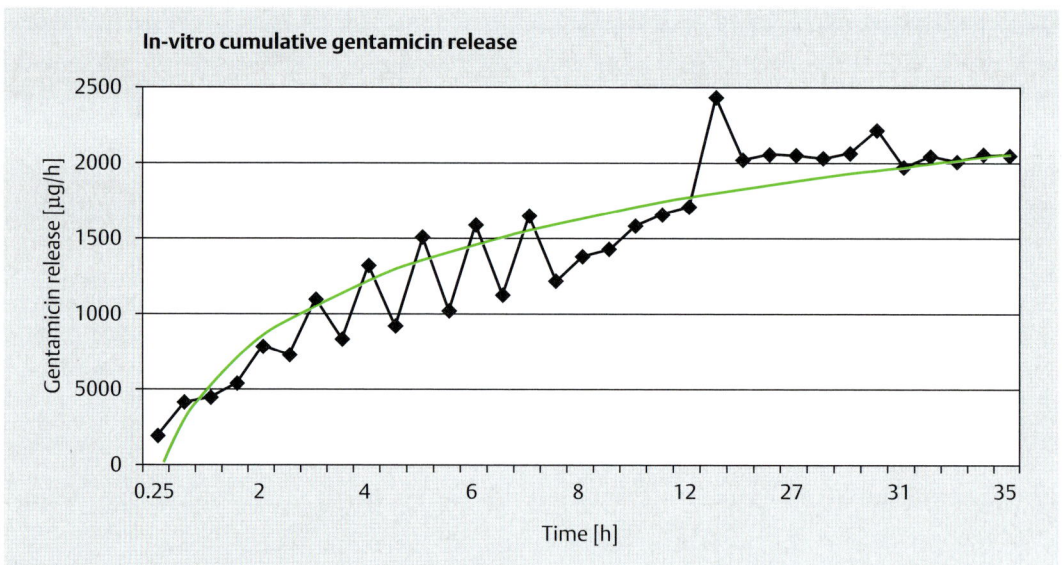

Fig. 8.**2b**   In-vitro release studies with polylactide-gentamicin pellets, method 1b (Walenkamp et al., 2007).

mal cement surface. With proper handling of the resulting hematoma, the local gentamicin concentration will increase immediately after implantation, to reach a peak level at about day three (Walenkamp, 1983; Walenkamp, 1997), (Fig. 8.**4a** and Fig. **14b**).

This maximum can be 50–100 fold the minimal inhibitory concentration (MIC) value of the causative bacteria. This high concentration will decrease rapidly, however, with increasing distance to the beads, and at 2–3 cms the effectivity will be largely reduced. Therefore, the beads must

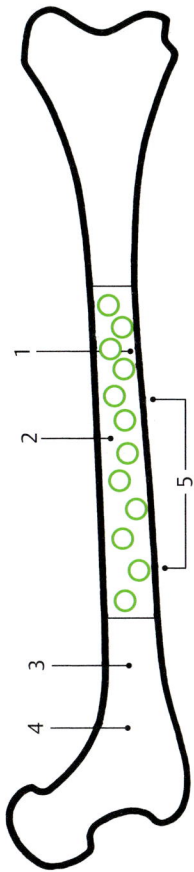

Dog	N beads	Days	Weeks	Hematoma (1)	Connective tissue (1)	Cancellous bone (2)	Cancellous bone (3)	Cancellous bone (4)	Cortical bone (5)
1	17	3	0.5	148		17.8		3.6	6.8
2	15	3	0.5	112		15.2		3.6	13
3	13	7	1	200		24	14.5	4	20.1
4	16	7	1	212		16.4		6.6	14.1
5	18	14	2	124		8.2	5.9	0.6	1.8
6	17	14	2	104		5.2	2.1	0.8	3.8
7	14	28	4	9.1	9.1	2.9		0.4	1.6
8	14	28	4		7.5	4.9		0.2	0.4
9	19	42	6		16.1	8.4	0.34	0.2	0
10	19	42	6		7.7	4.9	0.9	0.5	0
11	7	63	9		4.4	0.4	0.2	0.2	0
12	14	63	9		4.4	0.9	0	0	0
13	28	116	16.5		5.6	5.1	1	0.7	0
14	37	116	16.5		5.4	2.6	0.2	0.2	0
15	30	116	16.5		2.2	1.1	0.8	0	0

Fig. 8.3 Experiment performed by Wahlig (Wahlig et al., 1978) in 15 dogs. Gentamicin-PMMA beads were implanted in a femur for 3 – 116 days. Gentamicin concentrations (µg / mL) were measured in the hematoma and the resulting connective tissue (both 1), in cancellous bone (2), (3), (4), and in cortical bone (5). Note the decrease in concentration in relation to time and distance to the beads (figure and table constructed by the author, according to Wahlig et al., 1978).

be packed into the entire infected or contaminated area (Fig. 8.4b).

Elution of the antibiotic is only possible if there is a hematoma, as antibiotics are released from the PMMA carrier in exchange with water. Therefore, PMMA beads will be less effective in subcutaneous, lipophilic tissue. To ensure maximum antibiotic concentrations, the enveloping hematoma should not exceed the volume of the beads. On the other hand, drainage of the hematoma may result in loss of antibiotic. As in the case of collagen carriers, vacuum drains will also remove the colla-

gen, so they must be used as overflow drains from the beginning onwards.

PMMA beads can be applied as spacers in cavities of osteomyelitis and removed prostheses, respectively. They are easily removed after 2 – 4 weeks along the original incision, depending on the local anatomy. However, if they are inserted in soft tissue and / or in a stretched position, they subsequently will be encapsulated. The adhering granulation tissue will catch on the beads, which renders removal by just pulling on the chains an impossible or risky task. In this case, the beads

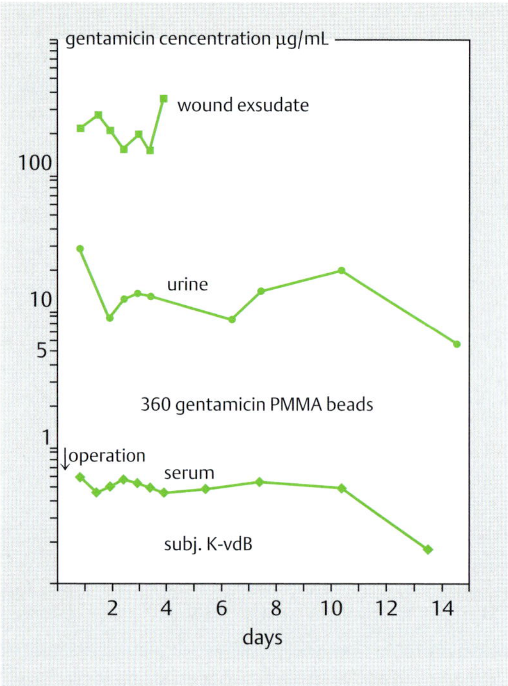

Fig. 8.**4a** The gentamicin concentrations in serum, urine and exsudate in a 65-year-old lady. After extraction of an infected total hip 360 gentamicin PMMA beads were implanted (Walenkamp, 1983).The exsudate concentration increased up to values 100 times the MIC value of the bacteria.

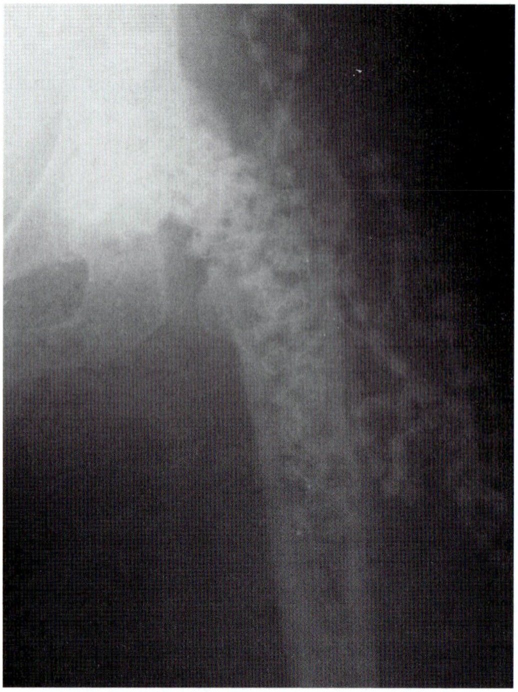

Fig. 8.**4b** Radiographic image after extraction of an infected total hip. The cavity is filled with antibiotic-loaded PMMA beads.

must be removed at an earlier stage. Permanent implantation of the beads is also possible. However, as there is always a risk of germs persisting on the beads (Von Eiff et al., 1997; Van de Belt et al., 2001; Neut et al., 2001), it is advisable to rather remove the beads.

If no reconstruction of the infected area is necessary, beads can also be inserted with the end of a chain protruding from the skin. In this case, the chain of beads can be extracted by simply pulling at the chain. In my experience, the best option is to start pulling 1 week after implantation, about 3 to 5 beads at a time, every other day. The chain should be implanted in a meander form, not stretched, and should protrude from the skin by a separate incision that is sufficiently wide. On chain removal, the end of every chain has to be inspected to check that the last bead has not slipped off.

Patients should not be sent home with beads in a joint cavity, because the chains may rupture. In case of reimplantation with a long-term interval, a spacer can be used. In osteomyelitic cavities, chains with beads may be removed after a longer period if they are not intra-medullary. In that case, they are fixed after 4–6 weeks.

PMMA beads are used as spacers in bone or joint when a reconstruction is postponed until the infection is cleared. Being able to wait and observe the healing process for a few weeks or months minimizes the risk of reinfection, according to the rule: "Heal the infection first, and reconstruct afterwards."

It is up to the experience of the clinician to decide, which calculated risk is acceptable in determining when and how to reconstruct.

So far, little experience has been gained in the use of resorbable antibiotic-loaded bone substitutes. Gentamicin-collagen and tobramycin-loaded calcium sulfate are amongst a few products currently available on the market. One of the best methods applied at the moment, is admixing of antibiotics by the surgeon himself into the autologous or homologous bone graft. In-vivo and in-vitro experiments as well as clinical trials demonstrate a protracted release of admixed antibiotics from bone grafts over several weeks (Buttaro et al., 2005a, Witsø et al., 1999, Buttaro et al., 2005b, Witsø et al., 2000, Witsø chapter 5, fig. 5.**1**). These results have promising implictions for prosthesis revision and osteomyelitic reconstructions.

Bone substitutes, such as hydroxylapatite, calcium sulphate, and tricalciumphosphate have to be removed completely in case of infection. Therefore coating or admixing with antibiotics by the producer or by the surgeon might be helpful.

Results

Results of prophylactic use are best documented in primary total hip prostheses. In experimental studies, admixed antibiotics have proven to be effective in protecting the prosthesis against infection from contaminated wounds, as well as against hematogenous infection for the period of 6 weeks after implantation (Elson et al., 1977; Blomgren and Lindgren, 1980). This may be a crucial period in which an unknown part of deep infections may be caused by concomitant pneumonia, decubitus, or urine infection in patients with decreased immune status.

The good results using antibiotic-loaded cement, as in the case of one-stage revisions with known or unknown infections, are due to the bactericidal effect on bacteria that are present in the entire wound bed after explantation of a prosthesis. This application can be regarded as borderland between prophylactic and therapeutic use.

In prophylactic as well as in therapeutic use, better results are to be expected from local antibiotic application than from systemic administration, because higher local antibiotic concentrations should kill more bacteria in tissues, even if tissue perfusion is impaired. This appears, however, to be difficult to prove in randomized clinical trials (RCT). The many clinical variables involved in osteomyelitis make clinical studies difficult to design and to evaluate.

A RCT to achieve approval by the Food and Drug Administration (FDA) in the United States failed to demonstrate significantly better results for the application of gentamicin PMMA beads in osteomyelitis versus parenteral antibiotic treatment. Participating surgeons worried about withholding additional parenteral antibiotics from the patients in the gentamicin beads group. Treatment with gentamicin beads alone was significantly cheaper (Blaha et al., 1993).

In a comparative RCT involving 77 open fractures, no significant difference could be demonstrated between local and perenteral antibiotic treatment (by man-made beads), due to the limited size of the study (Moehring et al., 2000).

Numerous open cohort studies have been published on the clinical results of treatment of osteomyelitis, prosthesis infection, and other orthopedic infections. Results, in general, are expressed as "healing percentages" in combination with a certain follow-up period. An infection will be considered as healed when all clinical symptoms have disappeared, including normalization of laboratory findings. It may be difficult to judge, if persistent pain is related to a low-grade persistent infection. The same applies for elevated infection parameters, such as the erythrocyte sedimentation rate (ESR) in rheumatoid patients or patients with other infections. Two proverbs express the pessimistic view on healing in osteomyelitis:

"Once osteomyelitis, always osteomyelitis" and "Osteomyelitis is a time bomb that always tics". However, literature and my own experience indicate that this pessimism cannot be justified any more. The treatment results in literature of aggressive surgical and medical interventions in early postoperative infection of prostheses, indicate that a healing percentage of 80–90% can be achieved. Most relapses will be recognizable a few months after systemic antibiotic therapy has been stopped.

In osteomyelitis, treatment results have improved over the years, increasing from 30–50% to 80–90% in the last century (Fig. 8.**5**).

Healing, however, should not be expressed as a healing percentage, but in terms of survival analysis, as in oncological treatment. We studied the healing rate in 100 consecutive patients with osteomyelitis (acute and chronic) and found 19 relapses. When these were treated with another treatment period (operations, eventually followed by postoperative systemic antibiotic treatment), the overall healing after 1–12 years was 92% (Walenkamp et al., 1998). The survival analysis showed that the relapses almost always occured

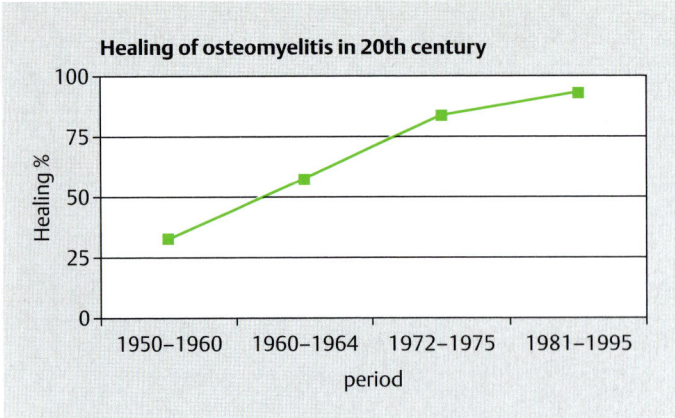

Fig. 8.5 Healing osteomyelitis improved in the 20th century. The graph is constructed by the author according to the literature.

in the first postoperative months and year. Also, experience since then shows that patients without healing can be identified early, and I dismiss patients from regular postoperative controls in the outpatient clinic after two years (Fig. 8.**6**).

In the beginning, when local antibiotic treatment of soft-tissue infections and osteomyelitis was introduced, there was considerable doubt amongst surgeons, whether the primary closure of the wound was permitted. It had always been advocated that infected wounds require open treatment after debridement. Closure after thorough debridement and implantation of a local antibiotic delivery system was a surgical revolu-

tion. Still, surgeons appear to have problems with this concept, as illustrated by the upcoming vacuum-assisted wound treatment.

Primary wound closure, which is necessary to keep the antibiotic inside the wound, however, has largely improved patient comfort and has significantly decreased the workload of nursing staff, as well as hospital stay, use of antibiotics, and the costs of treatment (Hoök and Lindberg, 1987).

References

Belt van de H, Neut D, Schenk W et al. Staphylococcus aureus biofilm formation on different gentamicin-loaded polymethylmethacrylate bone cements. Biomaterials 2001; 22: 1607–1611.

Belt van de H, Neut D, Uges DRA et al. Surface roughness, porosity and wettability of gentamicin-loaded bone cements and their antibiotic release. Biomaterials 2000; 21: 1981–1987.

Blaha JD, Calhoun JH, Nelson CL et al. Comparison of the clinical efficacy and tolerance of gentamicin PMMA beads on surgical wire versus combined and systemic therapy for osteomyelitis. Clin Orthop Relat Res 1993; 295: 8–12.

Blomgren G, Lindgren U. The susceptibility of total joint replacement to hematogenous infection in the early postoperative period: an experimental study in the rabbit. Clin Orthop Rel Res 1980; 151: 308–312.

Boda A. Antibiotic irrigation-perfusion treatment for chronic osteomyelitis. Arch Orthop Trauma Surg 1979; 95: 31–35.

Bruinewoud H. Ultrasound-induced drug release from polymer matrices. The glass transition temperature as a thermo-responsive switch (thesis). Technical University Eindhoven; 2005:167.

Buchholz H, Gartenmann H. Infektionsprophylaxe und operative Behandlung des schleichende tiefen In-

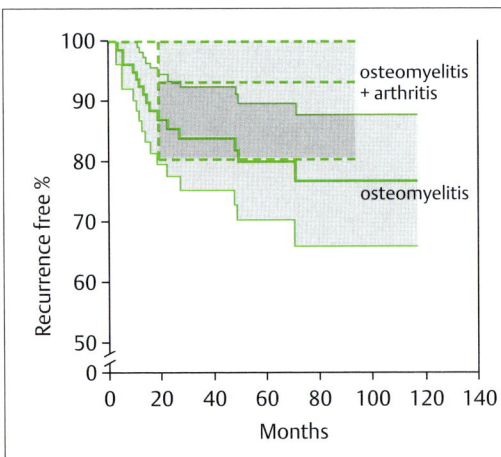

Fig. 8.**6** A survival analysis depicting the recurrence-free period after treatment of 100 patients with osteomyelitis (Walenkamp et al., 1998).

fektion bei der Totalen Endoprothese. Chirurg 1972;43:446–453.

Buttaro M, Gimenez MI, Greco G, Barcan L, Piccaluga F. High local levels of vancomycin without nephrotoxicity released from impacted bone allograft in 20 revision hip arthroplasties. Acta Orthop 2005; 76: 336–340.

Buttaro M, Pusso R, Piccaluga F. Vancomycin-supplemented impacted bone allografts in infected hip arthroplasty. Two-stage results. J Bone Joint Surg 2005; 87-B: 314–319.

Carrel A, Dakin, Daufresne, Dehelly, Dumas. Traitement abortif de línfection des plaies. Bull Acad de Med Paris 1915; 74: 361.

Coleman H, Bateman J, Dale G, Starr D. Cancellous bone grafts for infected bone defects. Surg Gynecol Obstet 1946; 83: 392.

Dakin H. On the use of certain antiseptic substances in the treatment of infected wounds. British Med J 1915; 2: 318.

Dreesman H. Über Knochenplombierung. Zentralbl f Chir 1896; 20: 55.

Eiff von C, Bettin D, Proctor R et al. Recovery of Small Colony Variants of Staphylococcus aureus following gentamicin bead placement for osteomyelitis. Clin Infect Dis 1997; 25: 1250–1251.

Elson RA, Jephcott AE, McGechie DB, Verettas D. Antibiotic loaded acrylic cement. J Bone Joint Surg 1977; 59-B: 200–205.

Elson RA, Jephcott AE, McGechie DB, Verettas D. Bacterial infection and acrylic cement in the rat. J Bone Joint Surg 1977; 59-B: 452–457.

Fitzgerald RH. Experimental osteomyelitis: description of a canine model and the role of depot administration of antibiotics in the prevention and treatment of sepsis. J Bone Jt Surg 1983; 65-A: 371–380.

Grace EJ, Bryson V. Modern treatment of chronic osteomyelitis with topical detergent antibiotic therapy. Surg Gynecol Obstet 1950; 91: 333–342.

Hedstrøm SA. The prognosis of chronic staphylococcal osteomyelitis after long-term antibiotic treatment. Scan J Infect Dis 1974; 6: 33–38.

Hoök M, Lindberg L. Treatment of chronic osteomyelitis with gentamicin-PMMA beads. A prospective study in Nepal. Trop Doct 1987; 17: 157–163.

Jenny G, Kempf I, Jaeger JH, Konsbruck R. Utilisation de billes de ciment acrylique à la gentamycine. Rev Chir Orthop Reparatrice Appar Mot 1977; 63: 491–500.

Kaarsemaker S, Walenkamp GH, vd Bogaard AE. New model for chronic osteomyelitis with Staphylococcus aureus in sheep. Clin Orthop Relat Res 1997; 339: 246–252.

Klemm K. Die Behandlung chronischer Knocheninfektion mit Gentamycin-PMMA-Ketten und Kugeln. In: Contzen H ed, Gentamycin-PMMA-Kette Gentamycin-PMMA-Kugeln Symposium München 12 November 1976: VLE Verlag; 1977: 20–27.

Klemm KW. Antibiotic bead chains. Clinical Orthop 1993; 295: 63–76.

Kühn KD. Bone Cements. Up-to-date comparison of physical and chemical properties of commercial materials. Springer-Verlag Berlin Heidelberg, 2000.

Löhr W. Die Behandlung der akuten und der chronischen Osteomyelitis der Röhrenknochen mit dem Lebertrangips. Arch Klin Chir 1934; 180: 206.

Moehring HD, Gravel C, Chapman MW, Olson SA. Comparison of antibiotic beads and intravenous antibiotics in open fractures. Clin Orthop Rel Res 2000; 372: 254–261.

Neut D, van de Belt H, Stokroos I et al. Biomaterial-associated infection of gentamicin-loaded PMMA beads in orthopaedic revision surgery. J Antimicrob Chemother 2001; 7: 885–891.

Papineau LJ. L'excision-greffe avec férméture retardée delibérée dans l'osteomyelite chronique. Nouv-Presse Med 1973; 2: 2753–2755.

Prigge E. The treatment of chronic osteomyelitis by the use of muscle transplant or iliac graft. J Bone Joint Surg 1946; 28: 576–593.

Sandberg Sørensen T, Ibsen Sørensen A, Merser S. Rapid release of gentamicin from collagen sponge: in vitro comparison with plastic beads. Acta Orthop Scand 1990; 61: 353–356.

Schurman DJ, Trindade C, Hirschman HP et al. Antibiotic-acrylic bone cement composites. J Bone Joint Surg 1978; 60-A: 978–984.

Voorhoeve A, Stöhr C. Ergebnisse bei der Behandlung der chronisch-eitrigen Osteomyelitis mit einem Palacos-gentamycin-Gemisch. MünschmedWschr 1973; 115: 924–930.

Wahlig H, Dingeldein E, Bergmann R, Reuss K. The release of gentamicin from polymethylmethacrylate beads. An experimental and pharmacokinetic study. J Bone Joint Surg Br 1978; 60-B: 270–275.

Wahlig H, Schliep HJ, Bergmann R, Hameister W, Grieben A. Über die Freisetzung von Gentamycin aus Polymethylacrylat. II. Experimentelle Untersuchungen in vivo. Langenbecks Arch Chir 1972; 331: 193–212.

Walenkamp GH. Chronic osteomyelitis. How I do it. Acta Orthop Scand 1997; 68: 497–506.

Walenkamp GH, Kleijn LL, de Leeuw M. Osteomyelitis treated with gentamicin-PMMA beads: 100 patients followed for 1–12 years. Acta Orthop Scand 1998; 69: 518–522.

Walenkamp GHIM. Gentamicin PMMA beads. A clinical, pharmacokinetic and toxicological study (thesis). KU Nijmegen; 1983.

Walenkamp GHIM, Bouma M et al. Pharmacokinetic study of gentamicin polylactide as a resorbable antibiotic delivery system in osteomyelitis. [in preparation] 2007.

Willenegger H. Therapeutische Möglichkeiten und Grenzen der antibakteriellen Spüldrainage bei chirurgischen Infektionen. Langenbecks Arch Chir 1963; 304: 670–672.

Winter L. Management of chronic osteitis and osteomyelitis with a coagulum of autogenous blood and penicillin and trombin. Int Chir 1951; 11: 510–524.

Witsø E, Persen L, Loeseth K, Bergh K. Adsorption and release of antibiotics from morsalized cancellous bone: in vitro studies of 8 antibiotics. Acta Orthop Scand 1999; 70: 298 – 304.

Witsø E, Persen L, Loeseth K, Bergh K. Cancellous bone as an antibiotic carrier. Acta Orthop Scand 2000; 71: 80 – 84.

(FR) Vancomycin Bone Cement – Experimental Data

Sebastien Parratte, Cédric Foucault, Michel Drancourt, Jean-Noël Argenson

Introduction and Background

According to Sir John Charnley, postoperative infection is the saddest of all complications after total hip arthroplasty. The use of peroperative antimicrobial prophylaxis and laminar airflow in surgical settings has reduced the risk of intra-operative infection to less than 1% after hip replacement and to less than 2% after knee replacement (Zimmerli et al., 2004). However, infections associated with prosthetic joints cause significant morbidity and remain a social, as well as an economic problem (Zimmerli et al., 2004). The overall annual costs of orthopedic implant-associated infections in the United States amount to $150–200 million and are about three times as much in other parts of the world (Van de Belt et al., 2001). To quote the French scientist Pasteur: "Environment is everything, bacteria are nothing." The methods of reducing infection after arthroplasty are based on this principle and include meticulous surgical technique, improved surgical environment using laminar flow, and the use of prophylactic systemic antibiotics (Argenson et al., 1992). In 1970, Buchholz and Engelbrecht (Buchholz and Engelbrecht, 1970) incorporated antibiotics in PMMA bone cement for the first time, to reduce the infection rate in orthopedic surgery. They assumed that the antibiotic will be released gradually, yielding higher local concentrations than can be achieved by systemic therapy. Gentamicin has been the most commonly used antibiotic, but resistance to this compound has increased in recent years (Argenson et al., 1994).

Major bacterial pathogens involved in infected arthroplasties, such as staphylococci and *Pseudomonas,* are now frequently resistant to gentamicin. In our experience, staphylococci account for 40–70% of the infections after total hip arthroplasty in Southern Europe, and 40% are resistant to gentamicin (Stein et al., 1998). Vancomycin, however, is effective against nearly all staphylococci and is, therefore, our agent of choice. We hypothesize that vancomycin in bone cement could be locally effective against bacteria – especially resistant staphylococci – growing in the biofilm that covers the prosthetic surface. Its application should provide upkeeping of the mechanical properties of bone cement, good elution characteristics, and maintenance of bacteriological properties during polymerization.

Perenteral vancomycin administration bears the risk of inducing renal and ear toxicity, as well as vascular allergic reactions. Furthermore, systemic administration of vancomycin may result in emergence of bacterial resistance. The addition of vancomycin in bone cement, however, may induce neither general toxicity nor resistance, since the amount of antibiotic in serum is negligible. The purpose of this paper is to confirm the biomechanical, bacteriological, and clinical implications in the use of vancomycin-loaded bone cement in hip and knee arthroplasty. In the first part, we analyze the mechanical and bacteriological properties on the basis of in-vitro and in-vivo studies (Fig. 9.1). The second part illustrates the clinical use of vancomycin in bone cement, as well as our clinical revision strategy for infected hip or knee prostheses, respectively.

Analysis of Mechanical Properties of Vancomycin-/Tobramycin-Loaded Bone Cements

Background

The purpose of this study was to investigate whether the tensile mechanical properties of four low-viscosity bone cements are affected when admixed with vancomycin and tobramycin (Argenson et al., 1994).

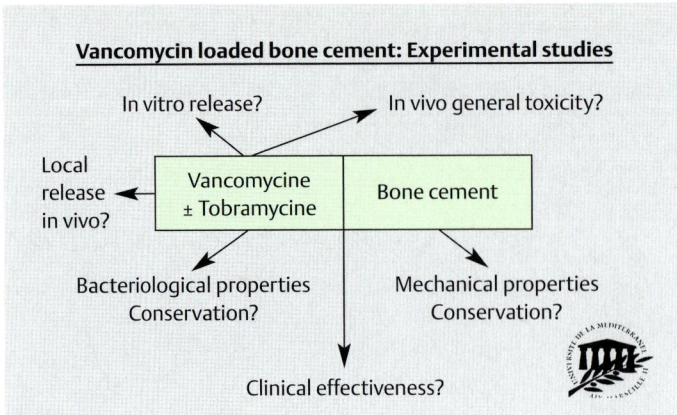

Materials and methods

Four low-viscosity cements were used throughout the study: CMW3, LVC (Zimmer), Palacos LV and Sulfix 60. For each cement, four tests were conducted: without antibiotics, with 2 g of vancomycin and 1 g of tobramycin, with 4 g of vancomycin and 2 g of tobramycin, and with 2 g of vancomycin alone. The antibiotic powder was added to the polymer powder and mixed thoroughly by hand. The powder and the monomer were then mixed according to the manufacturer's instructions for 2 minutes, at a rate of about 100 cycles per minute. For each test, several specimens were studied. After moulding, the specimens were machined according to DIN 53–455 on a Bridgeport CNC mill to a dumbell shape. Radiographic images were taken of each specimen, to visualize the internal void distribution and to detect large defficiencies in mechanical properties. Specimens with voids in the radius that would obviously lead to failure, were discarded. The specimens, 20 cm in total length, had a gauge length of 5 cm. After machining, all the specimens were stored at 21° C under a relative humidity of 20 % for a minimum of 6 weeks. For tensile testing, the specimens were fixed in an Instron Testing machine by two clamps 10 cm apart. A 5 cm displacement gauge was fixed to gauge length. The tension tests were performed at a crosshead speed of 25 m m/min. The data were collected by a computer and elastic modulus (MPa), tensile strength (MPa), and fracture strain were determined. A total of 78 specimens were tested. Each specimen came from a single mix of cement. Statistical analysis using the Student's t-test was used to compare the means of the tensile strength and fracture strain of the groups with and without antibiotic.

Results

Two of the 78 specimens lead to mechanical failures, due to the presence of large air voids (> 14 mm radius) in the region of the measuring area. A total of 76 specimens with voids of < 1 mm in the radius, were effectively tested. For these specimens the tension test could be conducted routinely.

Effect of antibiotic addition:

❖ addition of 2 g of vancomycin did not significantly affect the tensile mechanical properties of the four cements,

❖ addition of 2 g of vancomycin and 1 g of tobramycin significantly decreased the elastic modulus by 5–10 % except for Palacos, which was not affected,

❖ addition of 2 g of vancomycin and 1 g of tobramycin always decreased the tensile strengths of the cements, but the difference was only significant for the Sulfix (p = 0.001),

❖ addition of 2 g of vancomycin and 1 g of tobramycin did not significantly affect the fracture strain, except for Sulfix (p = 0.003), and

❖ addition of a double dose of antibiotic (vancomycin 4 g + tobramycin 2 g) did not significantly change the results obtained with a single dose.

Tensile properties of the four low-viscosity cements:

The tensile strength and fracture strain of Palacos LV and Sulfix 60 were significantly higher than those of CMW3 and LVC (Zimmer), without any antibiotics (P < 0.001; Student's *t* Test). After antibiotic addition, Palacos LV and Sulfix 60 consistently showed higher tensile strength and fracture strain, but this was not significant in all the cases. After antibiotic addition, Palacos LV always had a significantly higher tensile strength than the three other cements.

Discussion

The purpose of this study was to investigate the effect on the tensile properties of the cement after addition of antibiotics. Our results with vancomycin confirm that there is no significant effect on the tensile properties of the four low-viscosity cements studied. Simultaneous addition of vancomycin and tobramycin only affects the tensile properties of Sulfix, while its tensile strength and fracture strain remain much higher than for CMW3 and LVC (Zimmer). Lautenschlager (Lautenschlager et al., 1976) demonstrated the absence of deleterious effects of gentamicin powder up to 5 g on the tensile properties. These results also compare favorably with previous reports on diametral tensile strength obtained with gentamicin (Nelson RC et al., 1978). The in-vitro mechanical analysis of vancomycin addition in bone cement demonstrated acceptable effects on the tensile mechanical properties of four commonly used low-viscosity bone cements.

Chemical and Bacteriological Properties of Vancomycin-/Tobramycin-Loaded CMW1 Bone Cement

In-vitro elution

Background

Combining two antibiotics in antibiotic-loaded bone cement is common clinical practice (Hanssen et al., 2004; Hendriks et al., 2004; Jiranek, 2005). As the effect on elution characteristics is unknown, an in-vitro quantitative elution study was carried out. The purpose of this study was to determine the in-vitro elution kinetics of vancomycin and tobramycin in acrylic bone cement.

Materials and methods

To study the effect of vancomycin and tobramycin on their respective elution rates, an in-vitro elution study was designed. Three groups of five disks made of antibiotic-loaded CMW1 polymethylmethacrylate (PMMA) bone cement were prepared. One group contained only vancomycin. Tobramycin was added to the second group, and in the third group both antibiotics were combined. The amount of antibiotics added, was in keeping with the dosages applied in our clinic, i.e., 2 g of vancomycin per 40 g of CMW1 powder and 1 g of tobramycin per 40 g of cement powder. The antibiotics and cement powders were thoroughly mixed while in a dry state. The cement was manually mixed to form a dough, and then packed into standardized 28-mm-diameter 14-mm-thick machined polyethylene molds. When the cement had cured, the molds were removed, leaving five identical disks, each containing the same amount of vancomycin or tobramycin, respectively. For elution and sampling, each disk was fully immersed in a 40-mL mixed bath of human serum and trypcase soya at 37 °C in a covered beaker. The disks were removed at fortnightly intervals and each bath was stirred vigorously 10 times clockwise and 10 times counter-clockwise for the period of one year. Then a 5-mL sample was taken from each bath and frozen at – 20 °C until assayed for antibiotic content. Each disk was rinsed with 10 mL of normal saline and placed in a fresh 40-mL bath in a fresh beaker. Tobramycin and vancomycin concentrations in each sample were measured using fluorescence polarization immunoassay (Abbott TDxFLx; Abbott Laboratories, Abbott Park, IL).

Results

The elution rate of vancomycin from the disks in the vancomycin group is shown in Figure 9.**2**.

The three groups showed high early release rates with exponential decay. We observed a typical biphasic release curve with an initial peak release followed by a long tail of low release. After 8 months the amounts released were 2 – 10 % in the vancomycin group, 3 – 11 % in the tobramycin

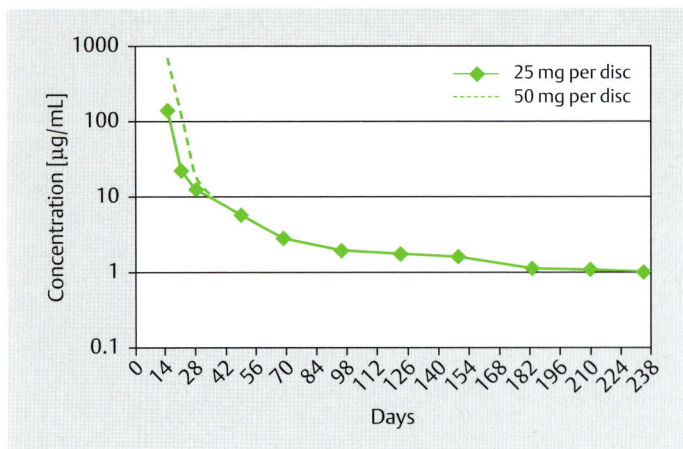

Fig. 9.2 The in-vitro vancomycin elution curve.

group and 5–12 % in the combined group, respectively.

Discussion

The results of our study show the characteristic high initial release and subsequent exponential decay for vancomycin that is commonly described in literature for other antibiotics (Penner et al., 1996; Seyral et al., 1994). Antibiotic release is well known to occur through a simple process, whereby exposed antibiotic on the cement surface dissolves into the surrounding fluid. Vancomycin release follows this principal (Kühn, 2000; Van de Belt et al., 2000; Bertazzoni et al., 2002; Kühn and Specht, 2003; Kühn et al., 2005). In our study, combining two different antibiotics in acrylic bone cement had no adverse effect on the in-vitro elution rates of both antibiotics. The use of vancomycin alone or in combination therapy in antibiotic-loaded bone cement may lead to a good antibiotic elution in vivo; however, this needs to be confirmed in further studies.

In-Vitro Antibacterial Activity of Vancomycin-/Tobramycin-Loaded CMW1 Bone Cement

Background

During polymerization 52 kJ of energy are released per mole MMA (Kühn, 2000). The polymerization heat may modify the antibacterial properties of the antibiotics (Beeching et al., 1986; Anagnostakos et al., 2005) – particularly of vancomycin. The aim of our study was to analyze the persistence of antibacterial activity around antibiotic-impregnated acrylic bone cement discs.

Material and methods

Two groups of three disks made of antibiotic-loaded CMW1 PMMA bone cement were studied. The antibiotic dosages were equivalent to those applied in our clinic; 2 g of vancomycin per 40 g of CMW1 powder and 1 g of tobramycin per 40 g of cement powder. The antibiotics and cement powders were thoroughly mixed while dry. The cement was manually mixed to form a dough, and then packed into standardized 28-mm-diameter 14-mm-thick machined polyethylene molds. Polymerization heat was registered at the surface of each disk. Each disk of vancomycin or tobramycin was placed on an agar plate inoculated with *Micrococcus luteus*. Inhibition zones were analyzed each day, until no antibiotic activity was left.

Results

The average maximum polymerization heat registered at the surface of each disk was 75 °C (minimum: 50 °C/maximum 90 °C). The vancomycin inhibition zone was statistically significant for an average of 50 days (minimum: 45 days/maximum: 56 days). The tobramycin inhibition zone was statistically significant for an average of 60 days (minimum: 53 days/maximum: 68 days).

Discussion

The results of our study demonstrated the persistence of antibacterial activity around antibiotic-impregnated acrylic bone cement discs. Polymerization heat did not affect the antibacterial properties of vancomycin in vancomycin-loaded bone cement.

In-Vivo Release Analysis of Vancomycin-Loaded CMW1 Bone Cement

Background

Perenteral administration of vancomycin may induce renal and ear toxicity, as well as vascular allergic reaction. Another problem of systemic administration of vancomycin is the emergence of bacterial resistance (Chohfi et al., 1998). The addition of vancomycin in bone cement may, however, induce neither general toxicity nor resistance. In fact, we assumed that vancomycin-loaded bone cement has a limited local action at the peroperative site with no general distribution. To confirm this hypothesis, we conducted an in-vivo study analyzing the concentration of vancomycin in blood, urine and locally.

Materials and methods

In this study 10 patients were included. The average age was 64 years. There were six total knee arthroplasties and four total hip arthroplasties. All the surgical procedures were performed by the same surgeon at the same center. The antibiotic dosages applied were 2 g of vancomycin per 40 g of CMW1 bone cement. The antibiotic was admixed to the cement using the method described above and the prosthesis was implanted. Subsequently, daily measurements of vancomycin concentrations were conducted during the first three postoperative days in blood, urine, and drains of each patient. The concentration of vancomycin in blood, urine and drain was also measured in a control group with systemic i.v. administration of vancomycin.

Table 9.**1** Mean vancomycin concentration in blood, urine and drain depending on the type of administration

	Bone cement administration	Intravenous administration
Blood	0.1–0.2 μg/mL	2–12 μg/mL
Urine	20–25 μg/mL	30–50 μg/mL
Drains	41–118 μg/mL	0.34–1.81 μg/mL

Results

The average in-vivo vancomycin concentrations in relation to the mode of administration are presented in Table 9.**1**.

Discussion

The results of our study confirmed that vancomycin-loaded bone cement had a limited local action at the peroperative site without general distribution. The concentrations in blood or urine were very low during the first three postoperative days and were undetectable after the third day. On the other hand, a persistence of effective local concentrations (1.2 mg/L) was observed after the third day. The measured concentrations exceeded the minimal inhibitory concentrations (MIC) of *Staphylococcus aureus* (0.8 mg/L). These results are comparable with the results of the Langlais study (Langlais, 2004) conducted using gentamicin. In the latter, concentrations in periprosthetic fluids were 20 times higher than the MIC, but were below the detection limit in blood after 24 hours and in urine after one week. The blood concentration was less than 1 mg/L, far below the ototoxic and nephrotoxic threshold (8 mg/L). The results of our study lead to the same conclusions for vancomycin.

Management Strategy for Infected Knee and Hip Arthroplasty

A standardized multidisciplinary protocol for infected knee or hip prostheses

1. Infection diagnosis

In our institution all infected prostheses are managed by a multidisciplinary team of orthopedic surgeons, bacteriologists, and radiologists. Diagnosis and future treatment regimens are managed by the surgeons and bacteriologists, depending on the findings on clinical and bacteriological examination. The management protocols are available online on the following website: http://ifr48.timone.univ-mrs.fr or on a Pocket PC form. A CT-scan is required, in case of severe bone destruction or very active infection. Standardized surgical bacteriological sampling is then performed at the operation site with a special "bone kit sample," including a periprosthetic liquid sample, a bone and soft tissue sample, and i.v. blood sample for biomolecular analysis. The main goal at this stage is to obtain a precise bacteriological diagnosis.

2. Surgical management

For early infections we use surgical lavage and debridement. This applies for infections of the hip occuring within 45 days and infections of the knee occurring within 30 days after implantation. In all other cases, two-stage revisions are indicated. For the hip, we perform a "short" two-stage revision, and for the knee it is a "long" two-stage revision, respectively. It is common practice at our institution to add antibiotics to spacers (Argenson et al., 1992; 1996, Parratte et al., 2004). The added antibiotics are always determined by the clinical microbiologist according to the individual bacterial susceptibility profile.

3. Surgical and bacteriological follow-up

The microbiologist manages a long-term antibiotherapy and controls the follow-up according to the protocol and susceptibility profile (Drancourt et al., 1996). Likewise, the surgeon controls the restitution of hip or knee function during the follow-up (Parratte, 2004).

Revision Strategy for Infected Hip Arthroplasty

Infection within 45 days

For the early hip infection we perform a surgical lavage, supplemeted with a long-term antibiotherapy according to the bacterial susceptibility profile. We control the clinical and biological remission.

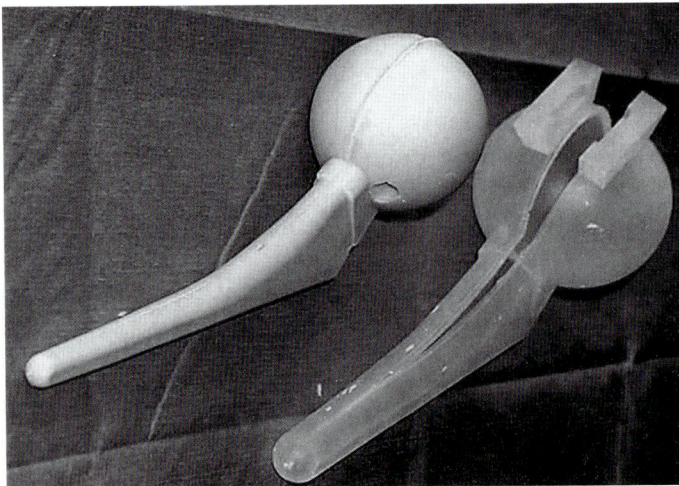

Fig. 9.**3a** Pre-modeled hip spacers.

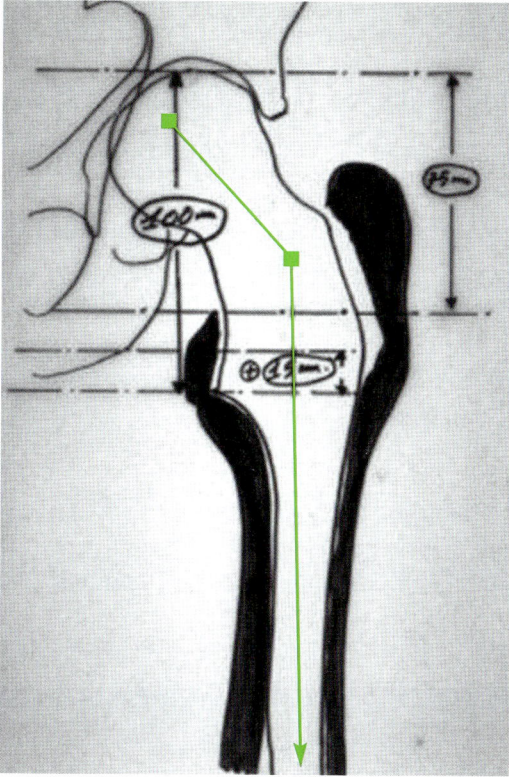

Fig. 9.**3b**   Custom-made hip spacer.

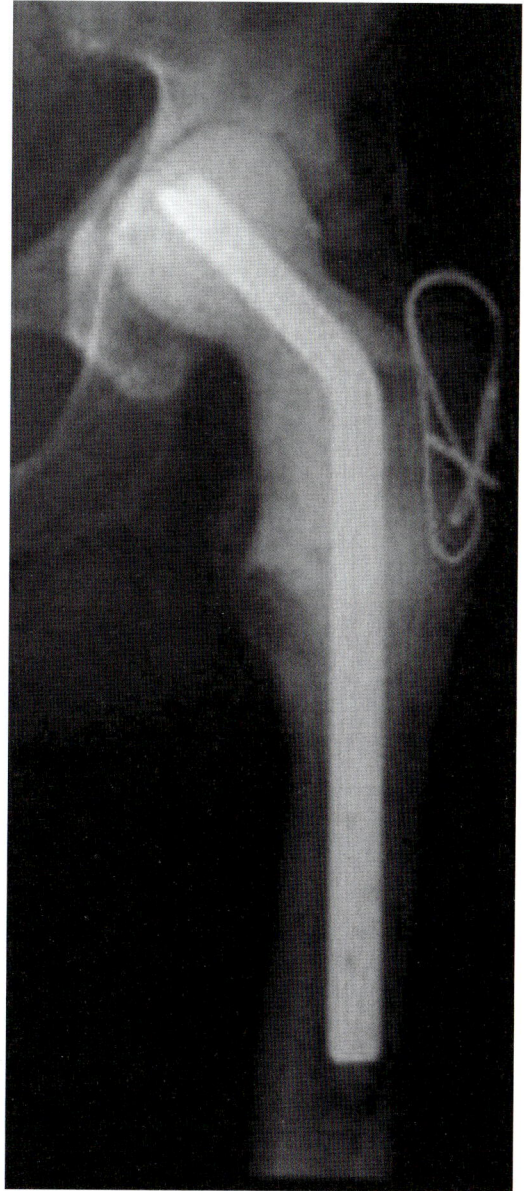

Fig. 9.**3c**   A modeled hip spacer.

Infection after 45 days

We perform a two-stage revision with delayed re-implantation of a new prosthesis. The time of delay depends on the type of bacteria and infection, but we strive to implement a short two-stage revision (with an interval of 6 – 8 weeks), whenever possible.

During the first stage, we remove all foreign material. We systematically collect standardized bacteriological surgical samples, as previously described. Debridement, involving removal of the hematoma, fibrous membrane, sinus tracts, and devitalized bone and soft tissue, is performed, followed by pulse lavage. An antibiotic-loaded bone spacer is applied according to the individual antibiogram. In the beginning, we used custom-made spacers. Now, with more experience, we prefer using a modeler (Figs. 9.**3a**, 9.**3b** and 9.**3c**).

When clinical and bacteriological parameters have returned to normal, the decision of reim-plantation is made together with the bacteriologist. We often do a CT-scan before reimplantation, to evaluate the acetabular and the femoral bone loss (Jacquier et al., 2004). For the femoral side we perform a "modified Exeter technique" with morcelized bone graft and a long cemented custom-made stem (Argenson et al., 1999). The stem is

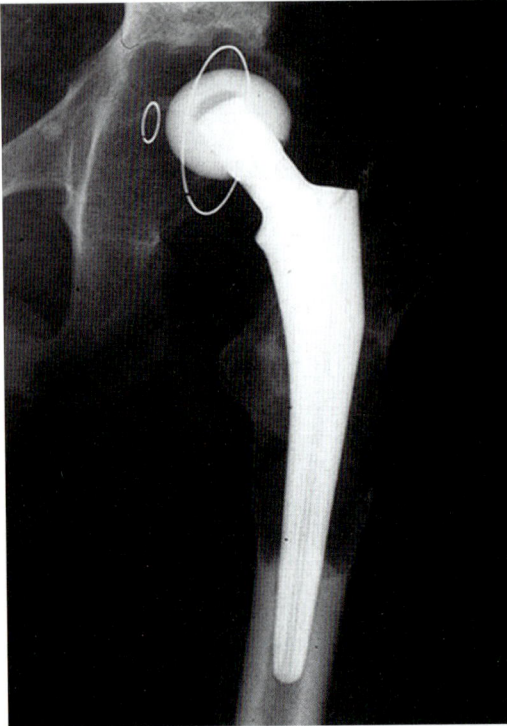

Fig. 9.**4a** A preoperative radiographic image of an infected hip (AP-view).

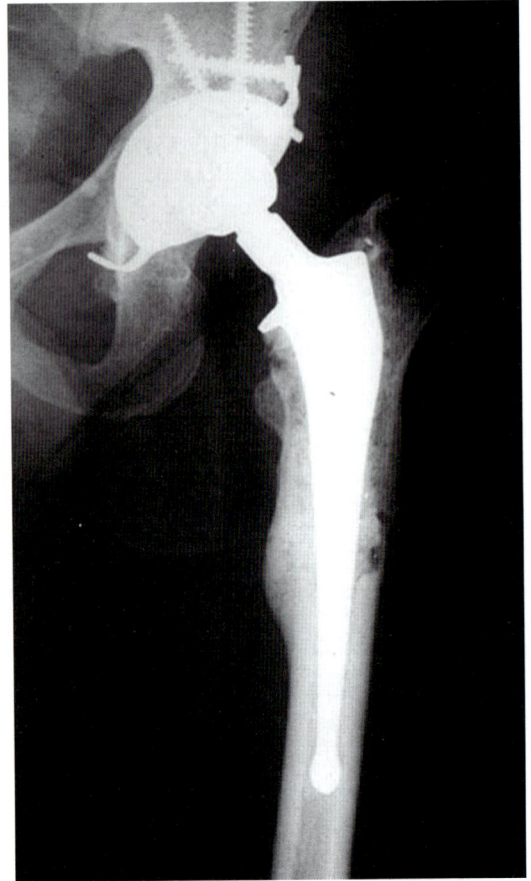

Fig. 9.**4b** A postoperative AP-view of an infected hip two-stage revision with "modified Exeter technique", using morcelized bone graft and a cementless cup.

longer than before to avoid fracture, and we use antibiotic-loaded cement according to the bacterial susceptibility profile (Figs. 9.**4a** and 9.**4b**).

Vancomycin is often used. For the acetabular side, we perform an impacted morcelized bone graft with a cementless cup (Argenson et al., 2004). The cup used in our series, combines the advantages of a "press-fit" cup and those of a reinforcement ring. The combination of this type of cup associated with morcelized bone graft seems reliable in achieving restoration of the bone stock, relocation of the hip center, and stability of the cup in infected total hip arthroplasty revision with loss of the bone stock (Argenson et al., 2004).

Revision Strategy for Infected Knee Arthroplastym

Background

We have recently performed a retrospective evaluation of the results of a multidisciplinary standardized management protocol for infected knee arthroplasty (Parratte et al., 2004). The protocol included surgical lavage for early infections (arthrotomy, debridement, washing), two-stage revisions with a long interval for late infections (removal of infected prosthesis, application of antibiotic mobile spacer and revision with a constrained prosthesis), salvage procedures (arthrodesis with a double orthogonal monobar external fixator) (Parratte et al., 2006), and amputations performed in cases of chronic infection associated with the destruction of the patellar tendon.

The series included 69 infected knee arthroplasties, managed in the same center according to the above mentioned protocol. The following questions were investigated: What are the infectious results using this management protocol? What are the advantages and the limitations of surgical lavage? Is a long two-stage reimplantation a good alternative? Is arthrodesis an effective procedure if the extensor mechanism is destroyed?

Materials and methods

All the patients were managed according to the protocol described above. A clinical evaluation was performed at follow-up by an independent observer. The first arthroplasties had been performed in other orthopedic clinics. Mean follow-up was 7 years (minimum: 1 year/maximum: 12 years). There was an equal gender distribution in the series. 85% of the patients presented at least one risk factor according to De Cloedt (De Cloedt et al., 1994). We observed general risk factors such as diabetes in 12%, rheumatoid polyarthritis in 6% or artheropathy, tumor, alcoholism, toxicomania. Local risk factors, such as previous surgery, were observed in 65% of the patients with a mean of 3 previous surgeries (1 to 9). Skin problems were observed in a third of the patients, bone defects in another third, and destruction of the extensor mechanism in 16 patients (22%). Identification of the pathogen was obtained in 95% of the patients. *Staphyloccocus aureus* was present in 33%, another staphyloccocus in 20% of the patients. A polymicrobial infection was seen in 15%. Other pathogens such as Streptococcus spp, *Pseudomonas aeruginosa*, Enterococcus spp were found in the other cases. Antibiotics were systematically added to bone cement as spacer and during reimplantation. Vancomycin was added in all cases in combination with another antibiotic according to the individual antibiogram. The antibiotic treatment regimen was managed by the microbiologist. The microbiologist performed a long-term double or triple antimicrobial chemotherapy according to the protocols previously described (Drancourt et al., 1993; Drancourt et al., 1997; Stein et al., 1998).

Results

We achieved a 75% remission rate, with a two-stage revision in 35 patients, and with conservative treatment in 14 patients. For 25% of the patients, arthrodesis (15 cases) and an amputation (2 cases) were required. We observed 95% lavage failure, when the lavage was performed after a 4-week delay and 47% failure for lavage within 4 weeks. Successful two-stage reimplantations were performed for 35 of the 38 patients (92%). The mean interval before reimplantation was 4 months in our series. We observed functional impairment such as stiffness or pain, in 80% of the patients. With regard to the arthrodesis, the fusion rate was 85% with a mean delay of 5 months.

Discussion

The infectious results of our series confirm the benefits of these management strategies for infected knee arthroplasties. However, we observed very poor results for surgical lavage, notably late lavage. The results of the long two-stage reimplantations were good in terms of follow-up, but we observed some limitations with regard to the functional outcomes. Arthrodesis with a double orthogonal monobar external fixator seems an effective procedure, when infected prosthesis is associated with destruction of the extensor mechanism (Parratte et al., 2006).

Conclusion

The results of our studies confirm the biomechanical, bacteriological, and clinical interest in the use of vancomycin-laoded bone cement in hip and knee arthroplasty. The addition of vancomycin to bone cement seems to be reliable and effective. We did not observe any general toxicity in our clinical studies. There seems to be only limited emergence of antibiotic resistance due to very poor release of vancomycin into systemic circulation.

With regard to infected hip and knee prostheses, a multidisciplinary strategy, including surgeons, microbiologists, and radiologists seems essential for an appropriate management of individual cases. Even if the infectious results of a two-stage procedure are good, the poor functional outcomes remain a problem. The evaluation of a one-stage procedure with the use of antibiotic-loaded cement in the case of non-aggressive bacteria should be performed in a prospective comparative study.

References

Anagnostakos K, Kelm J, Regitz T, Schmitt E, Jung W. In-vitro evaluation of antibiotic release from and bacteria growth inhibition by antibiotic-loaded acrylic bone cement spacers. J Biomed Mater Res B Appl Biomater 2005; 72: 373–378.

Argenson JN, Aubaniac JM, Curvale G, Groulier P, Drancourt M, Raoult D. L'infection ostéo-articulaire sur prothèse: Prévention, diagnostic, traitement. Presses Fontaine Poitiers 1992.

Argenson JN, Drancourt M, Huiskes R, Aubaniac JM. Ciment à la vancomycine dans les infections à staphylocoque sur prothèse de hanche: étude in vitro et clinique. Rev de Chir Orthop 1996; 87: 66–67.

Argenson JN, Gravier R, Aubaniac JM. Greffe morcelée impactée et tige cimentée dans les reprises de prothèses de hanche: évaluation de la reconstruction fémorale et des problèmes techniques. Rev Chir Orthop 2000; 86: 46–47.

Argenson JN, Parratte S, Flecher X, Aubaniac JM. Impaction Grafting for Acetabular Revision: Bringing Back the Bone. Orthopedics 2004; 27: 967–969.

Argenson JN, Verdonschot N, Seyral P, Raoult D, Huiskes R, Aubaniac JM. Mechanical properties and in-vivo activity of bone cement impregnated with Vancomycin: The Journal of Bone and Joint Surgery 1993; 75 Br: 235.

Argenson JN, Verdonschot N, Seyral P, Raoult D, Huiskes R, Aubaniac JM. The effect of Vancomycin and Tobramycin on the tensile properties of low-viscosity bone cements. European Journal of Experimental Musculoskeletal Research 1994; 3: 43–47.

Argenson JN, Verdonschot N, Seyral P, Raoult D, Huiskes R, Aubaniac JM. Ciment orthopédique et Vancomycine : diffusion, propriétés mécaniques, étude clinique. Rev de Chir Orthop 1994; 80: 167–168.

Beeching NJ, Thomas MG, Roberts S, Lang SD. Comparative in-vitro activity of antibiotics incorporated in acrylic bone cement. J Antimicrob Chemother 1986; 17: 173–184.

Belt van de H, Neut D, Schenk W, van Horn JR, van der Mei HC, Busscher HJ. Infection of orthopedic implants and the use of antibiotic-loaded bone cements, A review. Acta Orthop Scand 2001; 72: 557–571.

Belt van de H, Neut D, Schenk W, van Horn JR, van der Mei HC, Busscher HJ. Gentamicin release from polymethylmethacrylate bone cements and Staphylococcus aureus biofilm formation. Acta Orthop Scand 2000; 71: 625–629.

Bertazzoni, Minelli E, Caveiari C, Benini A. Release of antibiotics from polymethylmethacrylate cement. J Chemother 2002; 14: 492–500.

Buchholz HW, Engelbrecht H. Depot effects of various antibiotics mixed with Palacos resins. Chirurg 1970; 41: 511–515.

Chohfi M, Langlais F, Fourastier J, Minet J, Thomazeau H, Cormier M. Pharmacokinetics, uses, and limitations of vancomycin-loaded bone cement. Int Orthop 1998; 22:171–177.

De Cloedt P, Emery R, Legaye J, Lokietek W. Infected total knee prosthesis. Guidance for therapeutic choice. Rev Chir Orthop 1994; 80: 626–633.

Drancourt M, Stein A, Argenson JN, Zannier A, Curvale G, Raoult D. Oral Rifampicin plus Ofloxacin for treatment of staphylococcus infected orthopedic implants. Antimicrobial agents and chemotherapy 1993; 37: 1214–1218.

Drancourt M, Stein A, Argenson JN, Roiron R, Groulier P, Raoult D. Oral treatment of Staphylococcus spp. infected orthopedic implants with fusidic acid or ofloxacin in combination with rifampicin. J Antimicrob Chemother 1997; 39: 235–240.

Hanssen AD, Spangehl MJ. Practical applications of antibiotic-loaded bone cement for treatment of infected joint replacements. Clin Orthop Relat Res 2004; 427: 79–85.

Hendriks JG, van Horn JR, van der Mei HC, Busscher HJ. Backgrounds of antibiotic-loaded bone cement and prosthesis-related infection. Biomaterials 2004; 25: 545–556.

Jacquier A, Champsaur P, Vidal V et al. Évaluation des infections de prothèses totales de hanches au scanner. J Radiol 2004; 85: 2005–2012.

Jiranek W. Antibiotic-loaded cement in total hip replacement: current indications, efficacy, and complications. Orthopedics 2005; 28: 873–877.

Kühn KD. Bone cements, Up-to-Date comparison of Physical Properties and Chemical Properties of Commercial Materials. Springer Berlin 2000.

Kühn KD, Ege W, Gopp U. Acrylic bone cements: composition and properties. Orthop Clin N Am 2005; 36: 17–28.

Kühn KD, Specht R. Le Ciment Acrylique Osseux Historique, Characteristiques Chimiques et Proportietes Physiques Maitrise Orthopedique 2003; 126.

Langlais F: Antibiotic-loaded bone cements: from laboratory studies to clinical evaluation. Bull Acad Natl Med 2004; 188: 1011–1022.

Lautenschlager EP, Jacobs JJ, Marshall GW, Marks KE, Scwartz J Nelson CL. Mechanical strength of acrylic bone cements impregnated with antibiotics. J Biomed Mater Res 1976; 10: 837–845.

Nelson RC, Hoffman RO, Burton TA. The effect of antibiotic additions on the mechanical properties of acrylic cement. J Biomed Mater Res 1978; 12: 473–490.

Parratte S, Stein A, Sbihi A, Rochewerger A, Curvale G. Infected knee arthroplasty: results with a standardized multidisciplinary management. Rev chir orthop 2004.

Parratte S, Stein A, Sbihi A, Rochewerger A, Curvale. Knee arthrodesis with two monolateral external fixators: 19 cases with a mean follow-up of 7 years, Rev Chir orthop 2006 [In press].

Penner MJ, Masri BA, Duncan CP. Elution characteristics of vancomycin and tobramycin combined in acrylic bone cement. J Arthroplasty 1996; 11: 939–944.

Seyral P, Zannier A, Argenson JN, Raoult D. The release in vitro of Vancomycin and Tobramycin from acrylic bone cement. Journal of Antimicrobial Agent and Chemotherapy 1994; 33: 337–339.

Stein A, Bataille JF, Drancourt M et al. Ambulatory treatment of multidrug-resistant Staphylococcus-infected orthopedic implants with high-dose oral co-trimoxazole (trimethoprim-sulfamethoxazole). Antimicrob Agents Chemother 1998; 42; 3086–3091.

Zimmerli W, Trampuuz A, Ochsner PE. Prosthetic-Joint Infections, current concepts. N Engl J Med 2004; 351: 1645–1654.

(UK) Why cement the Total Hip?

Steffen Breusch, Henrik Malchau

Summary

This chapter gives a justification for the continued use of cement in total hip arthroplasty (THA). An overview of the evolution of cementing techniques and a definition of the current status of modern cementing techniques are presented. Excellent and consistent long-term results can be achieved for patients of all age groups when this strategy is implemented.

Introduction

It is difficult to measure success in patients having undergone THA. Clinical scores and patient-derived outcomes will vary from study to study and are rarely linked to implant fixation, at least in the short to mid-term. Long-term data and, in particular the overall re-operation rates, are important both to patient and surgeon. It has been the domain of the Scandinavian arthroplasty registries, to report revision rates for large cohorts of patients, thus providing representative data for their countries. Three main findings from the Annual Report 2004 from Sweden are of note. Firstly, the crude so-called revision burden (RB=revisions/ primary THA+revisions), calculated from 1992– 2004, was lowest for cemented implants with 9.8%. This compares favorably to the RB for hybrids (11.8%) and uncemented implants (26.4%), and also to the RB of many other countries with RB between 15–20% (United Kingdom, Norway, Denmark, United States). Secondly, with improved cementing techniques the RB for cemented implants was significantly reduced. Thirdly, uncemented fixation was associated with a higher risk of reoperation for all age groups.

Arguments for Cemented THA

Femoral stem survival is excellent in the long term, both for cemented and uncemented fixation (Aldinger et al., 2005; Berli et al., 2005; Malchau et al., 2000; Vervest et al., 2003; Williams et al., 2005). Implant survival rates of more than 95% after 10 years can be expected. Thigh pain is extremely rare in cemented fixation, but can have a negative impact on patient satisfaction and revision rates, despite otherwise excellent long-term fixation (Garcia-Cimbrelo et al., 2003). In addition, cemented femoral fixation provides versatility, partiularly in revision. In most cases where an acetabular revision is required in the presence of a well-fixed stem, a simple "cement-in-cement" revision can be performed, which facilitates the procedure (Howell et al., 2005). In case of infection, it is easier to remove cement than an ingrown uncemented femoral stem (Gehrke, 2005).

The issue of socket fixation remains controversial. The available literature is difficult to interpret and to compare. Studies of different implant types of small cohorts are important for our understanding of outcomes and they significantly influence surgeons' anchorage strategies and implant choices. However, published data need to be compared with care. In this context, one particular study may serve as an example. In 2002, Udomkiat (Udomkiat et al., 2002) reported an excellent twelve-year survival rate of 99.1% for a hemispheric porous-coated press-fit cup with "revision because of failure of fixation of the metal shell" as the end point. On closer look, the survival rate decreased to 95.3% with revision for any reason as the end point, and to 79.6% with exchange of the liner as the end point. In other words, the risk of requiring a further operative procedure was 20% within the first 10–12 years. The figures for reoperation rates – for any given reason – for cement sockets are not as high. Cemented cup survival is excellent in centers with a long tradition in cementing technique (Timperley et al., 2005). Also, across the Swedish Orthopedic Surgeons community, better survival of cemented sockets compared to uncemented fixation with conventional polyethylene (PE) have been registered. This explains the swing-back to cemented acetabular fixation. Given the universal agreement that wear-induced osteolysis is the main reason for implant loosening (Harris, 2001), cemented sockets also seem favorable in small acetabulas, e.g., in women, in developmental dysplasia, or congenital dislocation of the hip, respectively. In these cases, acceptable PE thickness is achieved, unless hard-on-hard bearings are used (for which only mid-term evidence is available). There is also some evidence that PE wear rates are less in cemented sockets when compared to uncemented devices (McCombe and Williams, 2004). It may well be that with improved PE and reduced particulate wear rates, revision rates will decrease for uncemented sockets as well, but the evidence so far is only short-term.

Finally, to qote the recent Annual Report 2004 from the Swedish Register, "uncemented fixation gives consistently poorer results regardless of age group".

Evolution of Cementing Techniques

The pioneer of cemented THA, Sir John Charnley, achieved an amazingly high operative standard based on dedication and thorough basic research. His concept, "low friction arthroplasty", still enjoys long term success with Kaplan-Meier survival rates of 85–90% after 20 years (Schulte et al., 1993; Neumann et al., 1994; Joshi et al., 1998). Other cemented stem designs showed a wide range between poor (Sutherland et al., 1982; Stauffer, 1982; Pavlov, 1987) and good results (Britton et al., 1996; Malchau et al., 1998; Havelin et al., 2000; Williams et al., 2004; Berli et al., 2005), both clinically and radiographically. However, it soon became obvious, that not only stem design, but also surgical and cementing technique, in particular, had to be considered as important factors influencing the outcome of cemented THAs. Beckenbaugh and Ilstrup (Beckenbaugh and Ilstrup, 1978) found a strong correlation between poor packing of cement and radiographic loosening. Other studies have also

shown higher loosening rates when cement filling of the medullary canal was incomplete (Stauffer et al., 1982; Kristiansen et al., 1985; Russotti et al., 1988). In this context, several authors postulated a poor prognosis based on flaws and deficiencies in the cement mantle, manufactured by the surgeon, as seen on the immediate post-operative radiograph (Ianotti et al., 1986; Roberts et al., 1986; Ritter et al., 1999).

Cement applications

In the first decade of cemented THAs cementing techniques were fairly crude (Table 10.**1**).

Femoral canal preparation was done by curetting out cancellous bone. Irrigation – if used at all – was limited and high viscosity was mixed and applied manually. However, it is important to note that even back then the first form of pressurized cement application was performed by "thumbing" down the cement from proximal to distal. Charnley (Charnley, 1970) had already emphasized the importance of achieving adequate cement pressure: "The cement is forced down the track of the medullary canal as a stiff dough, and the insertion of the point of the tapered stem of the prosthesis expands the stiff dough and injects it into the cancellous lining of the marrow space." This may offer an explanation why excellent long-term results have been achieved with so-called *first-generation* cementing techniques (Schulte et al., 1993; Neumann et al.; 1994; Joshi et al., 1998).

Cement containment and gun application

The introduction of a distal intramedullary cement restrictor allowed for cement containment and better pressurization, which resulted both in improved cement penetration (Markolf and Amstutz, 1976; Indong et al., 1978) and better clinical outcomes (Harris et al., 1982; Harris et al., 1986; Mulroy and Harris, 1990). Retrograde cement application via cement gun (Harris et al., 1986), generated higher cement pressures distally than proximally, a pattern which was reversed by finger packing (McCaskie et al., 1994; McCaskie et al., 1997). "Sustained cement pressurization" (Lee and Ling, 1981) further improved cement interdigitation (Bean et al., 1988) and provided a method capable of withstanding bleeding pressure, necessary to prevent blood entrapment, and to obtain a satisfactory cementing result (Askew et al., 1984; Benjamin et al., 1987).

Bone Lavage

A further significant step towards an improved cementing technique was the observation that bone lavage prior to cementation aided cement penetration (Halawa et al., 1978; Krause et al., 1982). Both bone lavage and cancellous bone quality (Halawa et al., 1982) were found to be significant factors with regard to improved mechanical shear strength (Bannister and Miles, 1988).

The combination of distal plug, retrograde cement application via gun, and bone lavage constitute the main factors responsible for the improved *second-generation* cementing techniques (Table 10.1).

Cement pressurization and pulsatile lavage

A further classification as *third-generation* techniques (Table 10.1) is probably more of academic and didactic interest. However, another important evolution of cementing techniques was certainly seen with the introduction of pulsatile bone lavage and pressurizing devices. This facilitated a more reproducible pressurizing technique (Lee and Ling, 1981; Breusch et al., 2000). Also, standardized vacuum cement mixing and the

use of stem centralizing devices are considered *third-generation* techniques. Vacuum mixing of cement has been shown to contribute to the long-term risk reduction of revision (Malchau et al., 2000). However, this may not be the case for all cement types (Breusch and Kühn, 2003). Distal stem centralizers, on the whole, clearly seem to be beneficial. They reduce the risk for stem tip-to-bone contact, which has been identified as a late failure mechanism due to osteolysis-induced periprosthetic fracture (Breusch and Malchau, 2005).

There may be dispute, as to whether the use of pulsatile lavage and pressurizing devices should be labeled *second-* or *third-generation* techniques. However, more thorough cleansing of the bone bed using pulsatile jet lavage has been shown to be significantly more effective than manual lavage (Breusch et al., 2000). Furthermore, the use of pressurizing devices to seal and contain cement at the femur and acetabulum, are proven steps to further improve cement pressurization and hence interdigitation. The routine use of pulsatile lavage and pressurizing devices should be considered mandatory elements of modern cementing techniques.

Table 10.1 Evolution of cementing techniques

First Generation	Second Generation	Third generation
Limited bone bed preparation	Bone bed preparation (bulb syringe irrigation / drying)	Thorough bone bed preparation (pulsatile lavage)
Unplugged femur	Distal cement restrictor (bone / plastic)	Improved distal cement restrictor
Stiff, doughy cement introduced by hand	Retrograde cement application via cement gun	Retrograde cement application via cement gun
Digital pressurization	Femoral and acetabular cement pressurization	Femoral acetabular and pressurizer
Hand mixing of cement	Open atmosphere cement mixing by hand	Vacuum mixing (centrifugation of bone cement)
		stem centralizers / cement spacers

Impact of Modern Cementing Techniques

Modern cementing techniques aim to improve the mechanical interlock between bone and cement in order to establish a durable interface. Cement interdigitation not only depends on bone preparation, but also on lavage and mode of cement application. Good interdigitation is a product of adequate cement penetration and resistance to bleeding. Another elegant method has been advocated, where bone cement is applied under vacuum suction and femoral drainage (Draenert et al., 1999), to reduce interface bleeding without the downside of intramedullary pressure increase. However, so far no long-term data using this technique have been published.

Pressurization and lavage of cancellous bone have been identified as the most significant factors with regard to enhanced cement interdigitation (Askew et al., 1984; Bannister and Miles, 1988; Halawa et al., 1978; Krause et al., 1982; Majkowski et al., 1993; Noble et al., 1982; Panjabi et al., 1986). They were also shown to be clinically highly effective. Several clinical studies, comparing patients before and after the introduction of modern cementing techniques, have confirmed the benefit of improved cement application techniques (Beckenbaugh and Ilstrup, 1978; Russotti et al., 1988; Britton et al., 1996; Malchau et al., 1998). The same benefit was also apparent in young patients (Barrack et al., 1992; Ballard et al., 1994; Mulroy and Harris, 1997; Howell et al., 2005). Also, if the risk for revision is taken as the measured outcome, the Swedish Hip Registry has provided important evidence to support this relationship (Malchau et al., 1998; Malchau et al., 2000; Annual Report, 2004). Probably one of the most significant findings was that the use of a dis-

tal intramedullary plug, pulsatile lavage, cement gun, and a proximal seal (representing modern generation cement techniques) reduce the risk of revision by approximately 20%, respectively. This is highlighted by a continuous improvement of implant survival in Sweden (Fig. 10.1). Currently, these techniques have to be considered as "gold standard" (Hashemi-Nejad et al., 1994; Breusch et al., 1999; Malchau et al., 2000), notably if used together with a well documented bone cement (Nilsen et al., 1996; Furnes et al., 1997; Malchau et al., 2000; Kühn, 2000; Kühn, 2005). Excellent outcomes with cements of higher viscosity, which seem more forgiving, have been reported (Havelin et al., 2000).

Key Points

- Modern cementing techniques are the key to long-term success.
- Improved outcome has been proven for:
  - meticulous bone preparation and preservation,
  - distal femoral plug (cement restrictor),
  - pulsatile lavage,
  - retrograde cement application via gun, and
  - sustained cement pressurization (pressurizer).
- There is evidence of improved outcome for:
  - vacuum mixing of bone cement, and
  - use of distal femoral stem centralizers.

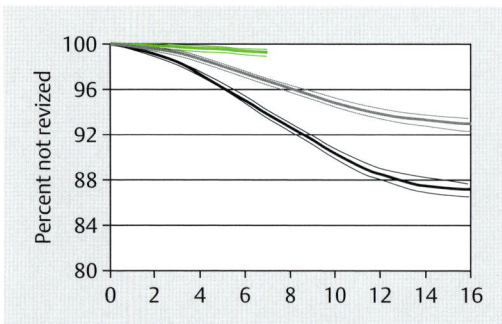

Fig. 10.1 Observed implant survival in three cohorts using different cementing techniques. There was significant improvement of implant survival with enhanced cementing techniques.
Green: Modern (n = 27.842),
Grey: Early (n = 19.100),
Black: Old (n = 20.404).

Conclusion

So far, it can be concluded from the literature that there is more than one reason for continuously advocating cemented THAs for all age groups. Performing a reproducible procedure with a high chance of long-term benefit to the patient and a low risk of reoperation, is not only desirable for the patient, but also has an enormous socio-economic impact on health care resources. Cemented THA carries the lowest revision burden.

"The best time to use cement, is the first time" (John Charnley, 1979).

References

Aldinger PR, Breusch SJ, Lukoschek M, Mau H, Ewerbeck V, Thomsen M. A ten- to 15-year follow-up of the cementless spotorno stem. J Bone Joint Surg Br 2003 Mar; 85 (2): 209–214.

Annual Report 2004. The Swedish National Hip Arthroplasty Register. www.jru.orthop.gu.se.

Askew MJ, Steege JW, Lewis JL, Ranieri JR, Wixson RL. Effect of cement pressure and bone strength on polymethylmethacrylate fixation. J Orthop Res 1984; 1: 412–420.

Ballard WT, Callaghan JJ, Sullivan PM, Johnston RC. The results of improved cementing techniques for total hip arthroplasty in patients less than fifty years old. J Bone Joint Surg 1994; 76-A: 959–964.

Bannister GC, Miles AW. The influence of cementing technique and blood on the strength of the bone-cement interface. Eng Med 1988; 17: 131–133.

Barrack RL, Mulroy RD, Harris WH. Improved cementing techniques and femoral component loosening in young patients with hip arthroplasty. A 12-year radiographic review. J Bone Joint Surg 1992; 74-B: 385–389.

Bean DJ, Hollis JM, Woo SL-Y, Convery FR. Sustained pressurization of polymethylmethacrylate: a comparison of low- and moderate viscosity bone cements. J Orthop Res 1988; 6: 580–584.

Beckenbaugh RD, Ilstrup DM. Total hip arthroplasty. A review of three hundred and thirty-three cases with long follow-up. J Bone Joint Surg 1978; 60-A: 306–313.

Benjamin JB, Gie GA, Lee AJC, Ling RSM, Volz RG. Cementing technique and the effect of bleeding. J Bone Joint Surg 1987; 69-B: 620–624.

Berli BJ, Schafer D, Morscher EW. Ten-year survival of the MS-30 matt-surfaced cemented stem. J Bone Joint Surg Br 2005 Jul; 87 (7): 928–933.

Breusch SJ, Berghof R, Schneider U et al. Der Stand der Zementiertechnik bei Hüfttotalendoprothesen in Deutschland. Z Orthop 1999; 137: 101–107.

Breusch SJ, Norman TL, Schneider U, Reitzel T, Blaha JD, Lukoschek M. Lavage technique in THA: Jet-Lavage Produces Better Cement Penetration Than Syringe-Lavage in the Proximal Femur. J Arthroplasty 2000; 15/7: 921–927.

Breusch SJ, Kühn KD. Knochenzement auf Polymethylmethacrylat Basis. Orthopädie 32. 2003 (1); 41–50.

Breusch SJ, Malchau H. (eds): The well cemented total hip arthroplasty. Springer Berlin, Heidelberg, New York, Tokyo 2005.

Britton AR, Murray DW, Bulstrode CJ, McPherson K, Denham RA. Long-term comparison of Charnley and Stanmore design total hip replacements. J Bone Joint Surg 1996; 78-B: 802–808.

Charnley J. Acrylic cement in orthopaedic surgery. E&S Livingstone Edinburgh, London 1970.

Charnley J. Low friction arthroplasty of the hip: Theory and practice. Springer Berlin, Heidelberg, New York, Tokyo 1979.

Draenert K, Draenert Y, Garde U, Ulrich Ch. Manual of cementing technique. Springer Berlin, Heidelberg, New York, Tokyo 1999.

Furnes O, Lie SA, Havelin LI, Vollset SE, Engesaeter LB. Exeter and charnley arthroplasties with Boneloc or high viscosity cement. Comparison of 1,127 arthroplasties followed for 5 years in the Norwegian Arthroplasty Register. Acta Orthop Scand 1997; 68 (6): 515–520.

Garcia-Cimbrelo E, Cruz-Pardos A, Madero R, Ortega-Andreu M. Total hip arthroplasty with use of the cementless Zweymuller Alloclassic system. A ten to thirteen-year follow-up study. J Bone Joint Surg Am 2003 Feb; 85-A (2): 296–303.

Gehrke T. Revision is not difficult! In: Breusch, Malchau (eds): The well cemented total hip arthroplasty. Springer Berlin, Heidelberg, New York, Tokyo 2005; 349–358.

Halawa M, Lee AJC, Ling RSM, Vangala SS. The shear strength of trabecular bone from the femur, and some factors affecting the shear strength of the cement-bone interface. Arch Orthop Trauma Surg 1978; 92: 19–30.

Harris WH, McCarthy JC, O'Neill DA. Femoral component loosening using contemporary techniques of femoral cement fixation. J Bone Joint Surg 1982; 64-A: 1063–1067.

Harris WH, McGann WA. Loosening of the femoral component after the use of the medullary-plug cementing technique. Follow-up note with a minimum five-year follow-up. J Bone Joint Surg 1986; 68-A: 1064–1066.

Harris WH: Wear and periprosthetic osteolysis: the problem. Clin Orthop Relat Res. 2001; (393): 66–70.

Hashemi-Nejad A, Goddard NJ, Birch NC. Current attitudes to cementing techniques in British hip surgery. Ann R Coll Surg Engl 1994; 76: 396–400.

Havelin LI, Espehaug B, Lie SA, Engesæter LB, Furnes O, Vollset SE. Prospective studies of hip prostheses and cements. A presentation of the Norwegian Arthroplasty Register 1987–1999. 67th Annual Meeting of the American Academy of Orthopaedic Surgeons, Orlando, USA, March 15–19, 2000.

Howell JR, Hubble MJW, Ling RSM. Stem design – the surgeon's perspective. In: Breusch, Malchau (eds): The well cemented total hip arthroplasty. Springer Berlin, Heidelberg, New York, Tokyo 2005; 180–189.

Ianotti JP, Balderston RA, Booth RE, Rothman RH, Cohn JC, Pikens GT: Aseptic loosening after total hip arthroplasty. Incidence, clinical significance, and etiology. J Arthroplasty 1986; 1: 99–107.

Indong Oh, Carlson CE, Tomford WW, Harris WH. Improved fixation of the femoral component after total hip replacement using a methacrylate intramedullary plug. J Bone Joint Surg 1978; 60-A:608–613.

Joshi RP, Eftekhar NS, McMahon DJ, Nercessian OA. Osteolysis after Charnley primary low-friction arthroplasty. A comparison of two matched paired groups. J Bone Joint Surg 1998; 80-B: 585–590.

Krause W, Krug W, Miller JE. Strength of the cement-bone interface. Clin Orthop 1982; 163: 290–299.

Kristiansen B, Jensen JS. Biomechanical factors in loosening of the Stanmore hip. Acta Orthop Scand 1985; 56: 21–24.

Kühn KD. Bone Cements. Up-to-date comparison of physical and chemical properties of commercial materials. Springer-Verlag Berlin Heidelberg, 2000.

Kühn KD. What is bone cement? In: Breusch S, Malchau H (ED): The well cemented total hip arthroplasty. Springer Verlag, Heidelberg 2005; 52–59.

Lee AJC, Ling RSM. Improved cementing techniques. Am Acad Orthop Surg Instr Course Lect 1981; 30: 407–413.

Majkowski RS, Miles AW, Bannister GC, Perkins J, Taylor GJS. Bone surface preparation in cemented joint replacement. J Bone Joint Surg 1993; 75-B: 459–463.

Malchau H, Herberts P. Prognosis of total hip replacement in Sweden: Revision and re-revision rate in THR. Presented at the 65th Annual Meeting of the American Academy of Orthopaedic Surgeons New Orleans, LA, February 1998.

Malchau H, Herberts P, Söderman P, Odén A. Prognosis of total hip replacement: Update and validation of results from the Swedish National Hip Arthroplasty Registry. 67th Annual Meeting of the American Academy of Orthopaedic Surgeons Orlando, USA, March 15–19, 2000.

Markolf KL, Amstutz HC. In vitro measurement of bone-acrylic interface pressure during femoral component insertion. Clin Orthop 1976; 121: 60–66.

McCaskie AW, Gregg PJ. Femoral cementing technique: current trends and future developments. J Bone Joint Surg 1994; 76B: 176–177.

McCaskie AW, Barnes MR, Lin E, Harper WM, Gregg PJ. Cement pressurisation during hip replacement. J Bone Joint Surg 1997; 79-B: 379–384.

McCombe P, Williams SA. A comparison of polyethylene wear rates between cemented and cementless cups. A prospective, randomised trial. J. Bone Joint Surg 2004. 86-B: 344–349.

Mulroy RD, Harris WH. The effect of improved cementing techniques on component loosening in total hip replacement. An 11-year radiographic review. J Bone Joint Surg 1990; 72-B: 757–760.

Mulroy RD, Harris WH. Acetabular and femoral fixation 15 years after cemented total hip surgery. Clin Orthop 1997; 18.

Neumann L, Freund KG, Sorensen KH. Long-term results of Charnley total hip replacement. Review of 92 patients at 15 to 20 years. J Bone Joint Surg 1994; 76-B: 245–251.

Nilsen AR, Wiig M. Total hip arthroplasty with Boneloc: loosening in 102/157 cases after 0.5–3 years. Acta Orthop Scand 1996 Feb; 67 (1): 57–59.

Noble PC, Espley AJ. Examination of the influence of surgical technique upon the adequacy of cement fixation in the femur. J Bone Joint Surg 1982; 64-B: 120–121.

Panjabi MM, Cimino WR, Drinker H. Effect of pressure on bone cement stiffness. Acta Orthop Scand 1986; 57: 106–110.

Pavlov PW. A 15 year follow-up study of 512 consecutive Charnley-Müller total hip replacements. J Arthroplasty 1987; 2: 151.

Ritter MA, Zhou H, Keating CM et al. Radiological factors influencing femoral and acetabular failure in cemented Charnley total hip arthroplasties. J Bone Joint Surg Br 1999 Nov; 81 (6): 982–986.

Roberts DW, Poss R, Kelley K. Radiographic comparison of cementing techniques in total hip arthroplasty. J Arthroplasty 1986; 1: 241.

Russotti GM, Coventry MB, Stauffer RN. Cemented total hip arthroplasty with contemporary techniques. A five-year follow-up study. Clin Orthop 1988; 235: 141–147.

Schulte KR, Callaghan JJ, Kelley SS, Johnston RC. The outcome of Charnley total hip arthroplasty with cement after a minimum twenty-year follow-up. The results of one surgeon. J Bone Joint Surg 1993; 75-A: 961–975.

Stauffer RN. Ten year follow-up study of total hip replacement: With particular reference to roentgenographic loosening of the components. J Bone Joint Surg 1982; 64-A: 983–990.

Sutherland CJ, Wilde AH, Borden LS, Marks KE. A ten-year follow-up of one hundred consecutive Müller curved-stem total hip replacement arthroplasties. J Bone Joint Surg 1982; 64-A: 970–982.

Timperley AJ, Howell JR, Gie GA. Rational for a flanged socket. In: Breusch, Malchau (eds): The well cemented total hip arthroplasty. Springer Berlin, Heidelberg, New York, Tokyo 2005; 209–213.

Udomkiat P, Dorr LD, Wan Z. Cementless hemispheric porous-coated sockets implanted with press-fit technique without screws: average ten-year follow-up. J Bone Joint Surg Am 2002 Jul; 84-A (7):1195–1200.

Vervest TM, Anderson PG, Van Hout F, Wapstra FH, Louwerse RT, Koetsier JW. Ten to twelve-year results with the Zweymuller cementless total hip prosthesis. J Arthroplasty 2005 Apr; 20 (3): 362–368.

Williams HD, Browne G, Gie GA, Ling RS, Timperley AJ, Wendover NA. The Exeter universal cemented femoral component at 8 to 12 years. A study of the first 325 hips. J Bone Joint Surg Br 2002 Apr; 84 (3): 324–34. Erratum in: J Bone Joint Surg Br 2002 Sep; 84 (7): 1091.

Diagnosis and Management of Infected Arthroplasty – The United Kingdom Experience

Paul Gaston

Introduction

Currently, there are very few orthopedic centers in the United Kingdom (UK) with a dedicated facility for the management of joint implant infections. Treatment tends to be provided by the surgeon and hospital, who undertook the primary operation. Most orthopedic surgeons deal with a small number of cases per annum. This chapter presents a summary of current management strategies for the treatment of infected arthroplasties, as practised in the United Kingdom. It cannot be said to be truly representative of all views on management held in this country, as it mostly draws on the teaching I have had from senior colleagues and partly from my own clinical experience.

My particular interest lies in techniques to aid the diagnosis of infection in arthroplasty, and I will concentrate on this in the first part of this chapter. The second part deals with clinical management including the use of antibiotic-loaded acrylic bone cement.

Pathogenesis and Diagnosis of Infection

Pathogenesis

Organisms have predilections for certain materials. Coagulase-negative staphylococci (CNS) have an affinity for polyethylene and become more pathogenic in contact with this surface. Organisms are most often introduced into the joint at the time of arthroplasty surgery. There they compete with host cells to colonize the implant – the so-called race for the surface (Gristina and Costerton, 1985), (Fig. 11.1).

Once established, they produce a glycocalyx "slime" or "biofilm" and form microcolonies. The organisms become sessile, with a very low rate of cell division, making most antibiotics much less effective. Daughter cells are shed ever-so-often producing flare-ups. It is very difficult for host immune cells or antibiotics to penetrate biofilm. Subsequently, the host forms a low-grade inflammatory reaction against the infection around the edge of the implanted biomaterials. This results in progressive loosening of the implant and bone loss.

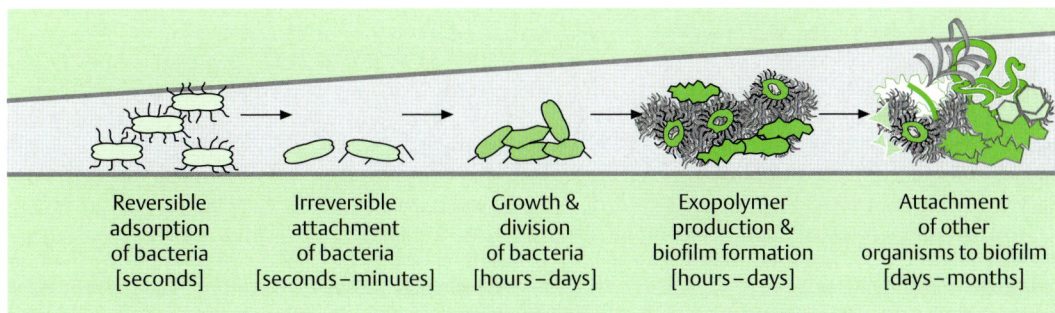

| Reversible adsorption of bacteria [seconds] | Irreversible attachment of bacteria [seconds – minutes] | Growth & division of bacteria [hours – days] | Exopolymer production & biofilm formation [hours – days] | Attachment of other organisms to biofilm [days – months] |

Fig. 11.1 Adherence of organisms to biomaterials (modified from Gristina and Costerton, 1985).

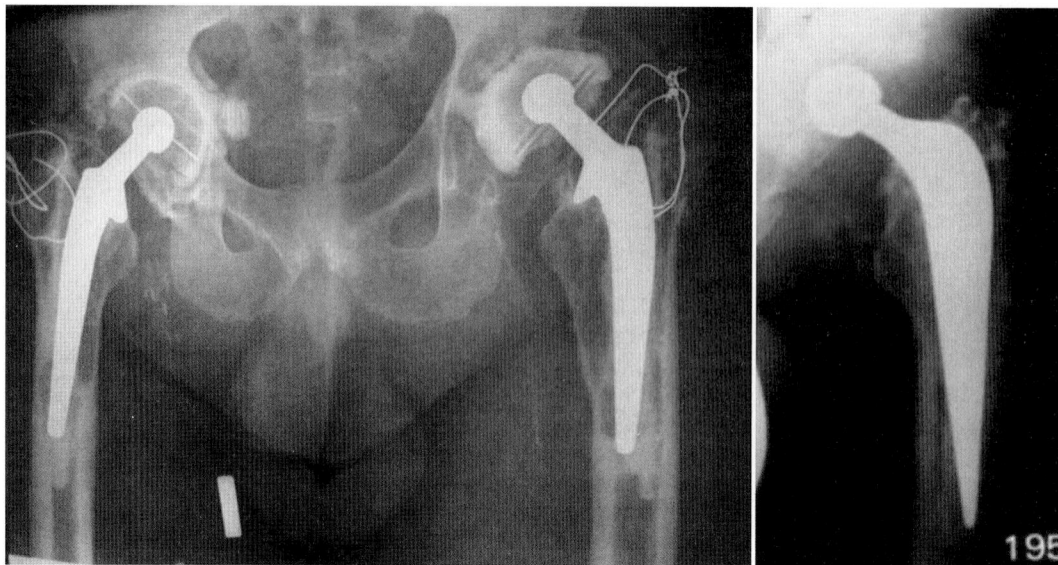

Fig. 11.**2**   Three loose hip replacements, of which only one is infected (arrow).

Reasons for difficulties in diagnosing infection

Most patients with infected joint replacements present with mechanical pain identical to that in aseptic loosening. In the radiographs above only one of the loose joints (arrow) is infected (Fig. 11.2). In the majority of patients, the pain results from the loosening process rather than from the infection itself.

A further major difficulty stems from the fact that bacteria such as skin commensals (e.g., coagulase-negative staphylococci), which normally are not pathogens in other areas of medicine, are the causative agents in this setting and are often disconted.

If a patient presents with a sinus overlying an infected joint replacement, the diagnosis of infection is certain. This is relatively rare. It can be very difficult to distinguish septic from aseptic loosening. Subsequently, many methods exist for the diagnosis of joint replacement infection. That so many tests are available is indicative of the fact that no one test is always diagnostically correct.

I will present a summary of the diagnostic tests in terms of when the results of investigations are available.
1. Diagnostic tests where results are available before revision surgery. (These help with management planning.)
2. Diagnostic tests where the results are only available after revision surgery. (These only help to confirm the diagnosis and guide the choice of systemic antibiotic if this is required.)

I will also present the results of a research study undertaken in Edinburgh looking at the accuracy of various tests for the diagnosis of infection in arthroplasty.

1. Results available before revision

Clinical features
Clinical features are often unreliable. Only 5% of patients with an infected joint replacement will have a temperature of 37.8 °C or more (Fitzgerald and Jones, 1985). However, there are some clinical features that may be of use. A history of wound healing problems and a feeling that the hip replacement has "never been right" after implantation, both raise the clinical suspicion of infection. On examination, the presence of sinuses is highly suggestive of infection (Petty et al., 1975). At operation, pus may be present. However this may be very localized. Joint infection can cause early loosening, and this may be another indicator.

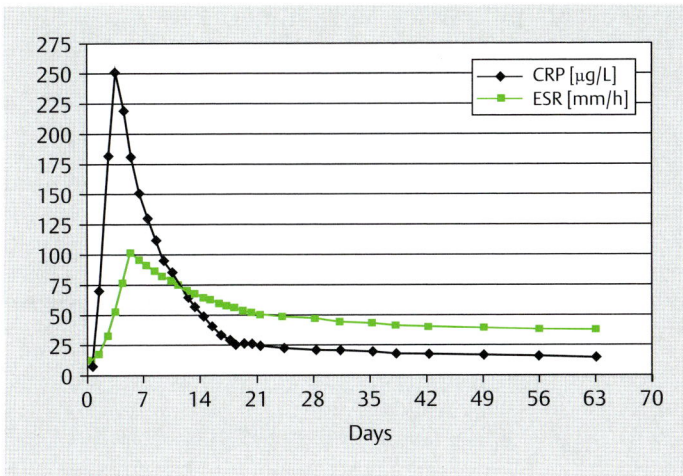

Fig. 11.**3** ESR and CRP after uncomplicated primary hip replacement.

Blood tests

After uncomplicated primary total hip replacement surgery the C-reactive protein (CRP) rises with a peak on the 2nd or 3rd day, but it is back to normal within 3 weeks (Shih et al., 1987). The erythrocyte sedimentation rate (ESR) rises more slowly and takes longer to return to normal (Fig. 11.**3**).

Full blood count, ESR and CRP have all been used for the diagnosis of infection in arthroplasty. The white cell count is most commonly normal and the CRP and ESR are frequently normal (Steckelberg and Osmon, 1994; Cuckler et al., 1991; Lieberman et al., 1993). In a series of 23 patients with proven deep infections of hip replacements Sanzen and Carlsson (Sanzen and Carlsson, 1989) found that the CRP was raised (>20 µg / L) in 19 patients. In only one of the 23 patients neither the CRP nor the ESR was raised.

Preoperative aspiration for microbiological culture

Joint aspiration can be of benefit, but reported sensitivities vary from 50–92% (Table 11.1). In a series of loose hip replacements Barrack and Harris (Barrack and Harris, 1993) reported 88% sensitivity and 50% specificity (large number of false positives). They had a very low number of infected patients (6 of 200 loose implants), which may render the value of their study less reliable. They concluded that aspiration should only be used for selected cases where there is a high index of suspicion of infection. Lachiewicz (Lachiewicz et al., 1996) reported 92% sensitivity and 96% specificity for hip aspiration in 142 loose hips, of which 19 were infected. (The higher proportion of infected cases makes this study more reliable for determining the accuracy of the diagnostic test.) He advocates selected aspiration on the basis of a raised ESR and / or if the hip had been in place for less than 5 years.

Table 11.1 Various reports on the diagnostic value of preoperative aspiration

	No. Infected No. Revized	Sensitivity %	Specificity %	Pos Pred Value %	Neg Pred Value %
Levitsky et al., 1991	9 / 72	67	96	75	93
Spangehl et al., 1999	35 / 202	86	94	67	98
Barrack and Harris, 1993	6 / 200	88	50	6	99
Phillips et al., 1983	11 / 136	91	82	30	99
Lachiewicz et al., 1996	19 / 142	92	97	n / a	n / a

In a more recent study, Williams and co-workers (Williams et al., 2004) from Sheffield, UK, found a high accuracy for preoperative aspiration in 273 revision hip replacements, of which 71 were infected (confirmed by intra-operative culture – the gold standard). They reported 80% sensitivity, 94% specificity, 81% positive predictive value, and the negative predicitive value was 93%. They found that tissue biopsies did not have superior results to simple needle aspiration. In a later report they noted that aspiration in the department of radiology produced the same level of diagnostic accuracy as aspiration in the operating theater (Ali et al., 2006).

Radiographic tests

Plain radiographs only occasionally indicate the presence of infection. Technetium isotope scans remain hot for at least one year after uncomplicated primary hip surgery. If they are negative ("cold") after one year, this is very reassuring and means that infection is unlikely. Persisting raised uptake after a year post operation suggests a pathological process within the joint replacement. However, this is not specific for infection (Levitsky et al., 1991a; Lieberman et al., 1993). To improve sensitivity and specificity, modifications of isotope scanning such as labeled white cell scanning have been used. This method was studied in 38 patients undergoing revision knee replacements, and was found to have a sensitivity of 83% and a specificity of 85% (Rand, 1990). This technique is difficult and only available in specialized centers.

2. Results available after revision

Histological techniques

Several studies have now shown that histology is of great value in diagnosing infection (Mirra et al., 1976; Athanasou et al., 1995; Feldman et al., 1995a). The presence of an acute infection, indicated by neutrophils (Fig. 11.4), as opposed to a chronic inflammatory response around a loosening joint replacement, can distinguish septic from aseptic loosening with accuracy in excess of 90%.

The criteria for diagnosing infection differ slightly in different papers in the literature. Athanasou (Athanasou et al., 1995) initially considered that an average count of 1 neutrophil per 10 high power fields picks up a high number of infected cases without increasing the false negative rate. On the other hand, other authors consider 5 or 10 as a positive result. The experienced pathologist can examine frozen sections intra-operatively, to give an *on-table* indication. These can be confirmed at a later stage with routine paraffin sections.

The major difficulty when using histology to diagnose infection arises in cases of inflammatory conditions such as rheumatoid arthritis. In these cases the histological picture can be confusing and less accurate.

Bacteriology

Bacteriological cultures of samples taken from around the joint replacement at the time of revision should be the gold standard for diagnosis of infection in this situation. However, in up to a fifth

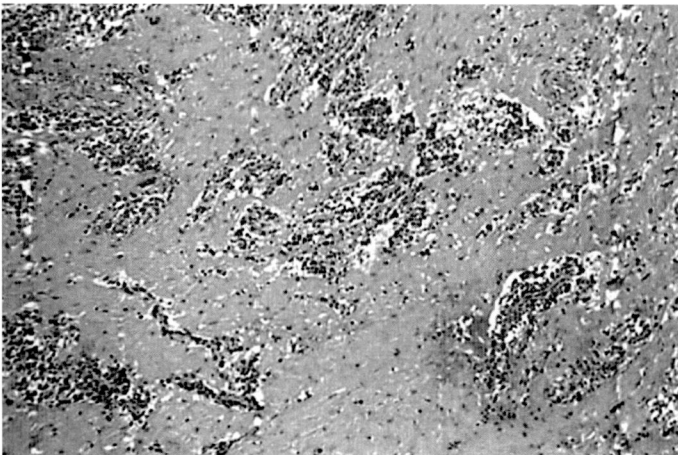

Fig. 11.4 A histology section of tissue from infected hip replacement showing marked neutrophilia.

of infected joint replacements no organisms are grown. Organisms in biofilms have particularly fastidious growth requirements. Delay in sample transport or preoperative/induction antibiotics may result in failure to grow organisms (Fitzgerald and Jones, 1985). Antibiotics should be stopped 2 weeks prior to sampling to improve the chance of a positive culture in a suspected infection.

If a single sample has been obtained and the sample grows a skin commensal such as CNS, it is difficult to know whether this is a pathogen or a contaminant. Multiple samples can help solve this dilemma. Bengston and Knutson (Bengston and Knutson, 1991) considered that there is a definite infection if 3 or more peroperative biopsies grow the same organism. In a study of 297 patients, Atkins and co-workers (Atkins et al., 1998a) showed that ideally six samples should be obtained. If there was growth from only one of the samples, then the chance of infection was very low. If, however, two or more of the samples grew the same organism, then there was a high chance of infection being present (97% specific and 71% sensitive). It was recommended that samples from the joint capsule, a swab from the joint fluid, samples from the membranes around both components, and samples from any further areas of interest should be obtained.

Experimental investigations

Modern molecular biology techniques may offer a new avenue. One is the polymerase chain reaction (PCR). Potential DNA is extracted from joint samples, and if present duplicated many times using "primers" that pick up only bacterial sequences (Fig. 11.5).

If bacterial DNA is present, then the sample is considered to be infected. Mariani (Mariani et al., 1996) reported the use of this technique with good sensitivity, but low specificity, i.e., a high false positive rate.

Edinburgh arthroplasty infection diagnosis study

In the Edinburgh Arthroplasty Unit, we undertook a research project to assess the diagnostic reliability of inflammatory markers (ESR and CRP), preoperative aspiration microbiology, and PCR to detect infection in 204 patients with loose, painful total joint replacements admitted for revision. As can be seen from the above discussion, there is no "gold standard" in the diagnosis of arthroplasty infection. For the purpose of this study we used specific criteria described by authors from the Mayo clinic (Hanssen and Rand, 1999) to decide whether the patient was infected or not. These were based on investigations where results were available after revision hip surgery.

Any one of the following criteria after revision assigned the patient as infected:
- the presence of a discharging sinus or pus in the joint,
- operative sample microbiology with:
  - 2 or more samples growing identical organisms, and
- operative sample histology showing:
  - acute inflammation.

The results of our study are summarized in Table 11.2.

The positive predictive value (PPV) and negative predictive value (NPV) of a diagnostic test are more useful than sensitivity and specificity in clinical practice. They allow the doctor to judge how likely any particular result is to be correct. In our study, if a single inflammatory marker (ESR or CRP) was raised, there was a 50/50 chance that the joint was infected. If normal, the joint was not infected 9 times out of 10. If 2 CRPs taken at different times were elevated, there was an 80% chance of infection. If both were normal, it was 94% certain that no infection was present. If the aspiration sample had positive microbiology, there was a 7 out of 10 chance that infection was present. If

	Sensitivity %	Specificity %	PPV %	NPV %
CRP >20	77	76	49	92
ESR >30	61	86	57	87
Aspiration	80	83	71	88
PCR	71	78	43	89

Table 11.2 Results of the Edinburgh Infection Diagnosis Study

PCR: Polymerase Chain Reaction

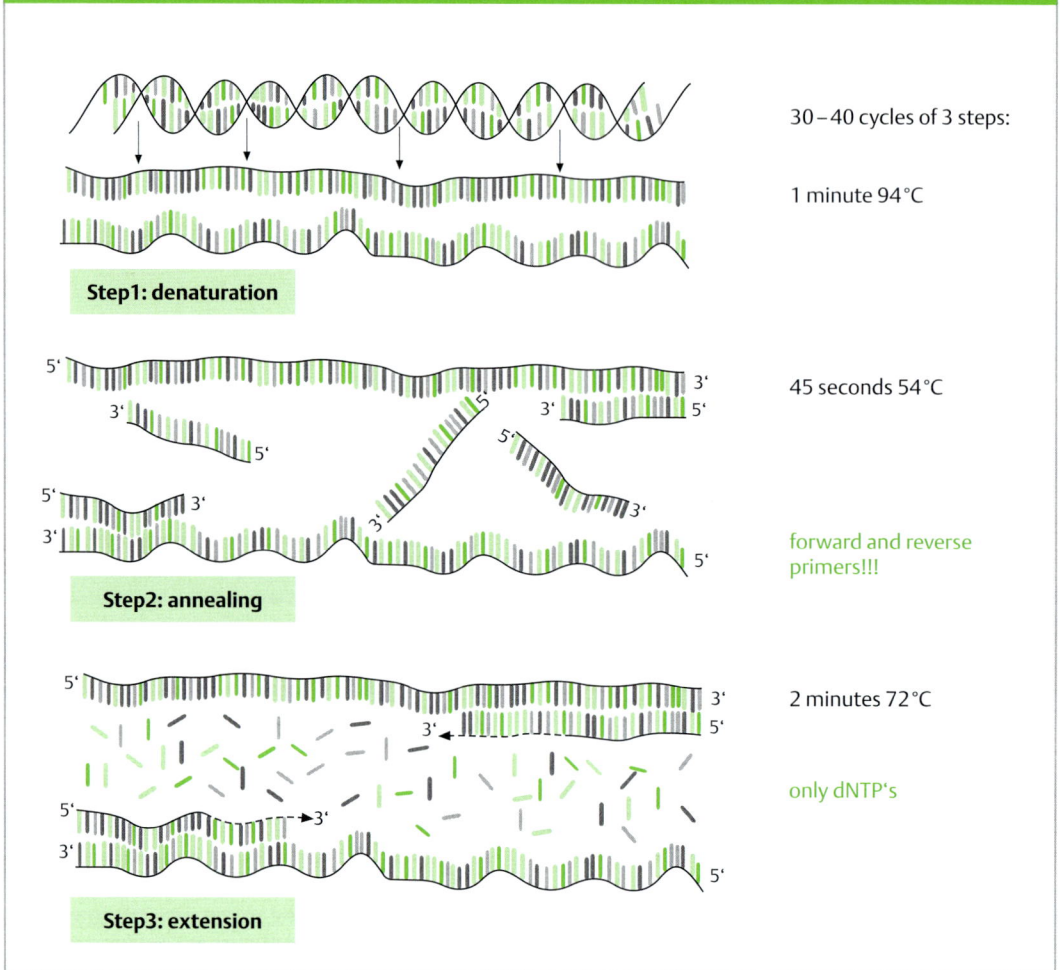

30–40 cycles of 3 steps:

1 minute 94 °C

Step1: denaturation

45 seconds 54 °C

forward and reverse primers!!!

Step2: annealing

2 minutes 72 °C

only dNTP's

Step3: extension

Fig. 11.**5**   The polymerase chain reaction.

joint aspiration was negative, there was a 9 out of 10 chance that no infection was present. In our study, PCR had a high false positive rate – a positive result was correct less than 50 % of the time.

Summary

Given the evidence presented above and the results of our local study, we use an investigation pathway for preoperative workup of loose painful joint replacements (Fig.11.**6**). Please note: this pathway is for guidance only and must be interpreted together with the overall clinical picture.

Management of Infected Arthroplasty

Traditionally, UK orthopedic surgeons have managed this problem by two-stage exchange, leaving the patient with either an excision arthroplasty or an antibiotic-loaded cement spacer for a variable period of time, until they are sure that the infection is cleared. Only then will they undertake re-

Investigation pathway

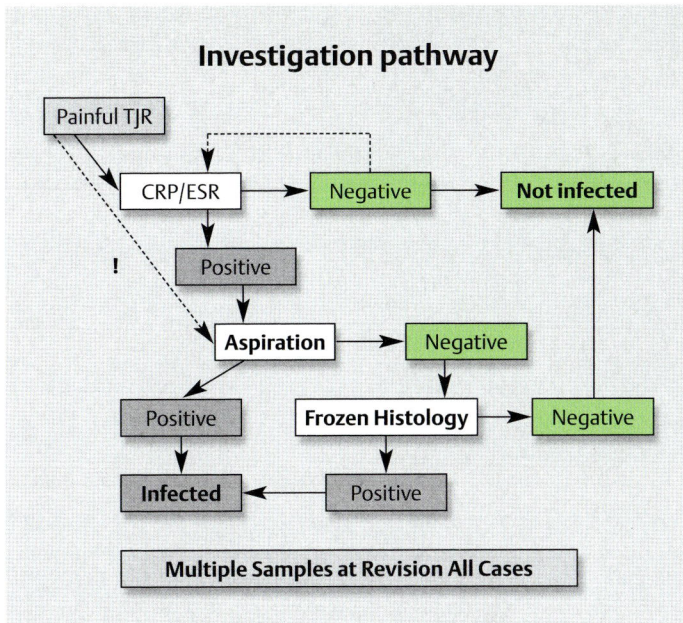

Fig. 11.**6**   An investigation pathway.

implantation of a new joint replacement. More recently there has been a trend to one-stage revisions for infection.

One-stage versus two-stage exchange

Most orthopedic surgeons would agree that for a successful one-stage revision operation for infected total joint replacement, certain criteria need to be met. These are the presence of a healthy patient, good soft tissues, and a "good" organism.

Cierny (Cierny et al., 2003) developed a classification system for osteomyelitis. Herein he includes an assessment of the patient divided into the following categories:

❖ A Healthy patient,
❖ B Local/Systemic compromise, e.g., peripheral vascular disease or diabetes, and
❖ C Treatment worse than disease.

For a successful one-stage exchange the patient must fall into group A.

There is debate as to whether or not the presence of a sinus is a contraindication for one-stage exchange. If the sinus can be excised as part of the debridement, then one-stage exchange may be appropriate. A similar view can be taken for the presence of pus/abscesses. If all purulent material can be removed, it may be possible to go ahead with a one-stage revision. If there is a large area of wound breakdown overlying an infected arthroplasty (Fig. 11.7), one-stage exchange is less likely to be successful.

Multiple previous operations on a particular joint also reduce the chance of success.

One factor that is crucial for one-stage exchange is that, prior to revision, the surgeon knows for certain that the joint is infected and which organism is causing the infection. As noted above, in UK practice an organism is often not grown from preoperative aspiration for microbiology culturing, even with repeated attempts to obtain positive cultures. This makes it very difficult to plan a one-stage exchange, as the clinician does not know which organism he is dealing with and has no sensitivities to guide the choice of antibiotic for the bone cement or postoperative systemic antibiotics. Under these circumstances one-stage exchange is impossible.

Certain organisms are also much more difficult to eradicate at one-stage exchange. Organisms with antibitotic resistance – the traditional methicillin resistant *Staphylococcus aureus* (MRSA) and the emerging multiply resistant *Staphylococcus epidermidis* (MRSE) often require several debridements, before clearance is achieved. Gram-nega-

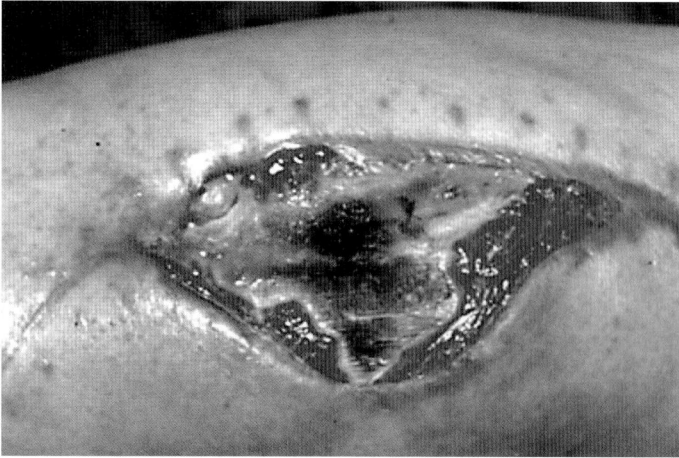

Fig. 11.**7** A chronically open wound over bipolar hemiarthroplasty.

tive species such as enterococci and pseudomonas are also notoriously difficult to eradicate, and it is probably sensible to ensure the infection is cleared, before a new joint replacement is implanted. The presence of multiple organisms can reduce the efficacy of one-stage exchange – it can be difficult to cover all organisms with the antibiotic-loaded bone cement.

Several UK surgeons have reported their results of one-stage revisions for infection, with varied levels of success. These include Elson (Elson, 1993) and Raut (Raut et al., 1995), who reported approximately 80% success for one-stage revisions for infection in two separate publications. These authors are experts in their field, undertaking a large number of revision operations per annum. As mentioned at the beginning of this chapter, most revisions for infection in the United Kingdom are undertaken by surgeons dealing with a small number of cases per annum. The majority of these surgeons tend to fall back on the traditional strategy for the management of arthroplasty infection – namely two-stage revision. In the hip, this commonly involves insertion of an antibiotic-loaded articulating spacer in an attempt to deliver high concentrations of antibiotic locally, and to keep the joint to the correct length (Fig. 11.**8**).

Choice of antibiotics in cement

In Edinburgh, we commonly use Palacos R+G cement (Heraeus) with gentamicin added by the manufacturer (Fig. 11.**9**).

Palacos R+G has been shown to have excellent antibiotic elution characteristics. However, the manufactured powder only contains gentamicin at 0.5 g per 40 g mix of antibiotic cement, a level, which most would consider inadequate for delivery of a high local concentration of antibiotic. More recently we have introduced a new cement for use in infected cases.

Copal contains higher concentrations of antibiotic with 1 g of gentamicin and 1 g of clindamicin per 40 g mix of cement. These 2 antibiotics have a synergistic effect in vivo, and this cement has been designed specifically for use in infected arthroplasty surgery.

Most surgeons also add an extra antibiotic to the bone cement preparation. The most commonly used is vancomycin. One reason for this is the lack of positive cultures and, therefore, the need to use a broad spectrum antibiotic – especially one that covers *coagulase-negative Staphylococcus* (CNS). As yet, we have no case of CNS resistant to vancomycin in Edinburgh. We use up to 4 g of vancomycin per 40 g mix of cement in spacers or beads at the first stage, and no more than 2 g per 40 g mix at reimplantation.

Systemic antibiotics

It is our usual practice to use systemic antibiotics in the management of infected arthroplasty. This is not the case in all centers in the United Kingdom. We use intravenous antibiotics in the initial phase after the first-stage operation for a variable

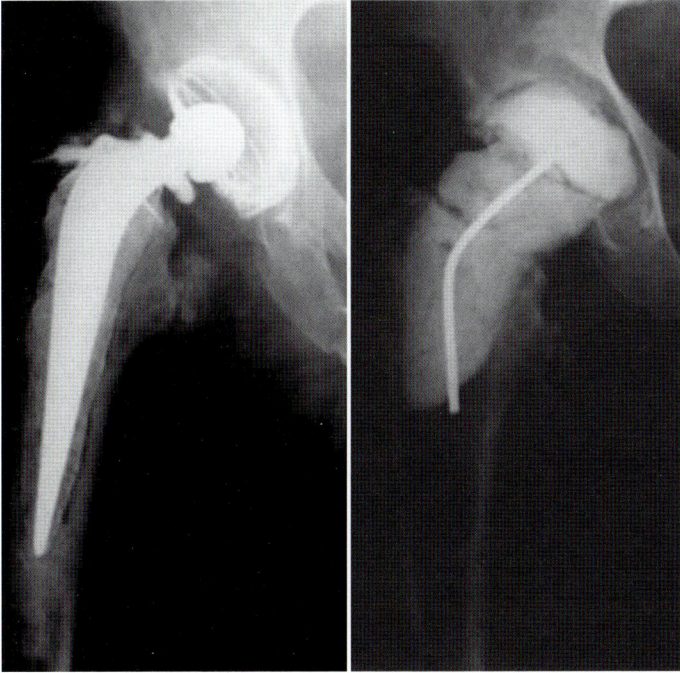

Fig. 11.**8**   An infected total hip replacement with a spacer in place after first-stage revision.

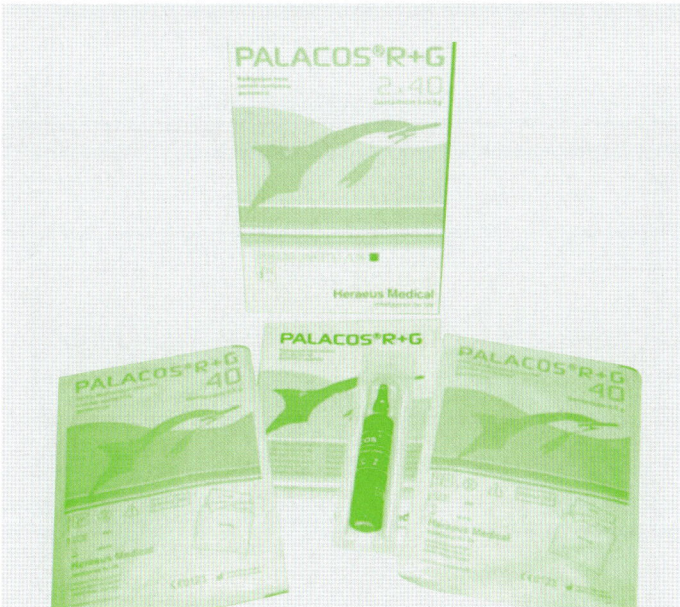

Fig. 11.**9**   Palacos R cement with gentamicin.

period, most often 2 weeks. If the organism is difficult or resistant, the period of intravenous antibiotics can be much longer, up to 6 weeks in duration. After the initial period of i.v. antibiotics, the patient is usually switched to a period of oral antibiotics, taking guidance from the consultant microbiologist. Our microbiologist has recently produced a set of guidelines for the use of systemic antibiotics in the management of infected arthroplasty (Table 11.3). These guidelines are adapted from a review by Zimmerli (Zimmerli et al., 2004).

Notes:

1. The choice of the antimicrobial depends on the susceptibilities of the isolated microorganism.
2. Patients with penicillin allergy (minor rash) can be treated with cefuroxime 1.5 g t.d.s. i.v. Patients with immediate hypersensitivity reactions to penicillin should be treated with i.v. vancomycin.
3. The vancomycin dose is to be calculated according to creatinine clearance, maintaining the trough levels between 15–20 mg/L.

Table 11.**3**   Antimicrobial treatment regimen of prosthetic joint infections according to pathogen, courtesy of Dr J Dave

Microorganism	Antimicrobial agent[1,2]	Duration	Followed by
Staphylococcus aureus or coagulase-negative staphylococci Meticillin-susceptible	Flucloxacillin[2] 2 g q.d.s. i.v. + Rifampicin 450 mg b.d. p.o./i.v.	2 weeks	Ciprofloxacin 500 mg b.d. p.o. + Rifampicin 300 mg b.d. p.o.
Staphylococcus aureus or coagulase negative staphylococci Meticillin-resistant	Vancomycin[3] 1 g b.d. i.v. + Rifampicin 300 mg b.d. p.o.	2 weeks	Ciprofloxacin 500 mg b.d. p.o. + Rifampicin 300 mg b.d. p.o. or Tecoplanin[4] 12 mg/kg o.d. i.v./i.m. or Doxycycline 100 mg b.d. p.o. or Cotrimoxazole 1 forte tablet t.d.s. p.o.
Streptococcus spp (except *S. agalactiae*)	Benzyl penicillin 1.2 g q.d.s. i.v. or Ceftriaxone 2 g o.d. i.v.	4 weeks	Amoxicillin 500 mg t.d.s. p.o.
Enterococcus species (penicillin-susceptible)	Gentamicin[5] 80 mg b.d. + Ampicillin/amoxicilin 2 g q.d.s. i.v.	2–4 weeks	Amoxicillin 500 mg t.d.s. p.o.
Nonfermenters (eg. *Pseudomonas aeruginosa*)	Ceftazidime 2 g t.d.s. i.v. + Gentamicin[5]	2–4 weeks	Ciprofloxacin 500 mg b.d. p.o.
Anerobes[6]	Clindamycin 600 mg q.d.s. i.v.	2–4 weeks	Clindamycin 300 mg q.d.s. p.o.
Mixed infections (without meticillin-resistant staphylococci)	Piperacillin-tazobactam 4.5 g t.d.s. i.v. or meropenem 1 g t.d.s. i.v.	2–4 weeks	Individual regimens according to antimicrobial susceptibilities

1 Choice of the antimicrobial agent depends on the susceptibilities of the isolated microorganisms; 2 Patients with penicillin allergy (minor rash) can be treated with cefuroxime 1.5 g t.d.s. i.v. Patients with immediate hypersensitivity reactions to penicillin should be treated with i.v. vancomycin; 3 Vancomycin dose to be calculated according to creatinine clearance, maintaining the trough levels between 15–20 mg/L; 4 Teicoplanin should be administered as loading dose 12 mg/kg rounded off to the nearest 200 at 12 hour intervals for the first 3 doses and then once a day; 5 Gentamicin treatment should be monitored with bi-weekly levels, aiming at trough levels <1 mg/L and peak levels 3–5 mg/L. Discuss dose alteration with the pharmacist or microbiologist in cases of renal impairment; 6 Alternatively, Gram-positive anerobes (e.g. *Propionibacterium acnes*) can be treated with benzyl penicillin 1.2 g q.d.s. i.v. or ceftriaxone 2 g o.d. i.v. and Gram-negative anerobes (e.g. Bacteroides species) with metronidazole 500 mg t.d.s. p.o./i.v.

4. Teicoplanin should be administered as loading dose 12 mg/kg rounded off to the nearest 200 at 12 hour intervals for the first 3 doses and then once a day.
5. Gentamicin treatment should be monitored with bi-weekly levels, aiming for trough levels <1 mg/L and peak levels 3–5 mg/L. Discuss dose alteration with the pharmacist or microbiologist in cases of renal impairment.
6. Alternatively, Gram-positive anerobes (e.g., *Propionibacterium acnes*) can be treated with benzyl penicillin 1.2 g, q.d.s. i.v. or ceftriaxone 2 g o.d., i.v. and Gram-negative anerobes (e.g., Bacteroides species) with metronidazole 500 mg t.d.s. p.o./i.v.

All antibiotics are stopped a minimum of 2 weeks before second-stage exchange. After the second stage, the patient is given only standard antibiotic prophylaxis for joint replacement surgery, i.e., 3 doses of third generation cephalosporin. In some difficult cases where doubt remains or for suppression of infection in patients unfit for major surgery, much longer courses of oral antibiotics are used, occasionally for life. The following shows our unit guidelines for the duration of treatment in various scenarios – please note that these are guidelines only (Table 11.**4**).

Length of interval between stages

Each case of joint replacement infection is dealt with on its own merits. As a rule, patients undergoing two-stage exchange have 2 weeks of intravenous antibiotics, followed by 4 weeks of oral antibiotics. Thereafter, they need to be off antibiotics for 2 weeks prior to the second stage. This means a minimum of 2 months between first- and second-stage operations. In practice, the interval is usually much longer. We use the CRP to monitor the response to treatment. As mentioned above, the CRP should fall to near normal levels in approximately 3 weeks if no infection is present. The CRP should be less than 20 on at least 2 occasions, at least 1 week apart before antibiotics can be stopped. Once systemic antibiotics have finished, it is important to continue to monitor the patient to look for clinical signs of recurrence of infection, and to repeat the CRP to ensure it does not begin to rise again. If the patient remains well with a quiet wound and CRP is less than 20, it is usually safe to proceed to the second stage. We do not routinely reaspirate before the second stage. If there are clinical signs of recurrence of infection, or there is a sharp elevation in CRP, we recommend a further wound/joint debridement rather than reimplantation, with a further period of systemic antibiotic treatment.

Results of two-stage treatment of infection

As part of the research into diagnosis of infection, I was able to study a subgroup of patients who underwent two-stage revision for infection. 32 patients (20 hips, 11 knees and 1 elbow) underwent such treatment in Edinburgh over a two-year period. These patients had systemic antibiotics for an average of 7 weeks after first-stage implant re-

Table 11.**4** Duration of treatment for prosthetic joint infections

Procedure	Duration of antimicrobial treatment
Debridement with retention	3 months for hip prosthesis 6 months for knee prosthesis
One-stage exchange	As above
2-stage exchange with long interval (≥6 weeks) with or without spacer	If interval is 4–6 weeks, Antibiotics are stopped at 2 weeks before planned reimplantation. If intraoperative samples culture is negative, stop antimicrobials. If not, continue antimicrobials for 3 months (hip prostheses) and 6 months (knee prostheses).
Implant removal without replacement	6 weeks
Long-term suppressive treatment	Long-term

moval and joint debridement. The average interval between stages was 16 weeks. 3 patients were lost to follow-up. The mean follow-up for the remaining patients was 2 years and 4 months. By this time, there were 4 proven recurrences (3/11 knees, 1/20 hips) giving a failure rate of 12.5%. Taking the "worst case scenario" where it is assumed that all those patients lost to follow-up also had had a recurrence of infection, our success rate was 78%. Success was defined as a healed wound with the patient not on antibiotics, and where the patient was happy with the relief of pain and overall function.

Other centers have better results after two-stage exchange. One unit with high expertise in this field is in Sheffield, lead by I Stockley. They employ a two-stage revision technique using high-dose local antibiotics in cement spacers and beads after the first stage, without using any systemic antibiotics. Similar criteria are used before the patient can proceed to second stage. They have achieved around 90% success in over 100 patients with this technique. Their work is due to be published in a detailed report later this year.

There is little evidence of the best results for management in the presence of difficult organisms such as MRSA/MRSE. Most surgeons in our unit would still advocate a two-stage revision strategy with a prolonged period of intravenous systemic antibiotics using vancomycin. A long interval phase is usually required to ensure eradication of infection.

Summary

Diagnosis of infection in arthroplasty is difficult, due to the presence of fastidious organisms growing in complex biofilms. Implant infections are commonly caused by organisms considered to be commensals, and are often dismissed as contaminants, e.g., CNS. Many diagnostic modalities exist for the detection of infection, but this is simply a reflection of the fact that there is no "gold standard" test in this field of practice. Research has shown that if a patient with a painful/loose joint replacement is suspected to have an infection, the first step is to check the inflammatory markers – ESR and CRP. If these are raised or suspicion remains, the next step is needle aspiration for microbiology. This may need to be repeated. At revision operation, it is important to send multiple samples to increase confidence in the results.

In the United Kingdom, two-stage exchange, with the use of antibiotic-loaded acrylic bone cement spacers, a period of systemic antibiotics, and a relatively long interval period before reimplantation of a new joint, is the common strategy for management of suspected/confirmed joint replacement infection. Single-stage exchange is advocated by some experts in specialist centers, but conditions must be favorable, including a healthy host, good soft tissues, and positive preoperative microbiology cultures of an organism sensitive to easily administered antibiotics. With either strategy, reported results vary with up to 20% recurrence rates at approximately 2 years.

References

Ali F, Wilkinson JH, Cooper JR et al. Accuracy of joint aspiration for the preoperative diagnosis of infection in total hip arthroplasty. J Arthroplasty 2006 Feb; 21 (2): 221–226.

Athanasou NA, Pandey R, de Steiger R, Crook D, Smith PM. Diagnosis of infection by frozen section during revision arthroplasty. Journal of Bone & Joint Surgery – British Volume 1995; 77: 28–33.

Atkins BL, Athanasou NA, Deeks JJ et al. Prospective evaluation of criteria for microbiological diagnosis of prosthetic joint infection at revision arthroplasty. The OSIRIS Collaborative Study Group J Clin Microbiol 1998a; 36: 2932–2939.

Barrack RL, Harris WH. The value of aspiration of the hip joint before revision total hip arthroplasty. Journal of Bone & Joint Surgery – American Volume 1993; 75: 66–76.

Bengtson S, Knutson K. The infected knee arthroplasty. A 6-year follow-up of 357 cases. Acta Orthop Scand 1991; 62: 301–311.

Cierny G, Mader JT, Penninck JJ. A clinical staging system for adult osteomyelitis. Clinical Orthopedics & Related Research 2003; (414):7–24.

Cuckler JM, Star AM, Alavi A, Noto RB. Diagnosis and management of the infected total joint arthroplasty. Orthopedic Clinics of North America 1991; 22 (3): 523–530.

Elson RA. Exchange arthroplasty for infection. Perspectives from the United Kingdom. Orthopaedic Clinics of North America 1993; 24 (4): 761–767.

Feldman DS, Lonner JH, Desai P, Zuckerman JD. The role of intraoperative frozen sections in revision total joint arthroplasty. J Bone Joint Surg Am 1995a; 77: 1807–1813.

Fitzgerald RH Jr, Jones DR. Hip implant infection. Treatment with resection arthroplasty and late total hip arthroplasty. American Journal of Medicine 1985; 78 (6B): 225–228.

Gristina AG, Costerton JW. Bacterial adherence to biomaterials and tissue. The significance of its role in clinical sepsis. Journal of Bone & Joint Surgery – American Volume 1985; 67: 264–273.

Hanssen AD, Rand JA. Evaluation and treatment of infection at the site of a total hip or knee arthroplasty. Review (141 refs). Instructional Course Lectures 1999; 48: 111–122.

Lachiewicz PF, Rogers GD, Thomason HC. Aspiration of the hip joint before revision total hip arthroplasty. Clinical and laboratory factors influencing attainment of a positive culture. Journal of Bone & Joint Surgery – American Volume 1996; 78: 749–754.

Levitsky KA, Hozack WJ, Balderston RA et al. Evaluation of the painful prosthetic joint. Relative value of bone scan, sedimentation rate, and joint aspiration. Journal of Arthroplasty 1991a; 6: 237–244.

Lieberman JR, Huo MH, Schneider R, Salvati EA, Rodi S. Evaluation of painful hip arthroplasties. Are technetium bone scans necessary? Journal of Bone & Joint Surgery – British Volume 1993; 75: 475–478.

Mariani BD, Martin DS, Levine MJ, Booth RE, Tuan RS. The Coventry Award. Polymerase chain reaction detection of bacterial infection in total knee arthroplasty. Clinical Orthopedics & Related Research 1996; 11–22.

Mirra JM, Amstutz HC, Matos M, Gold R. The pathology of the joint tissues and its clinical relevance in prosthesis failure. Clinical Orthopedics & Related Research 1976; 221–240.

Petty W, Bryan RS, Coventry MB, Peterson LF. Infection after total knee arthroplasty. Orthopedic Clinics of North America 1975; 6 (4): 1005–1014.

Phillips WC, Kattapuram SV. Efficacy of preoperative hip aspiration performed in the radiology department. Clinical Orthopaedics & Related Research 1983; 141–146.

Rand JA. The value of indium 111 leukocyte scanning in the evaluation of painful or infected total knee arthroplasties. Clinical Orthopedics & Related Research 1990; 179–182.

Raut VV, Siney PD, Wroblewski BM. One-stage revision of total hip arthroplasty for deep infection. Long-term follow-up. Clinical Orthopedics & Related Research 1995; (321): 202–207.

Sanzen L, Carlsson AS. The diagnostic value of C-reactive protein in infected total hip arthroplasties. Journal of Bone & Joint Surgery – British Volume 1989; 71: 638–641.

Shih LY, Wu JJ, Yang DJ. Erythrocyte sedimentation rate and C-reactive protein values in patients with total hip arthroplasty. Clinical Orthopedics & Related Research 1987; 238–246.

Spangehl MJ, Masri BA, O'Connell JX, Duncan CP. Prospective analysis of preoperative and intraoperative investigations for the diagnosis of infection at the sites of two hundred and two revision total hip arthroplasties. Journal of Bone & Joint Surgery – American Volume 1999b; 81: 672–683.

Steckelberg JM, Osmon DR. Prosthetic joint infections. In: Bisno AL, Waldvogel FA, eds., Infections asociated with indwelling medical devices. Washington D.C., American Scoiety of Microbiology Press 1994: 259–290.

Williams JL, Norman P, Stockley I. The value of hip aspiration versus tissue biopsy in diagnosing infection before exchange hip arthroplasty surgery. Journal of Arthroplasty 2004; 19 (5): 582–586.

Zimmerli W, Trampuz A, Ochsner PE. Prosthetic-joint infections. New England Journal of Medicine 2004; 351 (16): 1645–1654.

Management of Septic Joint Arthroplasty – The Hellenic Experience

Konstantinos N. Malizos, Nikolaos T. Roidis, Theophilos S. Karachalios, Lazaros A. Poultsides, Konstantinos A. Bargiotas

Introduction

Joint replacement surgery has become an essential component of modern medicine, setting new standards and offering a dramatically improved quality of life to patients that have been disabled for many years. Currently, more than 500,000 joint replacements are performed in the United States annually and more than 11.3 million patients have an artificial joint (Widmer, 2001; Isiklar et al., 1996; Darouiche et al., 2004). As the percentage of patients aged over 65 years is on the rise in industrialized countries, the number of patients requiring implants will continue to grow. By 2030, the estimated number of joint arthroplasties in the United States will exceed 1 million (Parvizi et al., 2004).

Joint arthroplasty has achieved its current status through a "trial and error" process and has lately become one of the safest and most effective surgical procedures. However, despite the otherwise successful outcome, lifelong durability is adversely affected by wear of contact surfaces, loosening of implant-to-bone interfaces, and notably by periprosthetic infections, which although less frequent remain one of the most feared and devastating complications, both for the patients and the treating physicians. Effective prophylactic measures have been successful in reducing the incidence of periprosthetic infection for total hip arthroplasties (THAs) or total knee arthroplasties (TKAs), occuring with a rate of 1.5–2.5 % for primary procedures. This is opposed to revision THAs or TKAs with a respective infection risk of 3.2 % or 5.6 % in long-term follow-up (Fitzgerald, 1995; Al-Maiyah et al., 2005; Hanssen, 1999; Parvizi et al., 2004).

Besides the institutional expenses and the indirect costs, treating an infected arthroplasty is devastating for the patient in terms of pain, suffering emotional burden, and additional morbidity. Even with successful treatment, patients often require 6–18 months before regaining the function they had before the onset of infection, and in some cases the joint mobility will remain permanently impaired (Spangehl et al., 2002; Huenger et al., 2005). It has been estimated that treatment of an infected THA requires twice the resources of a revision knee replacement for aseptic failure and results in a financial loss to the hospital of between $15 000 and $30 000 (Hebert et al., 1996). The attendant mortality was estimated in the 1970s and 1980s to range from 2.7 to 18 % in older patients (Berbari et al., 1998). More current studies have estimated the mortality attendant to surgical intervention for prosthetic joint infection (PJI) to be 0.4–1.2 % for 65-year-old patients and 2–7 % for 80-year-old patients. It has been estimated (Fisman et al., 2001) that there is a two-fold increase in the probability of death during the first 3 months after resection arthroplasty. (Lentino et al., 2003).

Diagnosis

The clinical presentation of a periprosthetic infection may vary from an acute septic postoperative complication, to an acute late hematogenous episode or to a late sub-acute or chronic infection with or without discharging sinus. The diagnostic approach in any of these clinical settings should include a high index of suspicion combined with a thorough history and physical examination. This should also be complemented by full blood work-up, radiographs, radionuclide studies, joint aspiration, and specialized histological evaluation of tissue specimens obtained at surgical intervention.

Management

A prosthesis-related infection is difficult to treat. Standard antibiotic protocols that are effective against other infections, generally fail to achieve cure in this particular situation. The immuno-incompetent zone around an implant, the reduced sensitivity of the bacteria growing in a biofilm, and the relatively poor availability of antibiotics from the blood stream at the site of infection probably all contribute to this fact. The mainstay of treatment is the removal of the infected prosthesis. Generally, antibiotic treatment is only expected to be successful after the removal of all foreign body materials. Usually, this is accompanied by thorough surgical debridement of the infected area at the time of the prosthesis removal. Subsequently, a prolonged course of systemic and local antibiotics aiming at the causative bacteria is applied. Local application is achieved by implanting antibiotic-releasing carriers such as antibiotic-loaded cement beads linked in chains or antibiotic-loaded bone cement spacers. This allows for antibiotic concentrations at a level that would cause side-effects if administered systemically.

Surgical treatment involves implantation of a new prosthesis either in one surgical procedure or in a second procedure. The treatment choice depends on:
1. the type of infection,
2. the severity of infection,
3. bacterial susceptibility/resistance to antibiotics,
4. whether or not the implant is loose,
5. the patient's general health, and
6. the condition of local soft tissue.

The different treatment modalities consist of suppressive antibiotics, debridement, i.e., thorough removal of infected tissue and lavage, revision in one or two stages, resection arthroplasty, arthrodesis, and amputation.

Nonsurgical management

Systemic antibiotics

Suppression of implant infection with antibiotics might be a management option in patients who are unable to undergo surgery, usually because of medical co-morbidities (Pavoni et al., 2004). However, the patient should be able to take antibiotics orally for a long period of time. Ideally, the antimicrobial agent should have bactericidal activity against surface-adhering, slow-growing, and biofilm-producing microorganisms. Since long-term antimicrobial therapy is needed, the microorganism should be susceptible to oral antimicrobial agents with good bioavailability (Zimmerli, 2004). Rifampin meets these requirements for staphylococci, but should never be administered alone, since staphylococci rapidly develop antimicrobial resistance (Giannoudis et al., 2005). Quinolones are excellent combination agents, because of their bioavailability, antimicrobial activity, and tolerability. Newer quinolones such as levofloxacin are effective against Gram-positive microorganisms (Trampuz et al., 2005). Other antimicrobial combination regimens are frequently needed, because of increasing resistance of staphylococci to quinolones. Fusidic acid, trimethoprim-sulfamethoxazole, minocycline, and linezolid can all be combined with rifampin; however, no data on these combination regimens have been reported. Also, few data are available on the treatment of Gram-negative bacilli. *In-vitro* studies and an animal model showed that ciprofloxacin had better efficacy against Gram-negative bacilli than beta-lactams.

Several studies have been undertaken, investigating the recurrence rate of infection with antibiotic suppression therapy. However, as the patient populations, the staging of the infection, and methods of treatment varied, the results are difficult to compare. One study of 33 infections around implants due to staphylococci, treated with surgical debridement and subsequent randomization to antibiotic therapy with ciprofloxacin alone or in combination with rifampicin, found 58% eradication by use of the single agent, as opposed to 100% of the combination (Zimmerli et al., 1998). The addition of rifampicin was thought to interfere with the glycocalyx, thereby potentiating the action of the antibiotic. Infection with methicillin-resistant *Staph. aureus* (MRSA) requires treatment with linezolid, a potent antibiotic available for oral use. Linezolid has eradicated MSRA in two reported cases with a follow-up of nine and eight months, respectively (Bassetti et al., 2001). The rates of eradication of antibiotic-resistant organisms with suppression therapy have been investigated and eradication was noted in 86% with a mean follow-up of five years. Here five recurrences occured, all within the first three years (Rao et al., 2003). Of these, three resulted from antibiotic-sensitive and two from antibiotic-resistant organisms.

Suppression therapy should be reserved for patients, in whom revision surgery is contraindicated, or who refuse major surgery, or where the prosthesis cannot be easily removed (Toms et al., 2006).

A few studies have described the management of unexpected positive intra-operative cultures when preoperative assessment had failed to show infection. In one study, a series of 31 patients was managed with a 6-week course of parenteral antibiotics. Follow-up of two years showed three persistent and two recurrent infections (Tsukayama et al., 1996). Based on these results, we believe a course of i.v. antibiotics administered for 6 weeks is advisable, when intra-operative cultures unexpectedly show positive results (Toms et al., 2006).

Surgical management of periprosthetic joint infection

Operative debridement

Operative debridement and retention of the prosthesis is the first surgical option in the case of acute infection in the early postoperative period (Type II) or for an acute hematogenous infection (Type III) at the site of a securely fixed and functioning prosthesis (Deirmengian et al., 2003), (Tables 12.1 – 3).

Suggested criteria for this treatment include:
1. a short duration of symptoms of infection, present for a few days or less than one week, since the duration of symptoms prior to debridement has been shown to affect outcome,
2. susceptible Gram-positive organisms, and
3. absence of prolonged postoperative drainage or a draining sinus tract, and
4. absence of prosthetic loosening or radiographic evidence of infection (Leone et al., 2005).

Table 12.**1**   Staging system for prosthetic joint infection

Category	Grading	Description
Infection type	I	Early postoperative infection (<4 weeks postoperatively)
	II	Hematogenous infection (< 4 weeks duration)
	III	Late chronic infection (>4 weeks duration)
Systemic host grade (medical and immune status)	A	Uncompromized (no compromizing factors)
	B	Compromized (1 – 2 compromizing factors)
	C	Significant compromise (>2 compromizing factors) or one of the following:
		■ Absolute neutrophil count <1000
		■ CD4 T cell count <100 – Intravenous drug abuse
		■ Chronic active infection at other sites
		■ Dysplasia or neoplasm of immune system
Local extremity grade	1	Uncompromized (no compromizing factors)
	2	Compromized (1 – 2 compromizing factors)
	3	Significant compromize (>2 compromizing factors)

Modified from: McPherson EJ, Woodson C, Holtom P, Roidis N, Shufelt C, Patzakis M. Periprosthetic total hip infection: outcomes using a staging system. Clin Orthop Relat Res 2002 Oct; (403): 8 – 15

Systemic host compromising factors (Medical and Immune)

- Age = 80 years

- Alcoholism

- Chronic active dermatitis or cellulitis

- Chronic indwelling catheter

- Chronic malnutrition (albumin = 3.0 g / dL)

- Current nicotine use (inhalational or oral)

- Diabetes (requiring oral agents and / or insulin)

- Hepatitic insufficiency (cirrhosis)

- Immunosuppressive drugs (methotrexate, prednisone, cyclosporine)

- Malignancy (history of, or active)

- Pulmonary insufficiency (room air arterial blood gas O2 < 60 %)

- Renal failure requiring dialysis

- Systemic inflammatory disease (rheumatoid arthritis, systemic lupus erythematosus)

- Systemic immune compromize from infection or disease (human immunodeficiency virus, acquired immunodeficiency virus)

Local extremity (wound) – compromizing factors

- Active infection present > 3 – 4 months

- Multiple incisions (creating skin bridges)

- Soft tissue loss from prior trauma

- Subcutaneous abscess > 8 cm^2

- Synovial cutaneous fistula

- Prior periarticular fracture or trauma around the joint (especially crush injury)

- Prior local irradiation to wound area

- Vascular insufficiency to extremity (absent extremity pulses, chronic venous stasis disease, significant calcific arterial disease)

- Chronic active dermatitis or cellulitis

Table 12.2 Systemic compromizing factors and local wound compromizing factors

Modified from: McPherson EJ, Woodson C, Holtom P, Roidis N, Shufelt C, Patzakis M. Periprosthetic total hip infection: outcomes using a staging system. Clin Orthop Relat Res 2002 Oct; (403): 8 – 15

- Acute infection with signs and symptoms = 14 – 28 days

- Stable implant with no signs or symptoms of loosening

- Clearly established diagnosis by isolating single microorganism from multiple specimens by aspiration or preferably by intraoperative culture during debridement

- Positive histopathologic results, preferably by frozen section

- Pathogen susceptible to oral, preferably bactericidal, antimicrobial agent

- Antimicrobial agent with proven effectiveness

- Patient able and willing to undergo long-term antimicrobial therapy

- Host A or B

- Local tissue conditions

Table 12.**3**   Criteria for treatment of orthopedic device-related infections with salvage of implant

Modified from: Widmer AF. New developments in diagnosis and treatment of infection in orthopedic implants. Clin Infect Dis 2001 Sep 1, 33 Suppl 2: 94 – 106

The reported rate for eradication of the infection has been between 26% and 71% following open debridement (Tsukayama et al., 1996). Arthroscopic irrigation and debridement (Dixon et al., 2004; Ilahi et al., 2005) within 48 hours from the onset of symptoms has been described as an alternative. Eight hips, infected with streptococci and treated accordingly, showed no recurrence of infection at a mean follow-up of 70 months. However, these results should not be extrapolated to infections with other organisms (Hyman et al., 1999). Statistical analysis of the indications for operative debridement showed improved quality, adjusted life expectancy, and cost-effectiveness when salvage revision surgery was performed in young healthy patients. Arthroscopic debridement was more beneficial in patients with reduced life expectancy (Fisman et al., 2001).

Single-stage revision with exchange of the implant
Single-stage revision with exchange of the implant is recommended in immunocompetent patients with an acute infection from identified bacteria susceptible to first-line antibiotics. The direct-exchange technique may be best reserved for a select number of patients and should be performed by surgeons with adequate experience. To be successful, this technique requires thorough

debridement, extending well into the medullary canal, followed by a prolonged postoperative course of parenteral antibiotics administered for a minimum of six weeks. Here, the key parameters to success appear to be a susceptible Gram-positive microorganism, use of antibiotic-loaded cement for fixation of the new prosthesis, and prolonged use of antibiotics after the revision surgery.

The rate of recurrence with this treatment at a minimum follow-up of ten years was 8.3% in 24 patients (Callaghan et al., 1999). A number of studies comparing single-stage versus two-stage exchange all favored the two-stage procedure. Elson had a 12.4% rate of failure with the single-stage method, compared to 3.5% with the two-stage procedure (Elson et al., 1993). Very similar results were reported by Garvin in a large study, with a recurrence rate of 10.1% and 5.6% of cases, respectively (Garvin et al., 1993). On the other hand, in single-stage procedures there is less surgical trauma with direct preservation of joint mobility, so that the functional outcome for the knee joint is better with less mechanical problems.

Local antibiotic delivery

Local antibiotic delivery carriers are capable of achieving extremely high local tissue concentrations when compared with those obtained with parenteral or oral antibiotic therapy. Antibiotic-loaded bone cement (ALBC) is the current "gold standard" for local antibiotic delivery in orthopedic surgery, despite some limitations (Evans et al., 2004; Stevens et al., 2005). Heating of the methylmethacrylate during polymerization may inactivate some antibiotics and limit the spectrum of applicable drugs. Also, the rate and dose of antibiotic elution from the cement is an important shortfall. Antibiotic elution is mostly a surface phenomenon. Antibiotics are released into the surrounding tissue in effective peak concentrations for only about 1 week, to successively diminish and become negligible after a relatively short period of time (Kühn 2000). Subsequently, the cement, if used as a spacer, becomes a foreign body, susceptible to colonization by microorganisms.

Over the last years, a number of alternative new technologies have been proposed for the local delivery of antibiotics as an adjunct to the parenteral and oral administration. The biodegradable antibiotic delivery materials have been classified into four broad categories: bone graft (Buttaro et al., 2005), bone graft substitutes or extenders, protein-based materials (natural polymers), and synthetic polymers. Antibiotic is absorbed to the surface of these materials and is then released into the wound environment (Garvin et al., 2005).

One of the most obvious concerns regarding extremely high levels of local antibiotics, is the potential for systemic toxicity – particularly in patients with abnormal renal function (Springer et al., 2004). The optimal antibiotic concentration required for efficacy against the pathogenic organisms varies, depending on their susceptibility, on the presence of biofilm, and on each specific antibiotic used. Some concern is expressed in the face of dose-dependent adverse effects on bone regeneration caused by many currently used antibiotics. There have been some recent observations regarding the use of pulsed electromagnetic fields (EMF) or ultrasound (US) as adjunctive methods to augment the efficacy of certain antibiotics. Here, the most exciting aspect is that these methods could not only be used to improve the efficacy of antibiotics for infection treatment, but also to enhance the process of bone restoration.

For those cases, where the cement is intended for permanent implant fixation, the addition of large quantities of antibiotics can jeopardize its mechanical properties and adversely influence the durability of arthroplasty (Parvizi et al., 2004).

The two-stage revision concept

Two-stage exchange revision

Two-stage exchange revision has become the most widely accepted treatment protocol for infected hip and knee arthroplasties (Urban et al., 2001; Haleem et al., 2004) and for infected shoulder and elbow arthroplasties (Sperling et al., 2001; Yamaguchi et al., 1998; Coste et al., 2004). The first step of this protocol requires the removal of the infected components and thorough debridement of scars, sinus tracts, interface membranes, and any pathological tissue from the joint space and the lumen of the diaphysis. The cavity is managed by introducing a temporary spacer made from an antibiotic-loaded bone cement mold. In all cases, where a Gram-positive microorganism has been identified, 3 g of vancomycin powder and 2 g of fucidic acid powder are added in every batch of bone cement (40 g). In cases, where there is a Gram-negative causative microorganism, we combine vancomycin with 3 g of imipenem per batch. Specific care is always taken to introduce part of the spacer into the medullary canal of the femur and the tibia.

The articulated spacer provides proper soft tissue and limb length between stages (Hsieh et al., 2004). This has several advantages including improved function, preservation of bone stock, prevention of soft-tissue contracture, and it is a source of local delivery of antibiotics (Hofmann et al., 2005; Durbhakula et al., 2004). The comparison of beads versus spacer was made in a retrospective review of 70 patients, managed with cement beads between stages and 58 who were treated with custom-made cement prostheses. The rate of eradication of infection was similar in both groups, with an overall rate of 95.3 %. However, the custom-made prosthesis was noted to provide higher hip scores, a reduced hospital stay and enhanced function between stages. At revision, there was reduced surgical time, reduced blood loss and transfusion requirements, respectively, as well as a lower rate of postoperative dislocation (Hsieh et al., 2004).

With the spacer in place, a minimum course of two weeks of intravenous antibiotics administration followed by six more weeks of oral antibiotics is given. Resolution of the infection is confirmed by the normal erythrocyte sedimentation rate (ES) and C-reactive protein (CRP) values. Three weeks after termination of the antibiotics another blood work-up is done. If ESR and CRP remain within the range of normal values, reimplantation of the arthroplasty is considered, provided that an examination of the wound area reveals absence of active infection, and an aspiration of the joint does not show bacterial growth (Ridgeway et al., 2005).

Despite its widespread acceptance (Barrack et al., 2000), two-stage revision bears several controversial aspects including the timing of the procedure, the use of antibiotic-loaded cement at the second stage, the role of allograft bone grafting, and the use of uncemented components. The ideal duration of antibiotic therapy between stages has not been established. We may go up to three months in selected cases, but a minimum of six weeks is more common practice (Hoad-Reddick et al., 2005).

As regards the timing of the second stage, recent studies have advocated revision between six weeks and three months after the first stage. Several authors believe that the use of antibiotic-loaded cement at revision reduces reinfection rates. Gentamicin-loaded cement was associated with eradication in 95% of patients after five years in Garvin et al.'s study (1994). Hanssen had a cure rate of 82% without antibiotic cement at the second stage, compared with 90% when an antibiotic was used (Hanssen et al., 1999).

Management of bone stock deficiency at revision is a major problem. Although bulk allograft use is a common scenario in revision surgery, there is a theoretical concern that using it after an infection may increase the rate of recurrence. Use of allograft in primary THA has been associated with an increased rate of infection – 6.8% compared to 0.2% with no allograft (Alexeeff et al., 1996). More recent studies of the use of allograft at revision for infection have reported recurrence rates of up to 7.5% (English et al., 2002).

With the increasing emergence of antibiotic-resistant microorganisms, studies have been conducted investigating their effect on the rates of reinfection, and looking at a possible trend toward poorer results in the presence of resistant bacteria. A recent report compared failure rates after two-stage revision between a group of 37 methi-

cillin-sensitive infections and a group of 9 MRSA infections. There was a 5.4% failure rate in the sensitive group as opposed to 11.1% of the group with a resistant infection. (Volin et al., 2004). The addition of rifampicin has been reported to increase the rate of eradication, regardless of antibiotic sensitivities.

The use of a cementless prosthesis at the second stage has been questioned, with early studies reporting reinfection rates as high as 18%, as well as additional cases of loosening. Other studies found similar reinfection rates between 12.5% and 18%. However, first-generation cementless implants were used in these series, and subsequent technological advances have improved the results in primary as well as in revision THA (Toms et al., 2006). More recent investigations have reported reinfection rates between 8% and 11% (Fehring et al., 1999). These more promising results demonstrate that modern cementless components can be used for second-stage revision, with the potential advantage of enhanced survival of the implant (Haddad et al., 2000; Kraay et al., 2005). Our preference in managing periprosthetic hip infections is to apply cementless implants at the second stage after a thorough debridement of the joint.

In each patient, multiple frozen sections and samples for cultures are obtained from the joint-spacer interface and as a guideline we follow the rule of the minimum, counting the polymorphonucleates (PMN) in 5 high power fields from each sample. If more than 5 PMNs are found in more than 5 samples, we will repeat the intermediate stage with another antibiotic-loaded cement spacer for two to three more months.

The results following reinfection after a two-stage revision for infection have been poor. A review of 34 such patients was associated with a 38% recurrence rate infection following a variety of operative interventions. There was a poor functional outcome in the majority of patients. The authors concluded that single-stage revision should not be performed in this situation, and that a two-stage exchange should only be recommended if the infection was due to the initial organism. As there are few studies on the management of this difficult problem, the ideal method of treatment remains still to be determined (Pagnano et al., 1997).

Resection arthroplasty or arthrodesis of the knee joint

Resection arthroplasty or arthrodesis of the knee joint (Bargiotas et al., 2006; VanRyn et al., 2002) should be reserved for seriously debilitated patients, whose general medical condition makes the revision surgery unsafe. This treatment option is also reserved for patients with recurrent infections and subsequently multiple surgeries or for those, in whom reimplantation of a knee prosthesis is not anticipated to yield a functioning joint. When this procedure is chosen, eradication of the infection with radical soft tissue debridement leaves a large bone defect and a soft tissue envelope with a scar. The type of fixation such as an IM nail, plates and screws, an external fixator, or a circular frame, depends on the size of the defect, the quality of the bone, and the possibility for primary wound closure. A successful fusion gives a stable infection-free limb with functional results inferior to revision TKA, which makes resection only a salvage procedure for selected indications.

For the hip joint, the removal of the spacers without reimplantation of a hip prothesis may be the choice for very few patients. We use this procedure only in patients, who either have a fungal infection as proven from histological findings of intra-operative samples, or who have a very large defect of the femur form previous failures, and the wound is full of scar tissue.

The Hellenic experience

In Greece, total joint arthroplasties are performed at 10 academic institutions, at 54 National Health System orthopedic departments and at 12 private hospitals. There is no arthroplasty registry in the country, and thus valid data can only be obtained from intradepartmental archives. A total of 6,500 hip arthroplasties and 5,500 knee arthroplasties are performed annually. There are no restrictions or minimum standard requirements for joint replacement procedures, as defined by The National Health System, and dedicated orthopedic surgery operative suites are available in more than 30% of the hospitals. According to the national literature, the reported incidence of infected hip arthroplasties is 1.5–2.4%, of infected knee arthroplasties is 2.8–2.9% and of infected hemiarthroplasties is ~2%. Three academic and one NHS department provide services for infected total joints on a regular basis, using up-to-date methods for diagnosis, well defined protocols for surgical management, and a thorough documentation of pathogens and clinical outcomes. However, a fair number of cases are sporadically treated at regional NHS and private hospitals. A recent survey showed that diagnosis is based on aspiration of the joint and on samples taken intra-operatively in 80% of the cases, while in the remaining cases the diagnosis is mainly based on the combination of clinical signs and imaging. Pathogens identified were *Staphylococcus aureus* in 45%, coagulase-negative staphylococci in 25%, other Gram-positive pathogens in 15% and other Gram-negative pathogens in 15%. Resistant pathogens (*multiresistant Staphylococcus aureus, multiresistant Staphylococcus epidermidis*) were found in 27% of the patients, with a few hospitals reporting a high incidence up to 60%. Two-stage revision arthroplasty for infection is performed in 75%, one-stage revision in 5%, and debridement and salvage of the prosthesis in 10% of the cases. These strategies comply with international standards. In one center, in particular, the infectiologists are very actively involved in the management, and antibiotic suppression strategies are used in a great number of patients. With respect to two-stage revision surgery, the average interval between the stages is 4 months (ranging from 6 weeks to 9 months), with antibiotic i.v. administration for 2–6 weeks, continued by oral administration for another 6 weeks. Local antibiotics are used in nearly all cases. Intra-operative preparation of spacers loaded with specific antibiotics after cultures or the knowledge of regional pathogen sensitivities to antibiotics are used in 60% of the cases. Antibiotic-loaded custom-made beads are prepared in a similar way in 20% of the cases, and commercially available spacers are used in 20% of the cases. In the few departments in which well defined protocols for diagnosis, surgical management, and antibiotic administration are used, the incidence of recurrence of infection is as low as 5%.

Conclusions and Future Perspectives

Orthopaedic implant-related infections should be renamed "orthopaedic biofilm infections", alternating between quiescent periods of biofilm growth and acute exacerbations caused by the release of planktonic bacteria. The acute phases should be treated with antibiotic therapy. Because orthopaedic biofilm infections share many etiologic factors with other biofilm infections, patients may benefit from insights that have been developed in other medical specialties. Infections may be controlled by very high concentrations of locally delivered antibiotics "on demand" by means of a novel ultrasonic-triggered release mechanism, and biofilm bacteria may be made more susceptible to antibiotics by the implementation of weak direct-current electric fields, or by ultrasonic energy delivered at particular wavelengths. Also, like all biofilm infections, orthopaedic infections may be prevented (Balaban et al., 2005) by the judicious use of specific signal analogs that block biofilm formation and lock potential pathogens in the planktonic mode-of-growth, in which they are susceptible to routine antibiotic therapy (Costerton, 2005).

References

Alexeeff M, Mahomed N, Morsi E, Garbuz D, Gross A. Structural allograft in two-stage revisions for failed septic hip arthroplasty. J Bone Joint Surg Br 1996; 78-B: 213–216.

Al-Maiyah M, Hill D, Bajwa A et al. Bacterial contaminants and antibiotic prophylaxis in total hip arthroplasty. J Bone Joint Surg Br 2005 Sep; 87 (9): 1256–1258.

Balaban N, Stoodley P, Fux CA, Wilson S, Costerton JW, Dell'Acqua G. Prevention of staphylococcal biofilm-associated infections by the quorum sensing inhibitor RIP. Clin Orthop Relat Res 2005 Aug; (437): 48–54.

Bargiotas K, Wohlrab D, Sewecke JJ, Lavinge G, Demeo PJ, Sotereanos NG. Arthrodesis of the knee with a long intramedullary nail following the failure of a total knee arthroplasty as the result of infection. J Bone Joint Surg Am 2006 Mar; 88 (3): 553–558.

Barrack RL, Engh G, Rorabeck C, Sawhney J, Woolfrey M. Patient satisfaction and outcome after septic versus aseptic revision total knee arthroplasty. J Arthroplasty 2000 Dec; 1 (8): 990–993.

Bassetti M, Di Biagio A, Cenderello G et al. Linezolid treatment of prosthetic hip infections due to methicillin-resistant Staphylococcus aureus (MRSA). J Infect 2001 Aug; 4 (2): 148–149.

Berbari EF, Hanssen AD, Duffy MC et al. Risk factors for prosthetic joint infection: case-control study. Clin Infect Dis 1998 Nov; 27 (5): 1247–1254.

Buttaro MA, Morandi A, Rivello HG, Piccaluga F. Histology of vancomycin-supplemented impacted bone allografts in revision total hip arthroplasty. J Bone Joint Surg Br 2005 Dec; 87 (12): 1684–1687.

Callaghan JJ, Katz RP, Johnston RC. One-stage revision surgery of the infected hip: a minimum 10-year follow-up study. Clin Orthop 1999; 369: 139–143.

Coste JS, Reig S, Trojani C, Berg M, Walch G, Boileau P. The management of infection in arthroplasty of the shoulder. J Bone Joint Surg Br 2004 Jan; 86 (1): 65–69.

Costerton JW. Biofilm theory can guide the treatment of device-related orthopaedic infections. Clin Orthop Relat Res 2005 Aug; (437): 7–11.

Darouiche RO. Treatment of infections associated with surgical implants. N Engl J Med 2004 Apr 1; 350 (14): 1422–1429.

Deirmengian C, Greenbaum J, Lotke PA, Booth RE Jr, Lonner JH. Limited success with open debridement and retention of components in the treatment of acute Staphylococcus aureus infections after total knee arthroplasty. J Arthroplasty 2003 Oct; 18 (7 Suppl 1): 22–26.

Dixon P, Parish EN, Cross MJ. Arthroscopic debridement in the treatment of the infected total knee replacement. J Bone Joint Surg Br 2004 Jan; 86 (1): 39–42.

Durbhakula SM, Czajka J, Fuchs MD, Uhl RL. Antibiotic-loaded articulating cement spacer in the 2-stage exchange of infected total knee arthroplasty. J Arthroplasty 2004 Sep; 19 (6):768–774.

Elson RA. Exchange arthroplasty for infection: perspectives from the United Kingdom. Orthop Clin North Am 1993; 24: 761–767.

English H, Timperley AJ, Dunlop D, Gie G. Impaction grafting of the femur in two-stage revision for infected total hip replacement. J Bone Joint Surg Br 2002; 84-B: 700–705.

Evans RP. Successful treatment of total hip and knee infection with articulating antibiotic components: a modified treatment method. Clin Orthop Relat Res 2004 Oct; (427): 37–46.

Fehring TK, Calton TF, Griffin WL. Cementless fixation in 2-stage reimplantation for periprosthetic sepsis. J Arthroplasty 1999; 14: 175–181.

Fisman DN, Reilly DT, Karchmer AW, Goldie SJ. Clinical effectiveness and cost-effectiveness of 2 management strategies for infected total hip arthroplasty in the elderly. Clin Infect Dis 2001; 32: 419–430.

Fitzgerald RH Jr. Total hip arthroplasty sepsis: prevention and diagnosis. Orthop Clin North Am 1992; 23: 259–264.

Fitzgerald RH Jr. Infected Total Hip Arthroplasty: Diagnosis and Treatment. J Am Acad Orthop Surg 1995 Oct; 3 (5): 249–262.

Garvin KL, Fitzgerald RH Jr, Salvati EA et al. Reconstruction of the infected total hip and knee arthroplasty with gentamicin-impregnated Palacos bone cement. Instr Course Lect 1993; 42: 293–302.

Garvin KL, Evans BG, Salvati EA, Brause BD. Palacos gentamicin for the treatment of deep periprosthetic hip infections. Clin Orthop 1994; 298: 97–105.

Garvin K, Feschuk C. Polylactide-polyglycolide antibiotic implants. Clin Orthop Relat Res 2005 Aug; (437): 105–110.

Giannoudis PV, Parker J, Wilcox MH. Methicillin-resistant Staphylococcus aureus in trauma and orthopaedic practice. J Bone Joint Surg Br 2005 Jun; 8 (6): 749–754.

Haddad FS, Muirhead-Allwood SK, Manktelow AR, Bacarese-Hamilton I. Two-stage uncemented revision hip arthroplasty for infection. J Bone Joint Surg Br 2000; 82-B: 689–694.

Hanssen AD, Rand JA. Evaluation and treatment of infection at the site of a total hip or knee arthroplasty. AAOS Instruct Course Lect 1999; 48: 111–122.

Haleem AA, Berry DJ, Hanssen AD. Mid-term to long-term follow-up of two-stage reimplantation for injected total knee arthroplasty. Clin Orthop Relat Res 2004 Nov; (428): 35–39.

Hebert CK, Williams RE, Levy RS, Barrack RL. Cost of treating an infected total knee replacement. Clin Orthop Relat Res 1996; 331: 140–145.

Hoad-Reddick DA, Evans CR, Norman P, Stockley I. Is there a role for extended antibiotic therapy in a two-stage revision of the infected knee arthroplasty? J Bone Joint Surg Br 2005 Feb; 87 (2): 171–174.

Hofmann AA, Goldberg T, Tanner AM, Kurtin SM. Treatment of infected total knee arthroplasty using an articulating spacer: 2- to 12-year experience. Clin Orthop Relat Res 2005 Jan; (430): 125–131.

Hsieh PH, Shih CH, Chang YH, Lee MS, Shih HN, Yang WE. Two-stage revision hip arthroplasty for infection: comparison between the interim use of antibiotic-loaded cement beads and a spacer prosthesis. J Bone Joint Surg Am 2004 Sep; 86-A (9): 1989–1997.

Huenger F, Schmachtenberg A, Haefner H et al. Evaluation of postdischarge surveillance of surgical site infections after total hip and knee arthroplasty. Am J Infect Control 2005 Oct; 33 (8): 455–462.

Hyman JL, Salvati EA, Laurencin CT, Rogers DE, Maynard M, Brause DB. The arthroscopic drainage, irrigation, and debridement of late, acute total hip arthroplasty infections: average 6-year follow-up. J Arthroplasty 1999; 14: 903–910.

Ilahi OA, Al-Habbal GA, Bocell JR, Tullos HS, Huo MH. Arthroscopic debridement of acute periprosthetic septic arthritis of the knee. Arthroscopy 2005 Mar; 21 (3): 303–306.

Isiklar ZU, Darouiche RO, Landon GC, Beck T. Efficacy of antibiotics alone for orthopaedic device related infections. Clin Orthop 1996; 332: 184–189.

Kraay MJ, Goldberg VM, Fitzgerald SJ, Salata MJ. Cementless two-staged total hip arthroplasty for deep periprosthetic infection. Clin Orthop Relat Res 2005 Dec; 441: 243–249.

Kühn KD, Bone Cements. Up-to-date comparison of physical and chemical properties of commercial materials. Springer-Verlag Berlin Heidelberg, 2000.

Leone JM, Hanssen AD. Management of infection at the site of a total knee arthroplasty. J Bone Joint Surg Am 2005 Oct; 87 (10): 2335–2348.

Lentino JR. Prosthetic joint infections: bane of orthopedists, challenge for infectious disease specialists. Clin Infect Dis 2003 May 1; 36 (9): 1157–1161.

McPherson EJ, Woodson C, Holtom P, Roidis N, Shufelt C, Patzakis M. Periprosthetic total hip infection: outcomes using a staging system. Clin Orthop Relat Res 2002 Oct; (403): 8–15.

Pagnano MW, Trousdale RT, Hanssen AD. Outcome after reinfection following reimplantation hip arthroplasty. Clin Orthop 1997; 338: 192–204.

Parvizi J, Wickstrom E, Zeiger AR et al. Frank Stinchfield Award. Titanium surface with biologic activity against infection. Clin Orthop Relat Res 2004 Dec; (429): 33–38.

Pavoni GL, Giannella M, Falcone M et al. Conservative medical therapy of prosthetic joint infections: retrospective analysis of an 8-year experience. Clin Microbiol Infect 2004 Sep; 10(9): 831–837.

Rao N, Crossett LS, Sinha RK, Le Frock JL. Long-term suppression of infection in total joint arthroplasty. Clin Orthop Relat Res 2003 Sep; (414): 55–60.

Ridgeway S, Wilson J, Charlet A, Kafatos G, Pearson A, Coello R. Infection of the surgical site after arthroplasty of the hip. J Bone Joint Surg Br 2005 Jun; 87 (6): 844–850.

Ryn van JS, Verebelyi DM. One-stage debridement and knee fusion for infected total knee arthroplasty using the hybrid frame. J Arthroplasty. 2002 Jan; 17 (1): 129–134.

Spangehl MJ, Hanssen AD. Management of the infected total knee replacement. Current Opinion in Orthopaedics 2002, 13: 23–29.

Sperling JW, Kozak TK, Hanssen AD, Cofield RH. Infection after shoulder arthroplasty. Clin Orthop Relat Res 2001 Jan; (382): 206–216.

Springer BD, Lee GC, Osmon D, Haidukewych GJ, Hanssen AD, Jacofsky DJ. Systemic safety of high-dose antibiotic-loaded cement spacers after resection of an infected total knee arthroplasty. Clin Orthop Relat Res 2004 Oct; (427): 47–51.

Stevens CM, Tetsworth KD, Calhoun JH, Mader JT. An articulated antibiotic spacer used for infected total knee arthroplasty: a comparative in vitro elution study of Simplex and Palacos bone cements. Journal of Orthopaedic Research 23 (2005): 27–33.

Toms AD, Davidson D, Masri BA, Duncan CP. The management of peri-prosthetic infection in total joint arthroplasty. J Bone Joint Surg Br 2006 Feb; 88 (2): 149–175.

Trampuz A, Zimmerli W. New strategies for the treatment of infections associated with prosthetic joints. Curr Opin Investig Drugs 2005 Feb; 6 (2): 185–190.

Tsukayama DT, Estrada R, Gustilo RB. Infection after total hip arthroplasty: A study of the treatment of one hundred and six infections. J Bone Joint Surg 1996; 78A: 512–523.

Urban JA, Garvin KL. Infection after total hip arthroplasty Curr Opin Orthop 2001; 12: 64–70.

Volin SJ, Hinrichs SH, Garvin KL. Two-stage reimplantation of total joint infections: a comparison of resistant and non-resistant organisms. Clin Orthop Relat Res 2004 Oct; (427): 94–100.

Widmer AF. New developments in diagnosis and treatment of infection in orthopedic implants. Clin Infect Dis 2001 Sep 1; 33 Suppl 2: 94–106.

Yamaguchi K, Adams RA, Morrey BF. Infection after total elbow arthroplasty. J Bone Joint Surg Am 1998 Apr; 80 (4): 481–491.

Zimmerli W, Trampuz A, Ochsner PE. Prosthetic-joint infections. N Engl J Med 2004 Oct 14; 351 (16): 1645–1654.

Zimmerli W, Widmer AF, Blatter M, Frei R, Ochsner PE. Role of rifampin for treatment of orthopedic implant–related staphylococcal infections: a randomized controlled trial. Foreign-Body Infection (FBI) Study Group. JAMA 1998; 279: 1537–1541.

Ⓘ Revision of Infected Hip Prostheses with Antibiotic-Loaded Preformed Cement Spacers – The Italian Experience

Carlo L. Romano, Enzo Meani

National Data and Organization

Joint replacement is one of the most successful procedures in orthopedic surgery that has been increasingly employed in Italy over the last years. To understand the relevance of septic complications after joint prosthetic surgery in Italy, a brief overview of the available data is worth giving.

According to a survey conducted by the Istituto Superiore di Sanità of the Italian Ministry of Health (www.ministerosalute.it), 285965 joint prostheses were implanted in Italy from 1999 to 2001, with an average increase of 15% – hip prostheses increased by 8%, knee prostheses increased by 45%. At that time, revision surgery accounted for approximately 8% of hip and 5% of knee prosthetic surgery, with a knee to hip ratio of 1/2. All the other joint replacements (mainly shoulder and ankle) amounted to approximately 2000 per year, with an increase of 15%, in three years.

The most recent data are reported by Torre and Romanini (Torre and Romanini, 2005).

According to these data approximately 120000 total joint replacements (TJR) are currently performed in Italy per annum: 78000 total hip replacements (THR) and 38000 total knee replacements (TKR), i.e., 65% and 31.6%, respectively of all TJR. Revision procedures account for approximately 10% of all prothesis implants. An increase of 18% for THR and of 85% for TKR, from the year 1999 until the end of 2003, reflects the increasing application of TJR.

Considering only direct costs (Diagnosis Related Groups, DRG reimbursements) the annual expenditure in Italy for TJR is approximately 900 million Euros, while estimated costs for rehabilitation are approximately 500 million Euros, per year.

The increasing number of joint replacements undertaken in our country leads to an estimated prevalence of joint prosthesis infection of more than 2600 new patients each year, with direct costs only for the surgical procedures amounting to approximately 90–100 million Euros, per year (Table 13.1). In other words, direct costs of septic complications of TJR correspond to approximately 10% of the total costs of TJR surgery.

Human, social, and economic costs of septic complications point out the need for a coordinated strategy on a national basis. To deal with bone and joint infection, an Italian scientific society was founded in Milan in 1996 (Gruppo Italiano di Infezioni Osteo-articolari, GISTIO). The GISTIO (www. gistio.it) is affiliated to the Italian Society of Orthopedics and Traumatology (SIOT) and is open to orthopedic surgeons, infectiologists, and microbiologists that are particularly involved in the field of bone and joint infections. The members meet on an annual basis and their official journal, the Quaderni di Infezioni Osteo-articolari, is published twice a year.

Also, there are specialized centers for bone and joint infections in different Italian Regions, however, without a coordinated distribution (Fig.13.1).

Table 13.**1** Estimated prevalence of infected TJR per year in Italy and related direct (surgical) costs

	Total TJR per year	New TJR infection cases per year
THR	78000	1404
TKR	38000	760
Hip revision	8000	400
Knee revision	2000	100
Other	2000	20
Total	**128000**	**2684**

Mean cost per revision surgery (DRG) € 18000, Total estimated cost (two-stage revision, only DRG) € 96624000.

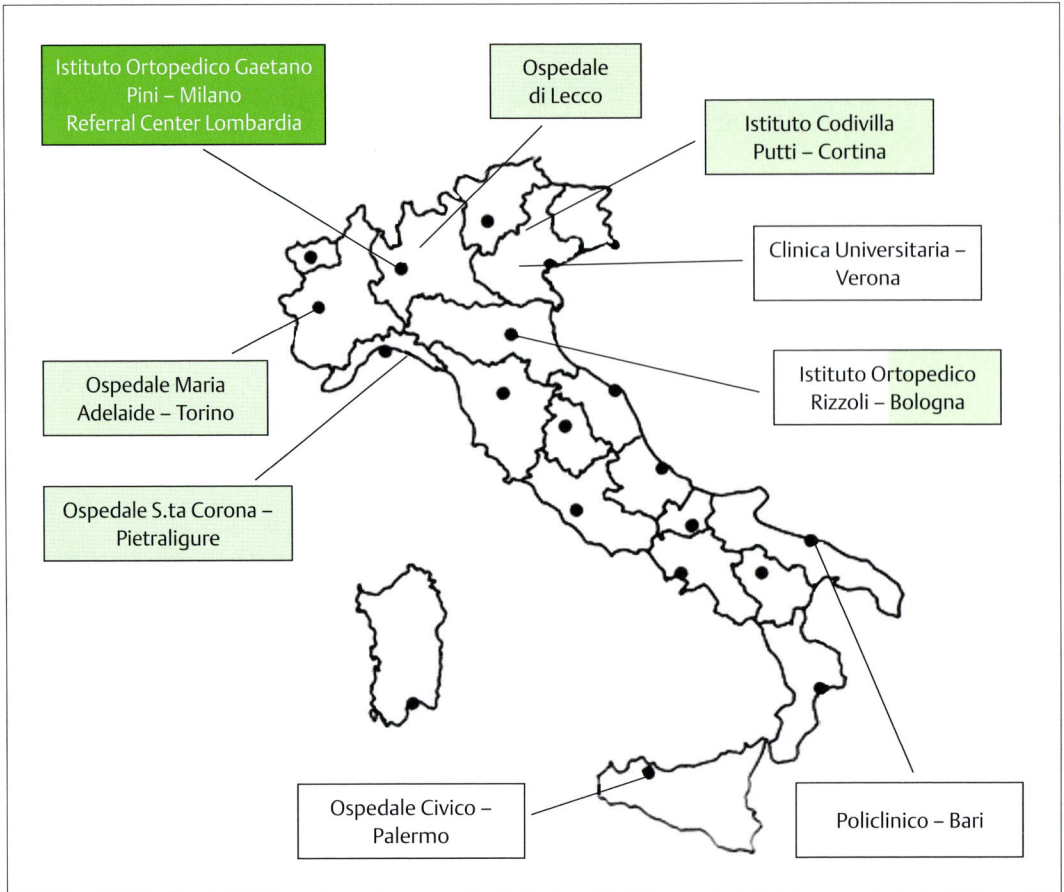

Fig. 13.1 Some of the Italian Orthopedic Centers particularly involved in the treatment of osteoarticular infections
dark green = regional referral center
light green = specialized department
white = specialized individual surgeons

The G. Pini Orthopedic Institute is the only referral Center for bone and joint infection in the Lombardia Region (9 million inhabitants), and it also receives approximately 15–20% of patients from other Italian regions.

Few analytical data are available on the medical (type and length of antibiotic therapy) and surgical treatments (Girldestone, single-stage or two-stage revision) employed most frequently in our country for prosthetic infections. According to various scientific presentations in specialized meetings and to personal knowledge, two-stage revision with custom-made or pre-formed antibiotic-loaded cement spacers, followed by cemented or cementless revision prosthesis, seems the preferred choice amongst the vast majority of surgeons involved in the treatment of chronic prosthetic infections in Italy.

The antibiotic-loaded bone cement market represents approximately 10% of the Italian market of bone cements. At the moment about 800 preformed antibiotic-loaded spacers are sold in Italy, each year.

In the near future, the implementation of an improved coding system for treatment strategies on a regional and national level should yield more detailed data regarding the current treatment approach to prosthetic infections in our country.

Revision of Infected Hip Prostheses using Antibiotic-Loaded Preformed Cement Spacers and Cementless Revision Prostheses

Infection after total hip arthroplasty is a serious complication, and several treatment strategies have been proposed (Carlsson et al., 1978; Buchholz HW et al., 1981; Bittar et al., 1982; McDonald et al., 1989; Duncan et al., 1993; Ivarsson et al., 1994; Nestor et al., 1994; Younger et al., 1997; Fehring et al., 1999, Kühn 2000).

Two-stage reimplantation using an interval spacer of antibiotic-impregnated bone cement has been investigated previously as a method to eradicate infection and prevent limb shortening (Duncan et al., 1993; Ivarsson et al., 1994; Younger et al., 1998; Fehring et al., 1999).

Preformed antibiotic-loaded spacers (Spacer G, Tecres Spa, Italy [Fig. 13.**2**]) offer known mechanical resistance (Baleani et al., 2003; Affatato et al., 2003), predictable antibiotic release (Bertazzoni et al., 2004), and reduced surgical time (Magnan et al., 2001), while long-stem shapes allow to overcome the frequent occurrence of proximal femoral bone loss, provide immediate primary stability, and allow partial weight bearing (Romano and Meani, 2004).

Medium-term results of a consecutive series of patients with chronically infected total hip arthroplasty, treated according to a protocol that included two-stage revision using preformed antibiotic-loaded cement spacers and cementless modular long-stem revision prostheses, supplemented with prolonged systemic antibiotic therapy after first and second stage, are reported.

In the years 2000–2006, 98 patients, affected by chronic septic hip prosthesis, underwent two-stage hip revision in our department. The first 46 consecutive patients were included in the study. The follow-up period ranged from 18–60 months after revision (mean: 42 months).

In all patients, the infected prosthesis was removed and a preformed antibiotic-loaded spacer (Spacer G, Tecres Spa, Italy) was implanted. The Spacer G is a preformed "off the shelf" antibiotic-loaded hip spacer made of polymethylmethacrylate. It is available in three different head sizes and with two stem sizes – a short one with 260 mm and a long one with 360 mm. The decision for either spacer may be made intra-operatively. The inner part of the spacer features a stainless steel rod that increases mechanical resistance. The cement is preloaded by the manufacturer with gentamicin with a concentration of 1.9 %.

8–12 weeks after implantation, the spacer was removed and the patients underwent reconstruction using cementless modular prostheses and *non*cemented cups.

All the patients received systemic antibiotic treatment with two antibiotics for six weeks after the first and the second stage, based on the results of the antibiogram.

18 men and 28 women were included. The average age at the time of the operation was 55.3 years (range: 18 to 79 years). 28 patients were Type B hosts according to the Ceirny-Mader classification system (Calhoun et al., 1994).

20 of the initial prosthetic components were cemented, 20 were uncemented and 6 were hybrids (femoral stem cemented, cup uncemented). Preoperative limb shortening ranged from 0 to 60 mm.

The interval between the previous index operation and the revision ranged from 1–8 years. 13 patients had undergone a previous revision operation and in the remaining patients, all but 6 had at least one previous failed debridement.

Specimens for culture were obtained from wound drainage in 24 patients, from hip aspirate in 19 patients, and intra-operatively only in 3 patients.

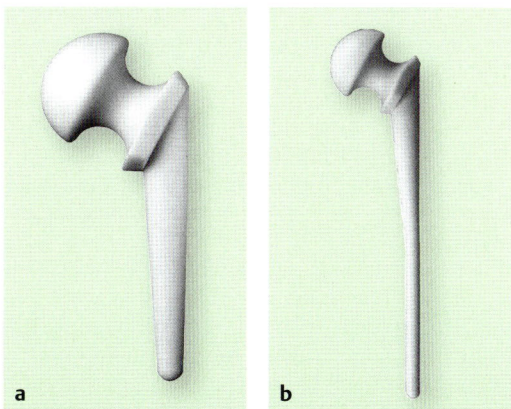

Fig. 13.**2** Preformed antibiotic-loaded spacers (Spacer G, Tecres Spa, Italy)
A) short (260 mm) and
B) long-stemmed (360 mm) spacers come in three different head sizes (not shown).

All the hips in this series were treated with resection arthroplasty through a lateral approach, with the patient in supine position. In 32 cases, a large femoral-window opening or a transfemoral approach was necessary to remove a solidly fixed cemented or cementless femoral component or cement mantle.

After prosthesis removal and meticulous debridement of femoral bone and soft tissues, the Spacer G (Tecres Spa, Italy), a preformed cement spacer containing gentamicin 1.9%, was inserted. In all the patients, the spacer was fixed only proximally to prevent implant rotation, with one pack of antibiotic-loaded cement (Cemex Genta, Tecres Spa, Italy) containing gentamicin 1.9% admixed with vancomycin 5%. The vancomycin powder was thoroughly mixed with the cement powder into a fine consistency before the addition of the liquid monomer. If gentamicin-resistant strains were present, vancomcin was added to the spacer with the drilling technique, described by Bertazzoni (Bertazzoni et al., 2004).

After spacer implantation and reduction, the osteotomy was reapproximated around the antibiotic cement spacer with resorbable sutures, and no metallic cerclages or plates were used for further synthesis. No bone grafts were used at the time of spacer implant. Thirty-two patients had severe proximal femoral bone loss that required the use of a long-stem cement spacer, and nine patients received autologous (three) or homologous (six) bone grafts with autologous platelet-rich-plasma.

Postoperatively, patients were allowed touch-down weight bearing for one month, followed by partial weight bearing on the operated extremity with two crutches until reimplantation.

All the patients received a minimum of six weeks of organism-specific antibiotics postoperatively and returned for clinical follow-up at the completion of their antibiotic course.

Routine laboratory studies were obtained including complete blood count with differential, erythrocyte sedimentation rate (ESR), and C-reactive protein (CRP). Patients were scheduled for removal of the spacer and revision arthroplasty 2–4 weeks after completion of intravenous antibiotics or 8–12 weeks after spacer implantation. Patients with successful eradication of their infection, as evidenced by complete blood count with differential and CRP within the normal ranges, underwent the second stage of their reconstruction. If clinical suspicion for persistent infection

remained, despite negative laboratory studies, joint aspiration before reimplantation was performed for cultural examination, as well as a white blood cell count. In all cases, intra-operative cultures were obtained at the time of the second-stage procedure.

At revision, the hip was exposed through the same lateral incision, and all the spacers were removed without difficulty.

Touch-down weight bearing was allowed for 6 weeks, followed by 50% weight bearing for another 6 weeks. Full weight bearing and abductor strengthening were permitted at 12 weeks after surgery. After operation, perenteral antibiotics were administered for 6 weeks. After each procedure closed suction drainage was inserted and removed again after 48 hours.

All the patients underwent enoxaparin 0.4 mL/d treatment for 30 days after surgery to prevent thromboembolic complications and celecoxib 200 mg/d was administered for 14 days after revision surgery to prevent heterotopic ossifications (Romano et al, 2003).

Our primary outcomes included eradication of infection, spacer stability and integrity, and implant stability.

Failure of treatment was defined as a recurrence of infection, determined by the occurrence of clinical signs of infection (redness, swelling, pain, fistulae), at any given time at follow-up.

Preoperative and postoperative hematologial studies included the determination of ESR, white blood cell count, and CRP level. Plain radiographs included anteroposterior and translateral views of the hip joint.

Radiographic examination was performed at two, six and twelve months postoperatively, followed by yearly intervals thereafter. The radiographic results were compared to determine femoral component subsidence and signs of osteolysis.

Hip function was recorded using the method of Merle d'Aubigne (Merle d'Aubigne et al., 1965). In this scoring system, 6 points were awarded for the following: pain, walking ability, and movement range. This amounted to a total score of 18 for a normal hip. A rating of 17–18 was considered excellent; 15–16, good; 13–14, fair; and < 13, poor. Clinical failure was defined as a Merle d'Aubigne hip score of < 13. Preoperative and most recent postoperative scores were compared using the Wilcoxon signed-rank test.

Heterotopic ossification (HO) was quantified, using the classification of Brooker (Brooker et al., 1973).

The spacer dislocation and use of allograft were also noted and included in the analysis. Complications, including persistent infection, fractures, implant instability, subsidence or proximal migration, and revision were noted.

Results

The 46 patients included in this study were followed up for an average of 42 months (range, 18 – 60 months). Two patients were lost to follow-up at, respectively 24 and 34 months postoperatively.

The average preoperative hip score by Merle d'Aubigne was 4.9 points (range: 3 – 12 points). Before operation, ESR averaged 82 mm/h (range: 12 – 155 mm/h), and CRP levels averaged 72 mg/L (range: 5 – 258 mg/L). ESRs, CRP levels, or both were high in 44 patients.

The following organisms were identified: *Staphylococcus aureus* in 20 patients and *Staphylococcus epidermidis* in 18 patients (methicillin-resistant staphylococcus strains: 22), *Pseudomonas aeruginosa* in 8 patients, *Escherichia coli* in 2 patients, *Enterobacter cloacae* in 1 patient, *Serratia marcescens* in 1 patient. No microorganisms were isolated in two patients. 6 patients showed a mixed flora. 24 of the 50 isolated strains were gentamicin-resistant.

The duration of the first stage of the operation averaged 165 minutes (range: 125 – 220 min). Blood transfusions averaged 4.5 units of blood.

The interval between the first and second-stage operation ranged from 9 – 15 weeks.

During the interval, most patients had tolerable pain in the hip; 30 patients had no pain, 14 patients had mild pain, and 2 patients had moderate pain.

36 patients were able to walk with partial weight bearing and 10 walked with touch-down weight bearing. 1 patient, who had a femoral nerve palsy, walked with a knee brace.

At the time of revision surgery, intra-operative specimens were positive in one patient *(coagulase-negative Staphylococcus* [CNS]*)*, without clinical signs of infection recurrence.

A cementless femoral component was implanted in all of the 46 revised hips (Profemur R modular long-stem Wright-Cremascoli or S-ROM Johnson&Johnson DePuy). Acetabular revisions were performed with uncemented components in all of the cases.

The duration of the second-stage operations averaged 175 minutes (range: 130 – 250 min). Blood transfusions averaged 4.2 units (range: 3 – 12 units) of blood. The closed suction drain was removed at 2 days after the second-stage operation. The total drainage ranged from 210 – 650 mL (average: 470 mL).

No clinical evidence of infection recurrence was noted at the time of the latest follow-up in 43 of 44 patients (97.7%) Two patients were lost to follow-up. The patient with infection recurrence was affected by a severe rheumatoid arthritis. 3 years post-revision, cup loosening became evident which, on intra-operative cultural examination, proved to be an infection recurrence due to CNS.

At the latest follow-up, all the remaining acetabular components were stable and none of the femoral components were revized. In 42 hips, the femoral stems were fixed by bone ingrowth and good proximal bone remodeling was achieved (Figs. 13.**3a – f**).

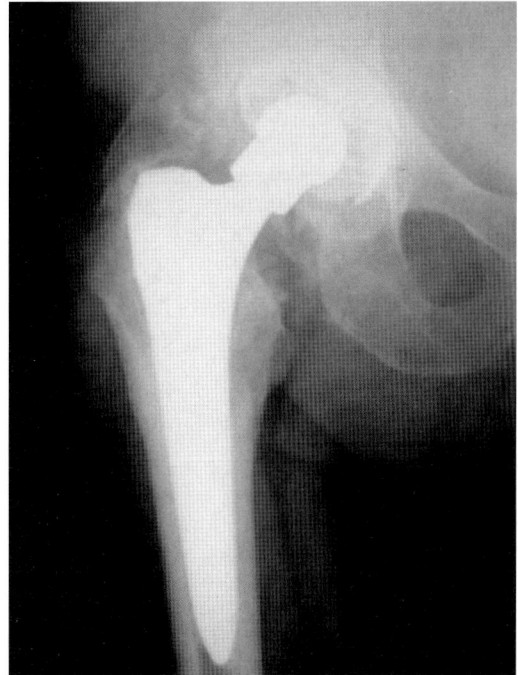

Fig. 13.**3a** A 54-year-old man, who had persistent infection with a draining sinus in previously failed revision surgery.
Preoperative plain radiograph.

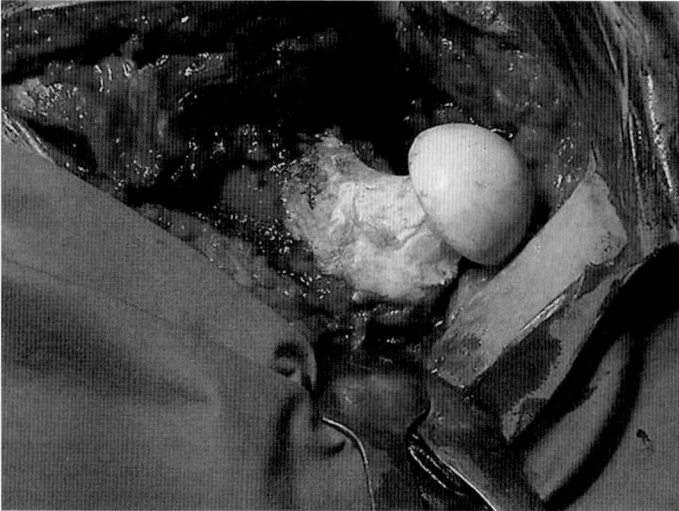

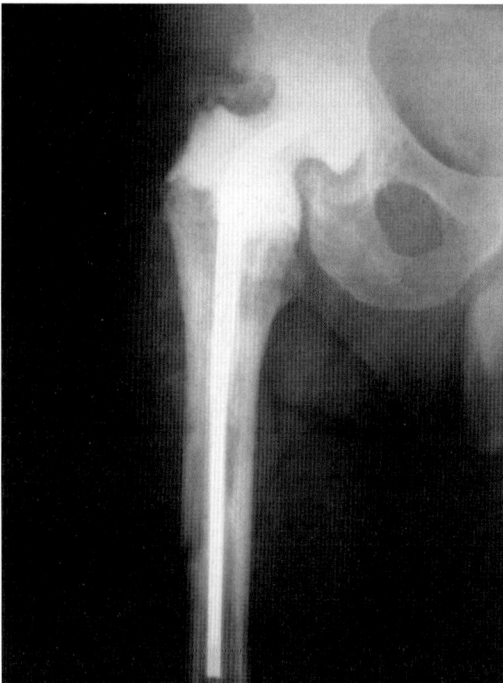

Fig. 13.**3c** Radiographic view of the spacer in situ.

The remaining 4 femoral stems subsided by 2 to 5 mm, but they were stabilized by stable fibrous ingrowth. All 9 hips that received morcelized autologous (3 patients) or homologous (6 patients) bone grafts and platelet-rich plasma, showed complete healing within 6 months with bone ingrowth.

Overall, the hip score was improved to an average of 13.8 points (range 10–16 points). 26 patients (55%) had excellent or good results, 14 patients had fair results, and 4 patients had poor results. The short operated limbs were lengthened a mean of 19 mm (range: 0–35 mm).

Postoperative complications included 9 spacer cranial dislocations that required no treatment, but prevented weight bearing, 1 femoral nerve palsy, partially recovered after 12 months, and 2 revision prosthesis dislocations that required open reduction and change of the modular neck offset. No grade 3 or 4 HO occured.

Four patients had side effects during antibiotic treatment including gastrointestinal tract dysfunction in one patient, temporary liver dysfunction in two patients, and bone marrow depression in one patient. These side effects were resolved after temporary withdrawal of antibiotics.

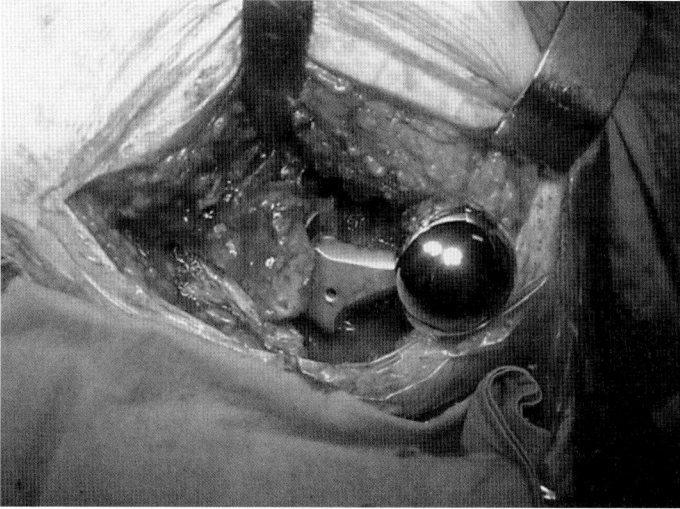

Fig. 13.**3d** Revision with a modular cementless implant and a large (38 mm) metal-on-metal ball and socket at 76 days after spacer implantation.

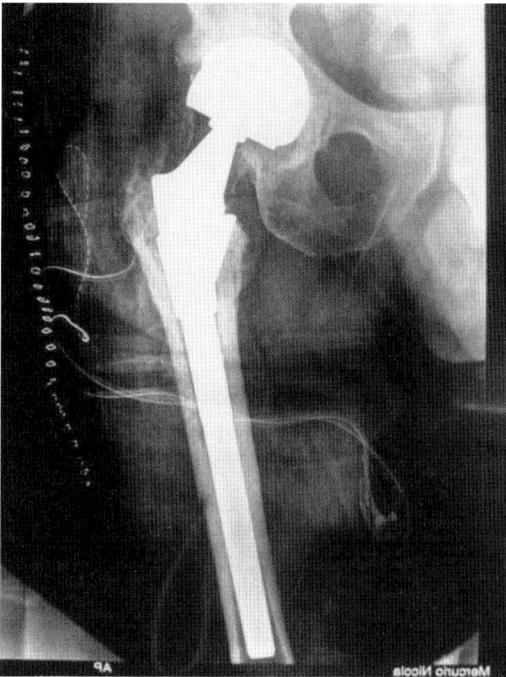

Fig. 13.**3e** Early postoperative radiographic image.

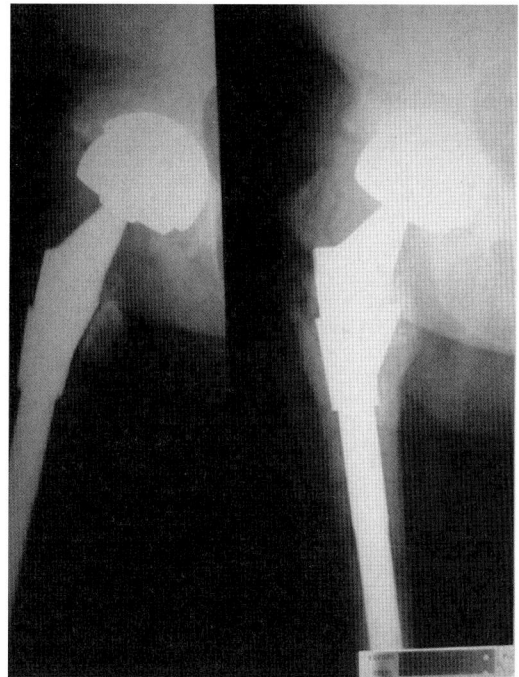

Fig. 13.**3f** Control after two years.

Discussion

Duncan and Beauchamp (Duncan and Beauchamp, 1993), who introduced the concept of the interval spacer in a two-stage procedure for the treatment of infected THA, developed a more refined interval spacer with a metal-on-polyethylene bearing prosthesis of antibiotic-loaded acrylic cement (Prostalac). The eradication rate of infection was 94%. The merits of Prostalac were decreased hip pain and the ability to walk between the two stages. The Spacer G preformed cement spacer allows for early weight bearing and (protected) walking, pain-free hip mobility, and predictable local antibiotic release, whilst concurrently offering the following advantages: reduced operation time, availability in different sizes such as long-stem spacers.

In this context, long-stem preformed spacers appear to be particularly useful, considering the frequent occurrence of proximal femoral bone loss in hip infection surgery, either due to the loosening of the prosthesis, the septic process, surgical debridement, or intraoperative fractures (Glassman et al., 1987; Cameron, 1991; Peters et al., 1993; Younger et al., 1995; Aribindi et al., 1999; Chen et al., 2000; Miner et al., 2001). Also, in these challenging cases, long-stem spacers provide primary stability and mechanical resistance, thus allowing partial weight bearing, whilst also maintaining the range of movement and limb length (Romano and Meani, 2004).

Dislocation of the spacer components was the main complication in the presented series of patients (19%) and, although it did not require any treatment, the limb length was shortened and weight bearing was impossible. Concurrent acetabulum bone loss and/or muscle insufficiency and the fixed offset of the spacer are the main reasons for the relatively high rate of this complication in our series. Patients should be informed adequately, prior to spacer implant, of the possibility of this complication that does not seem to affect the final results, but that can significantly reduce walking ability during the second-stage interval. It should be noted that, even if there is spacer dislocation, the spacer nevertheless is helpful in preventing further limb shortening, and in assuring local antibiotic delivery, while filling the dead space after prosthesis removal.

Dislocation of the revision prosthesis occured in two patients (4%) both of whom required open reduction and change of modular neck offset.

Although this is a relatively low rate, compared to other studies, in which revision prosthesis dislocation rates range from 10.2–31% (Engh et al., 1988; Engelbrecht et al., 1990; Miner et al., 2001), both cases in our series had spacer dislocation prior to revision surgery. If there is spacer dislocation, we now recommend earlier revision (6–8 weeks after spacer implant), whenever possible and the use of larger (36 mm or more) metal-on-metal socket balls. With this strategy, no dislocation after revision was observed in our most recent series of 43 patients.

Cementless revision arthroplasty provided a higher success rate than the cemented revision in a similar follow-up of aseptic loosenings in various studies (Engh et al., 1988; Engelbrecht et al., 1990; Lawrence et al., 1994; Moreland and Bernstein, 1995) and long-term survivorship of antibiotic-loaded cemented prosthesis was shown to be rather low (Buchholz et al., 1981). In revision of infected hip prostheses, however, the cementless system may have a possible disadvantage, because antibiotics can only be admixed to cement. On the other hand, one may argue that if the antibiotic in the cement spacer did not provide sufficient local antibiotic levels during a two to three months period, this will be achieved even less with the necessarily lower levels of antibiotics added to cement that is used to fixate a revision prosthesis.

So far, relatively few studies have reported the results of two-stage reimplantations using cementless components in an infected hip. Nestor et al. (1994) reported an 18% rate of recurrent infection in their study of 34 cementless revisions for the treatment of infected total hip prostheses. They concluded that cementless revision does not improve the rate of resolution of infection. On the other hand, Fehring (Fehling et al., 1999) and Haddad (Haddad et al., 2000) reported an 8% recurrence rate in their studies.

Eradication of infection was achieved in 97.7% of patients in our series and, using our protocol (local and systemic antibiotic treatment), cementless revision appears safe and effective in eradicating infection and allowing good stability on the medium term. Our results are better than the 80–95% eradication rates reported in the literature for chronic infection (Carlsson et al., 1978; Buchholz et al., 1981; Garvin et al., 1994; Lieberman et al., 1994). We are now extending our series of patients and follow-up periods to verify these very encouraging preliminary data. Our results are also remarkable, if one considers that 13 (28%) of our patient population had had at least one failed previous revision procedure and that 28 (55%) were Cierny-Mader B-type hosts.

Staphylococcus aureus and *Staphylococcus epidermidis* are the predominant organisms of infection after joint arthroplasty. *Methicillin-resistant Staphylococcus* (MRS) has been identified as an important pathogen in patients, who have an infection at the site of a joint prosthesis. This was also the case in our series, with a relative prevalence of 47%. Vancomycin is the most potent agent against MRS (Frommelt and Kühn, 2005; Kühn, 2000). Gentamicin is potent against enterobacteriaceae and *Psedomonas aeruginosa*, which are common pathogens of infection after joint arthroplasty. Nevertheless, many Gram-positive and Gram-negative organisms are resistant to gentamicin. In our series, 48% of isolated strains were gentamicin-resistant. Therapeutic levels of vancomycin and gentamicin have been found in vitro and in drainage fluid, after application of vancomycin or gentamicin-loaded cement (Hill et al., 1977; Kuechle et al., 1991; Levin, 1975; Marks et al., 1976; Murray, 1984; Nelson et al., 1993; Masterson et al., 1998; Duncan and Masri, 1995).

Levels of vancomycin in serum, after the application of vancomycin-loaded cement, have been shown to be negligible, and an association between the use of vancomycin in cement and the isolation of vancomycin-resistant enterococci has not been shown (Masterson et al., 1998; Duncan and Masri, 1995).

It has been claimed that a drain should not be inserted to spare the antibiotic-rich periprosthetic fluid (Younger et al., 1998). We think, however, a drain should be inserted to prevent a hematoma, which could provide a medium for organism growth. Also, drain insertion decreases the dead space caused by the hematoma. In the present study, a closed suction drain was inserted in all patients, and we found that drain insertion was not correlated with infection recurrence.

Systemic antibiotic administration was performed for approximately six weeks after the first- and second-stage operation. The antibiotic choice was based on the cultural examination and the antibiogram. In all cases, two antibiotics were administered perenterally during the first 3 or 4 weeks and then taken orally. As no comparative studies exist, it is not possible to derive any conclusion, whether this prolonged systemic antibiotic treatment was a useless over-treatment. On the contrary, we suggest it may have played a role in the overall good success rate in this series of patients. Four of our patients (9%) had side effects due to antibiotics, including temporary liver dysfunction and bone marrow depression. These side effects might be related to postoperative intravenous antibiotics or antibiotics used in the cement spacer (or both). However, the safety of the antibiotic delivery from the cement spacer is established (Duncan and Masri, 1995) and the side effects resolved after temporary withdrawal of intravenous antibiotics in all the patients.

We observed no side effects due to the use of autologous or homologous morcelized bone graft. To our knowledge, this is also the first report on the use of platelet-rich plasma in revision surgery in previously infected hip prosthesis. It was shown in different studies (Tonelli et al., 2005) that platelet-rich plasma locally provides growth factors that are able to promote and accelerate bone healing, both in animals and in humans. It was not the aim of this study to demonstrate a quicker or larger bone growth in patients, treated with platelet-rich plasma in two-stage cementless revision of septic hip prosthesis, however our data point out the safety of this technology in this particular application. Here further studies are needed, given the frequent occurrence of bone loss in revision surgery in infections.

Summary

46 patients with infected total hip arthroplasty were treated with two-stage revision, using a preformed antibiotic-loaded cement spacer and uncemented modular hip revision prosthesis. Systemic antibiotic therapy was administered for 6 weeks after the first and the second operation. 32 patients had severe femoral bone loss that required the use of a long-stem cement spacer and necessitated the use of bone grafts in 9 patients at revision. At a mean follow-up of 3.5 years (minimum 1.5 – maximum 5 years) no clinical or laboratory signs of infection recurrence were observed in 97.7% of the patients. In 9 patients there was cranial dislocation of the spacer, which prevented weight bearing, but did not require further treatment.

Preformed antibiotic-loaded spacers and uncemented modular hip revision prostheses appear to be an effective solution for infected total hip prostheses. Long-stem antibiotic-loaded spacers and long-stem revision prostheses are helpful in preventing proximal femoral bone loss.

References

Affatato S, Mattarozzi A, Taddei P et al. Investigations on the wear behaviour of the temporary PMMA-based hip Spacer-G. Proc Inst Mech Eng 2003; 217 (1): 1–8.

Aribindi R, Paprosky W, Nourbash P et al. Extended proximal femoral osteotomy. AAOS ICL 1999; 48: 19.

Baleani M, Traina F, Toni A. The mechanical behavior of a pre-formed hip spacer. Hip International 2003; 13 (3): 159–162.

Bertazzoni Minelli E, Benini A, Magnan B, Bartolozzi P. Release of gentamicin and vancomycin from temporary human hip spacers in two-stage revision of infected arthroplasty. J Antimicrob Chemother 2004; 53 (2): 329–334.

Bittar ES, Petty W. Girdlestone arthroplasty for infected total hip arthroplasty. Clin Orthop 1982; 170: 83.

Brooker A, Bowerman J, Robinson R. Ectopic ossification following total hip replacement: incidence and a method of classification, J Bone Joint Surg. Am 1973; 55: 1629.

Buchholz HW, Elson RA, Engelbrecht E et al. Management of deep infection of total hip replacement. J Bone Joint Surg Br 1981; 63: 342.

Calhoun JH, Cierny G, Holtom P et al. Symposium: current concepts in the management of osteomyelitis, Contemp Orthop 1994; 28: 157.

Cameron HU. Use of a distal trochanteric osteotomy in hip revision, Contemp Orthop 1991; 23: 235.

Carlsson AS, Joseffson G, Lindberg LT. Revision with gentamicin-impregnated cement for deep infections in total hip arthroplasties. J Bone Joint Surg Am 1978; 60: 1059.

Chen W-M, McAuley JP, Engh C et al. Extended slide trochanteric osteotomy for revision total hip arthroplasty, J Bone Joint Surg 2000; 82-A: 1215.

Duncan CP, Beauchamp CP. A temporary antibiotic-loaded joint replacement system for management of complex infections involving the hip. Orthop Clin North Am 1993; 24: 751.

Duncan CP, Masri BA. The role of antibiotic-loaded cement in the treatment of an infection after a hip replacement. Instr Course Lect 1995; 44: 305.

Engelbrecht DJ, Weber FA, Sweet MB, Jakim I. Long-term results of revision total hip arthroplasty. J Bone Joint Surg Br 1990; 72: 41.

Engh CA, Glassman AH, Griffin WL, Mayer JG. Results of cementless revision for failed cemented total hip arthroplasty. Clin Orthop 1988; 235: 91.

Fehring TK, Calton TF, Griffin WL. Cementless fixation in two-stage reimplantation for periprosthetic sepsis. J Arthroplasty 1999; 14: 175.

Frommelt L, Kühn KD. Antibiotic-loaded Cement. In: Brausch S, Malchan H. The well-cemented total hip arthroplasty. Springer Berlin Heidelberg New York 2005; 86–92.

Garvin KL, Evans BG, Salvati EA et al. Palacos gentamicin for the treatment of deep periprosthetic hip infections, Clin Orthop 1994; 298: 97.

Glassman AH, Engh CA, Bobyn JD. A technique of extensile exposure for total hip arthroplasty, J Arthroplasty 1987; 2: 11.

Haddad FS, Muirhead-Allwood SK, Manktelow AR, Bacarese-Hamilton I. Two-stage uncemented revision hip arthroplasty for infection. J Bone Joint Surg Br 2000 Jul; 82 (5): 689–694.

Hanssen AD, Rand JA. Evaluation and treatment of infection at the site of a total hip or knee arthroplasty, J Bone Joint Surg 1998; 80A: 91.

Hill L, Kienerman L, Trustey S, Blowers R. Diffusion of antibiotics from acrylic bone-cement in vitro. J Bone Joint Surg Br 1977; 59: 197.

Ivarsson I, Wahlstrom O, Djerf K, Jacobsson SA. Revision of infected hip replacement: Two-stage procedure with a temporary gentamicin spacer. Acta Orthop Scand 1994; 65: 7.

Kuechle DK, Landon GC, Musher DM, Noble PC. "Elution of vancomycin, daptomycin, and amikacin from acrylic bone cement". Clin Orthop1991; 264: 302.

Kühn KD. Bone Cements. Springer Heidelberg 2000.

Lawrence JM, Engh CA, Macalino GE, Lauro GR. Outcome of revision hip arthroplasty done without cement. J Bone Joint Surg Am 1994; 76: 965.

Levin PD. The effectiveness of various antibiotics in methyl methacrylate. J Bone Joint Surg Br 1975; 57: 234.

Lieberman JR, Callaway GH, Salvati E et al. Treatment of the infected total hip arthroplasty with a two-stage reimplantation protocol. Clin Orthop 1994; 301: 205.

Magnan B, Regis D, Biscaglia, Bartolozzi P. Preformed acrylic bone cement spacer loaded with antibiotics. Use of two-stage procedure in 10 patients because of infected hips after total replacement. Acta Orthop Scand 2001; 72 (6): 591–594.

Marks KH, Nelson CL, Lautenschlager EP. Antibiotic-impregnated acrylic bone cement. J Bone Joint Surg Am 1976; 58: 358.

Martell JM, Pierson RH 3d, Jacobs JJ et al. Primary total hip reconstruction with a titanium fiber-coated prosthesis inserted without cement. J Bone Joint Surg Am 1994; 75: 554.

Masterson EL, Masri BA, Duncan CP. Treatment of infection at the site of total hip replacement. Instr Course Lect 1998; 47: 297.

McDonald DJ, Fitzgerald RH Jr, Listrup DM. Two-stage reconstruction of a total hip arthroplasty because of infection. J Bone Joint Surg Am 1989; 71: 828.

Merle d'Aubigne R, Postel M, Mazabraud A et al. Idiopathic necrosis of the femoral head in adults. J Bone Joint Surg Br 1965; 47: 612.

Miner TM, Momberger NG, Chong D et al. The extended trochanteric osteotomy in revision hip arthroplasty: a critical review of 166 at mean 3-year, 9-month follow-up. J Arthroplasty 2001; 16: 188.

Moreland JR, Bernstein ML. Femoral revision hip arthroplasty with uncemented, porous-coated stems. Clin Orthop 1995; 319: 141.

Murray WR. "Use of antibiotic-containing bone cement". Clin Orthop 1984; 190: 89.

Nelson CL, Evans RP, Blaba JD et al. A comparison of gentamicin-impregnated polymethylmethacrylate bead implantation to conventional parenteral antibiotic therapy in infected total hip and knee arthroplasty. Clin Orthop 1993; 295: 96.

Nestor BJ, Hanssen AD, Ferrer-Gonzalez R, Fitzgerald RH Jr. The use of porous prostheses in delayed reconstruction of total hip replacements that have failed because of infection. J Bone Joint Surg Am 1994; 76: 349.

Peters PC, Head WC, Emerson RH. An extended trochanteric osteotomy for revision total hip replacement. J Bone Joint Surg 1993; 75-B: 158.

Romano CL, Duci D, Romano D, Mazza M, Meani E. Celecoxib versus indomethacin in the prevention of heterotopic ossification (HO) after total hip arthroplasty. J Arthroplasty 2004 Jan; 19 (1): 14–18.

Romano CL, Meani E. The Use of Pre-Formed Long Stem Antibiotic-Loaded Cement Spacers for Two-Stage Revisions of Infected Hip Prosthesis. Multimedia Education Center American Academy of Orthopaedic Surgeons San Francisco CA March 10–14, 2004.

Saleh K, Holtzman J, Gavini A et al. Reliability and intra-operative validity and preoperative assessment of standardized plain radiographs in predicting bone loss at revision hip surgery, J Bone Joint Surg 2001; 83-A: 1040.

Tonelli P, Mannelli D, Brancato L, Cinotti S, Morfini M. Counting of platelet derived growth factor and transforming growth factor-beta in platelet-rich plasma used in jaw bone regeneration. Minerva Stomatol 2005; 54 (1–2): 23–34.

Torre M, Romanini E. Registro nazionale protesi d'anca: stato dell'arte. Proceedings 4° Convegno annuale "National Action Network Italia" Istituto Superiore di Sanità, Roma 13 december 2005.

Younger AS, Duncan CP, Masri BA. Treatment of infection associated with segmental bone loss in the proximal part of the femur in two stages with use of an antibiotic-loaded interval prosthesis. J Bone Joint Surg Am 1998; 80: 60.

Younger AS, Duncan CP, Masri BA, McGraw RW. The outcome of two-stage arthroplasty using a custom-made interval spacer to treat the infected hip. J Arthroplasty 1997; 12: 615.

Younger TI, Bradford MS, Magnus RE et al. Extended proximal femoral osteotomy. A new technique for femoral revision arthroplasty. J Arthroplasty 1995; 10: 329.

Treatment of Infected Prostheses – The Dutch Experience

Geert H. I. M. Walenkamp

Introduction

Surgical treatment of infections involving sequestrectomy, excision of granulation tissue or abscesses and removal of hardware, such as prostheses, may result in a cavity. Such a cavity is seen as one of the causes for nonhealing of orthopedic infections, and many treatment protocols for orthopedic infections aim at reducing the size of the cavity. In the sixties and seventies, the application of a suction drainage system to clean cavities in osteomyelitis and prosthetic infections was common practice in the Netherlands (Willenegger, 1963). Often, two drains were used in a hip cavity to introduce Ringer's solution, and two more large-sized drains were applied to drain the fluid and exsudate (Fig. 14.1).

It was not necessary to add antibiotics to the fluid, as the effect was mainly mechanical. The intention was to keep the suction drainage system for 6 weeks. However, these systems appeared to be not very effective – drains often blocked and leaked, which meant intensive nursery care. Patients were bedridden and the period of 6 weeks was seldom feasible. After a period of ten days, there was an increased risk of Gram-negative superinfections (Walenkamp, 1983). In the wound itself the fluid followed a straight course between in- and outlet drain, so the cleaning effect of the wound was not very effective. Today, these suction drainage systems are only used in special cases, such as in septic arthritis as a distension suction system.

In 1977, polymethylmethacrylate (PMMA) beads with gentamicin became available in the Netherlands, and I was able to study its safety and effectivity in the treatment of orthopedic infections. Safety was evaluated with regard to renal, cochlear, and vestibular functions, and the effectivity was compared with a historical control group of patients, as well as in a small prospective randomized controlled trial (RCT) (Walenkamp, 1983; Walenkamp et al., 1986). Since 1982, I use gentamicin PMMA beads as standard therapy in my clinical work at the Orthopedic Department of the Maastricht university hospital. In 25 years, I have treated all kinds of orthopedic infections at the septic unit – notably osteomyelitis (Walenkamp, 1997; Walenkamp et al., 1998) and infected prostheses. The following chapter is based on experience in the treatment of early or late infections of about 60 total knee prostheses (TKP) and 150 total hip prostheses (THP). This experience is representative of the daily practice of my fellow orthopedic surgeons in the Netherlands. I will discuss mainly the practical and tech-

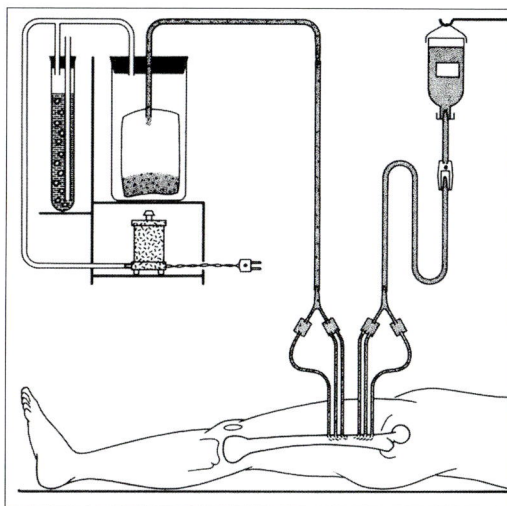

Fig. 14.1 Schematic representation of a suction drainage system commonly used in the treatment of orthopedic infections, before gentamicin PMMA beads became available at the end of the seventies (Walenkamp 1983).

nical aspects of these infections. I will also try to provide a treatment schedule for prosthesis infections, based on the pharmacokinetic understanding of local antibiotic treatment that has been described more extensively in chapter 8 in this book.

Early Postoperative Infections

In early postoperative deep infections of prostheses, we assume that the contamination and infection is limited to the hematoma in the wound, and does not involve the prosthesis-(cement)-bone interface. When the infection is only superficial and limited to the skin and superficial subcutaneous layers, the infection can be treated with high-dose intravenous antibiotics only – without operation. However, if there is an extensive subcutaneous infection or the suspicion of a deep infection, operative debridement becomes necessary, since i.v. antibiotics alone cannot penetrate sufficiently into a large hematoma, abscess, or avital tissues.

Successful treatment of early postoperative infections is related to the length of treatment delay. If debridement and antibiotic therapy are initiated within the first 2–4 postoperative weeks, the healing rate, which varies a lot in the literature, seems to be 60–80% (Gillespie, 1990; Hanssen and Spangehl, 2004; Trebse et al., 2005). Unfortunately, the distinction between aseptic and septic wound healing problems is generally not easily made, so that unnecessary treatment delays often cannot be avoided in this critical early postoperative period.

When the superficial wound is debrided, the fascia has to be opened if there is any doubt that the infection is not limited only to the subcutaneous layer. Intraarticular granulation and avital tissue is removed, and the wound is washed by pulse lavage (Ringer's solution without antibiotic admixture). The prosthesis remains in place if stable, as in the treatment of early osteosynthesis infections. We do not always remove polyethylene or ceramic inserts, to avoid damage of the components.

In a next step, local antibiotic carriers are inserted in the form of PMMA beads or resorbable gentamicin collagen. The number of beads is limited by the space available. In a hip 120–180 beads can be placed around the neck of the femoral component, in a knee 90–120 are placed into the suprapatellar bursa region (Fig. 14.2). Wound closure is watertight to keep the antibiotic inside. Drains are inserted to limit the volume of the hematoma. These are removed as soon as possible. To avoid cracks in the chains and beads, patients are not allowed to walk. Systemic antibiotics are added intravenously.

The beads are removed after 2 weeks and the same procedure is repeated if there is any doubt about healing, i.e., another debridement is performed and antibiotics are administered for another 2 weeks. After one or two of these treatment periods the i.v. antibiotic therapy is stopped, and the patients are dismissed on oral antibiotics (for another 3–6 months). When a relapse of the in-

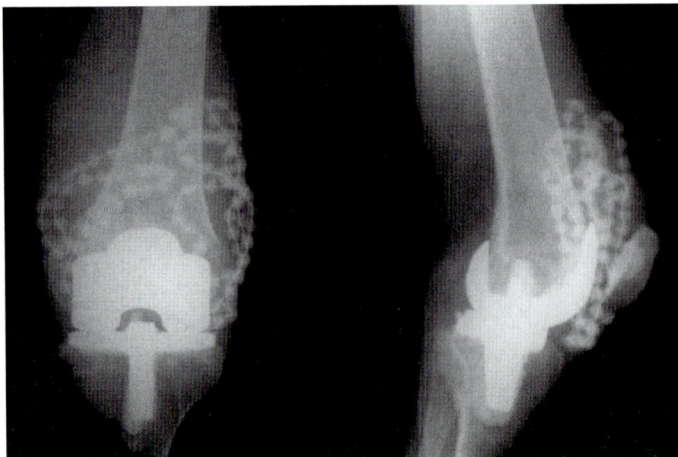

Fig. 14.**2** Radiographic images of gentamicin beads implanted in early postoperative infections treated with the prosthesis in situ.

fection occurs after stopping the antibiotics, the prosthesis has to be removed.

Resorbable antibiotic carriers can be used instead of beads to avoid a second operation. One of these carriers is collagen, commercially available as gentamicin collagen (Ipsen et al., 1991; Kanella-kopoulou and Giamarellos-Bourboulis, 2000). The resorption of the collagen within 4–6 weeks, however, may cause a disturbing secretion for 3–4 weeks. This is difficult to distinguish from a purulent secretion, and it may also cause a fistula to the prosthesis. Collagen should, therefore, only be used in deep joints or cavities if the tissue layers can be closed securely. Some of the antibiotic-loaded collagen combinations release their antibiotics too quickly (Sørensen et al., 1990). If a high local antibiotic concentration for more then a few hours is intended, carriers with a protracted release of the gentamicin should be used.

PMMA beads, as well as collagen with gentamicin are commercially available as a standard combination, but can be supplied custom-made with vancomycin, as well as clindamycin, if necessary.

Late Infection

In case of a late infection of the prosthesis, the infection also affects the bone-cement or prosthesis-bone interface, so it is always deep. In this case, the prosthesis has to be removed.

The removal of the prosthesis is often a demanding procedure, especially on the femoral side. Special instruments are needed as well as expertise (Gehrke, 2005). In difficult cases, a window has to be made in the femoral cortex. Uncemented prostheses are not always easier to extract. Despite infection there is often no loosening, and some types of prostheses have such a tight bond to bone that fragmentation of the proximal femur is inevitable. This applies especially to titanium alloy (Zweymüller, Symax) or madriporic-structured prostheses (Lord).

After removal of all components, the acetabulum and the femur are debrided using the same instruments as used to prepare the reimplantation of the prosthesis. This provides good bone debridement. Also, the size of the next prosthesis and the need for special reinforcements, such as bone grafts or special prostheses, can be assessed. Subsequently, PMMA beads are implanted in the entire infected area: 300–360 beads in THP, and

120–180 beads in TKP, in chains of 60 beads each. The fascia over the beads is closed watertight, and a drain is placed in the center. Beads are only placed in the subcutaneous tissue if there is an abscess cavity. A second drain is placed in the subcutaneous tissue. Intravenous antibiotic therapy starts during the operation itself, as soon as deep tissue samples for culture have been taken. The choice of the antibiotic is based on the per-operatively identified bacteria.

Postoperatively, a good "hematoma management" is necessary to create an optimal balance between the removal of too much hematoma, on the one hand and keeping the gentamicin inside, on the other hand. If the hematoma is too large, the concentration of the gentamicin decreases. In a THP revision, the deep drain is therefore used as a syphoning drain – without suction – for one postoperative day to avoid loss of too much blood, and is removed after a short subsequently period of suctioning. The subcutaneous drain is removed on the second postoperative day or later, so that a subcutaneous hematoma can be avoided.

As described in early postoperative infections, debridement with a 2-weeks period of local treatment can be repeated a few times if necessary. The concentration of local antibiotics decreases after 2 weeks to less effective values, so they should be replaced.

In any case, it is not easy to decide if there is appropriate healing. Provided that antibiotic-loaded PMMA beads are used and with proper hematoma management, the wound must be dry after 1 week. If there is still secretion, there may be a persistent infection. Other parameters to decide if healing is appropriate are mainly the C-reactive protein (CRP) value, body temperature, and decrease of induration of soft tissues. Combined, these offer the best immediate information. The erythrocyte sedimentation rate (ESR) reacts much too slowly, to be helpful in the decisions that have to be taken in the given short time frame.

After removal of the beads, two main questions have to be answered with regard to the further treatment:

1. Will a prosthesis be reimplanted?

Reimplantation should only be performed if a patient is mentally and physically able to cope with a possible relapse of the reimplanted prosthesis. If the patient hardly survived the first treatment of an infected prosthesis, it is better not to reimplant. Also, the bone stock must be good enough to accept the prosthesis with or without extensive reconstructions. The more reconstruction is needed at reimplantation, the more we want to be sure that the infection has been successfully eradicated.

2. If so, when?

Reimplantation can be performed during the same hospital stay, after a few weeks of local antibiotic treatment as a short-term two-stage revision.

If a longer period in between seems to be better, the patient is sent home for 3–12 months, constituting a long-term two-stage revision.

Girdlestone and Arthrodesis

If no reimplantation is meant to follow in the hip, an empty space is left after removal of the beads. It is not necessary to fill the space with a muscle graft, to perform an arthrodesis, or to maintain traction for a few weeks. Patients are mobilized with two crutches, permitting for weight bearing. Most of the patients are able to walk with two crutches if they are capable and fit enough. Unfortunately, this is often not the case. Walking with a Girdlestone hip takes up al lot of energy and strong hands and arms are needed (Fig. 14.3a).

A Girdlestone hip, in general, causes a shortening of 4–8 cms of the leg, and an exorotation of about 45–90 degrees (Garvin and Hanssen, 1995; Hanssen and Spangehl, 2004). Due to muscle shortening, the patient has to help with his hands in order to move the leg. Sometimes, the contact of the proximal femur and the pelvis causes considerable pain, necessitating a secondary muscle interposition.

In some patients there is extensive periarticular calcification (PAO), (Fig. 14.3b).

This constitutes a second clinical type of Girdlestone: a stable, less shortened hip that allows weight bearing without crutches. PAO is more frequent in hip prostheses and in men. In Girdlestone hips, the stiffness allows for better walking. Sitting, however, is more difficult.

In knees and ankle joints, an arthrodesis has to be performed if a definite solution without pros-

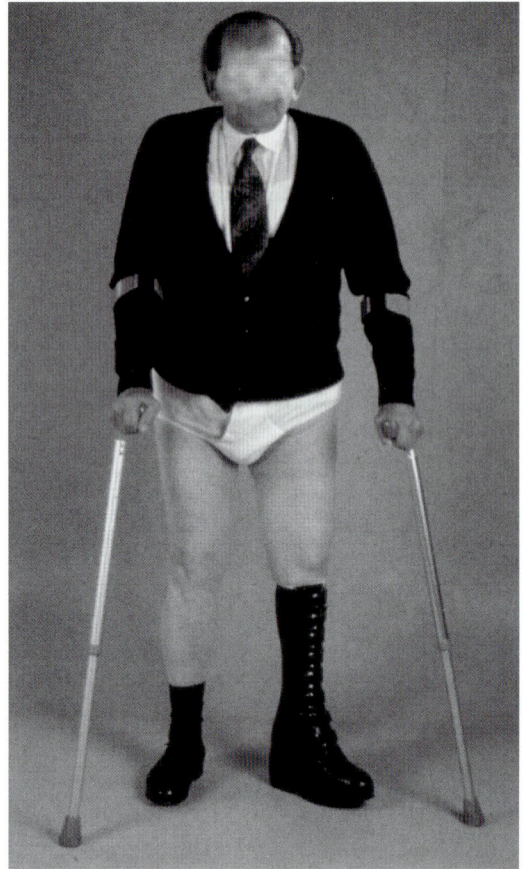

Fig. 14.**3a** A patient with a Girdlestone at the left side.

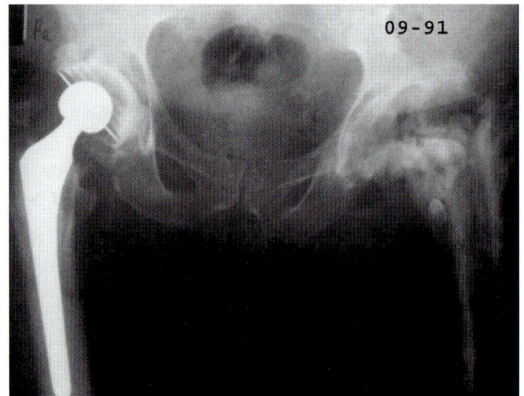

Fig. 14.**3b** Periarticular calcifications create a relatively stable hip, but shortening and exorotation remain.

thesis is wished. A Girdlestone-like situation could be a solution in the shoulder, elbow, and wrist if necessary, with the aid of an orthotic support.

Short-Term Two-Stage Reimplantation

After a number of treatment periods of 2 weeks each, reimplantation can follow if healing is appropriate. Beads are extracted, and after final reaming, the prosthesis is reimplanted, if necessary, with a bone graft (Figs.14.**4**). If bone cement is used, it is antibiotic-loaded. A few years ago, we also started using *non*cemented prostheses as implants in infection revisions. In the future, pros-

theses with antibiotic-loaded coatings may be preferable, when available.

Bone grafts can be admixed with antibiotics that show protracted elution, both in in-vitro studies and in in-vivo experiments (chapter 5). This allows admixture of an individualized choice of antibiotics.

One week after reimplantation, the antibiotic therapy is switched from intravenous to oral administration (if possible). There is no evidence, how long antibiotics should be given after reimplantation. We apply antibiotics for 6–12 weeks, but take into account the improvement of laboratory tests (ESR), the virulence of the germ, and soft-tissue involvement.

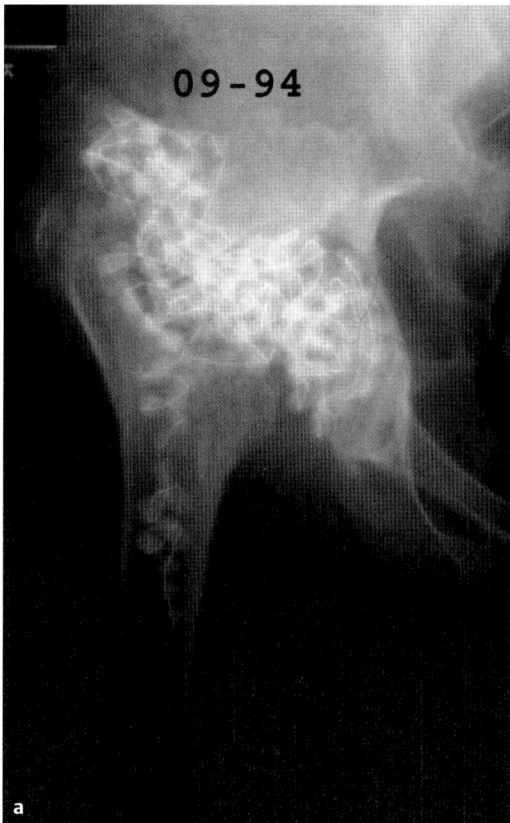

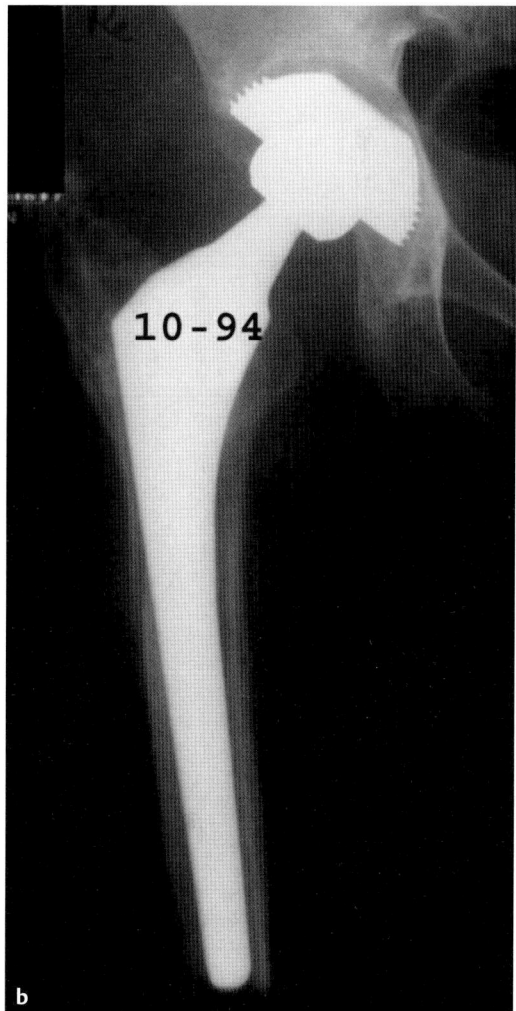

Fig. 14.**4a, b** Radiographic images of a short-term two-stage revision: reimplantation after 2 weeks of local treatment in a patient with a low grade infection.

Long-Term Two-Stage Reimplantation

In these patients, beads are removed and the hip is left either without interposition, or a spacer may be implanted. A spacer keeps the soft tissues at length. This facilitates late reimplantation and improves postoperative function, especially in knees (Hanssen and Spangehl, 2004; Anagnostakos et al., 2006). We found, however, that the antibiotic concentration in spacers is inferior to that created by PMMA beads. So we do not use spacers for the infection treatment itself, but only as temporary replacement during the long interval period.

As in short-term treatment, we change the administration of systemic antibiotics at 1 week postoperatively to oral. 6 weeks after the oral antibiotic has been stopped, a punction of the joint is cultured. If no microorganisms are grown, reimplantation is planned and performed as soon as possible (Fig. 14.5). We have already determined beforehand during debridement, which type and size of prosthesis is to be used, and if special reconstructions and grafts are required.

At the final operation, the spacer is removed and tissue cultures are taken from the wound. Then the reimplantation is carried out. Continued treatment with systemic antibiotics is not necessary if the cultures remain negative. But because the final bacteriological result will take some time, up to 2 weeks, patients are temporarily treated with antibiotics until the final results are

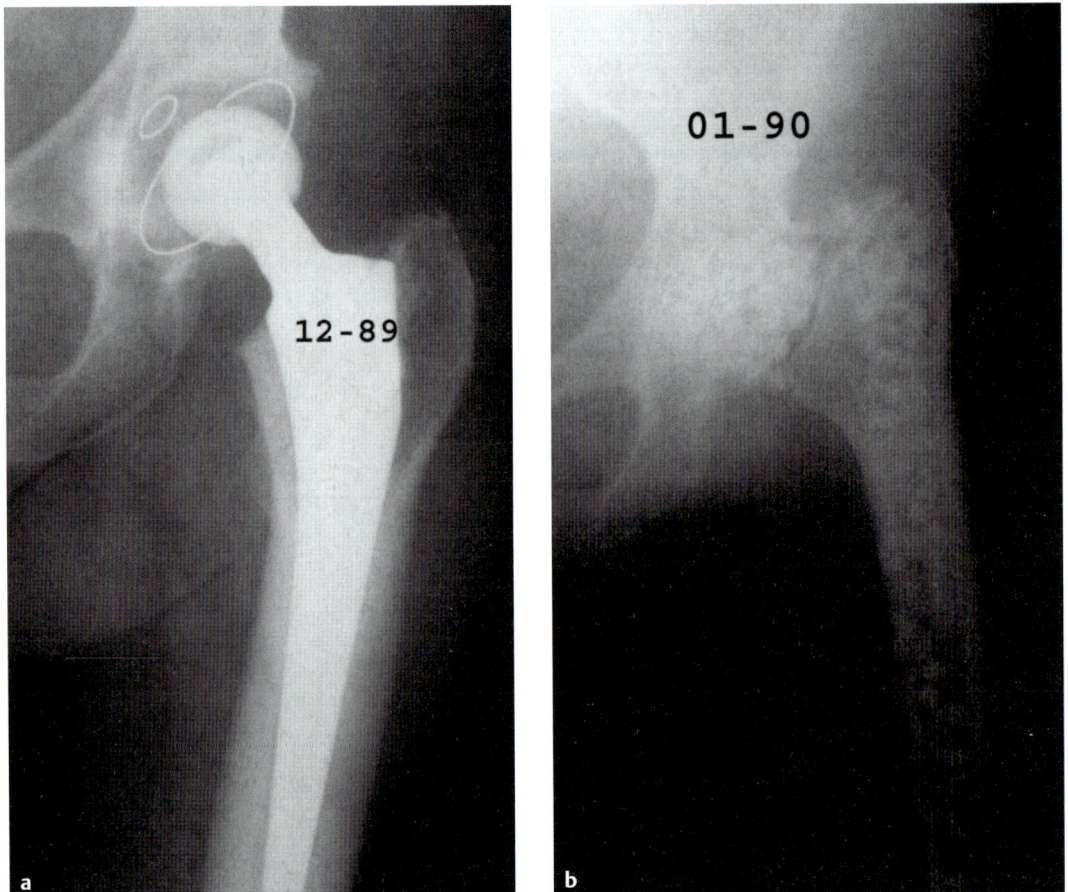

Fig. 14.**5a–e** Successive radiographic images of a long-term two-stage revision in a patient with a more virulent infection and doubtful healing after 2 weeks of treatment with gentamicin beads. Treatment took place before spacers were available, so shortening occured during the Girdlestone period.

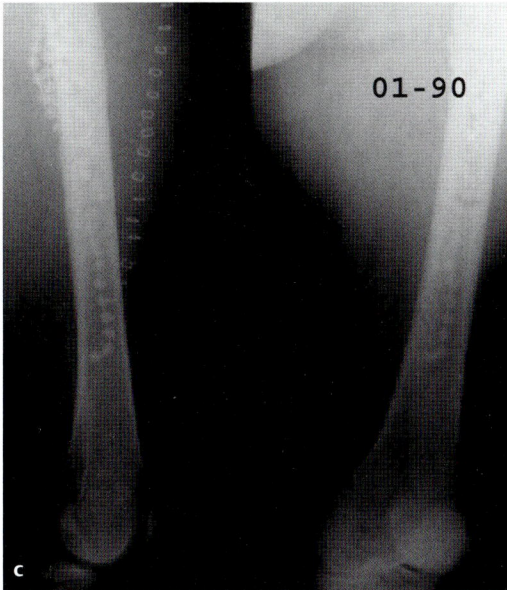

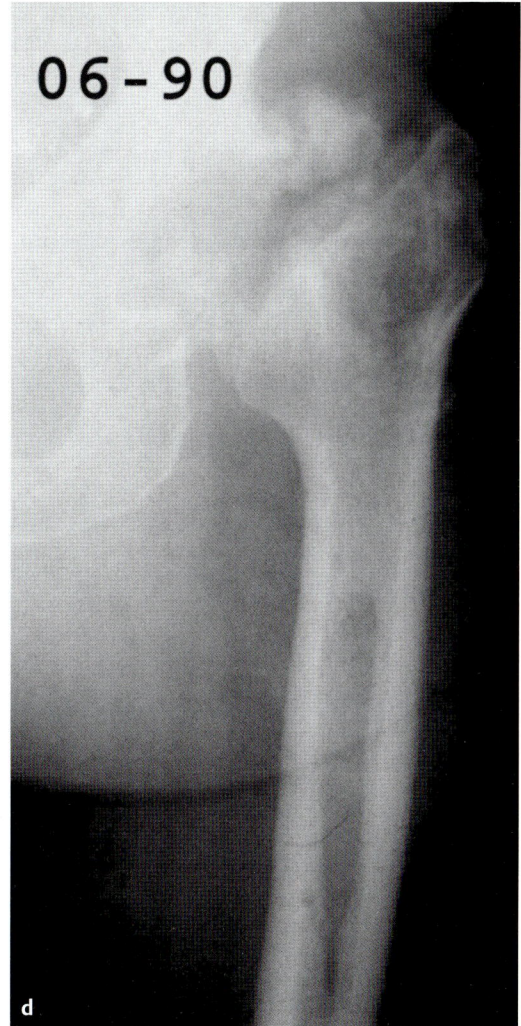

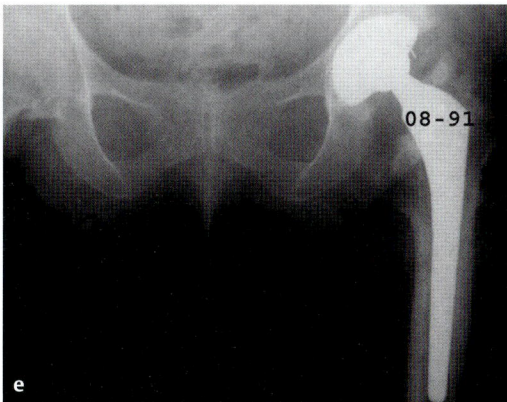

Fig. 14.**5a – e** (cont.)

known. If cultures appear to be (unexpectedly) positive, then again a 6 – 12-weeks antibiotic treatment will follow to avoid reinfection (Toms et al., 2006).

One- or Two-Stage Reimplantation?

Several articles and reviews have shown that the success rate of a two-stage revision of infected prostheses is better than a one-stage – about 90% versus 80% if antibiotic-loaded cement is used

(Garvin and Hanssem 1995). Good results of one-stage revisions are mainly described by specialized clinics, such as the Endoclinic in Hamburg (Buchholz et al., 1981, Gehrke, 2005) or the Hip Centre in Wrightington (Raut et al., 1996). These results are possible, mainly because sophisticated preoperative bacteriological diagnostics, patient-individualized antibiotic admixtures in bone cement, and surgeons with extensive experience are available.

In most countries, two-stage exchange is the customary procedure (Jackson and Schmalzried,

139

2000; Hanssen and Spangehl, 2004; Tos et al., 2006). In France, a retrospective review of the results of 14 orthopedic teaching centers showed that the healing percentage in 349 patients after more then 2 years follow-up was 88% in one-stage procedures, and 85% in two-stage procedures. With one-stage procedures, the healing rate of a moderate infection was 90%, as compared to 70% in severe infections. An important finding was that the amount of stages correlated with the complication rate. There were 9% mechanical complications in a one-stage procedure and 20% in a two-stage revision (Vielpeau and Lortat, 2002; Langlais, 2003). In a survey looking at the results of revision with reimplantation of the infected total hip, several authors found the same: The best results are achieved with the use of antibiotic-loaded bone cement in a two-stage procedure (91–93%), the worst in a one-stage reimplantation without antibiotic-loaded bone cement (58–59%). When a one-stage reimplantation is performed using antibiotic-loaded bone cement, the result is 82–86% (mainly data from the Endoclinic, Hamburg). The same healing percentage is achieved in a two-stage procedure without antibiotic-loaded cement, which, however, is not the same as not using cement (Garvin and Hanssen, 1995; Langlais, 2003). Sufficient data are not yet available to verify whether reimplantation with a noncemented prosthesis is safe. However, it seems justified in a two-stage procedure if the infection is cleared before reimplantation.

In the Netherlands, complicated revisions of infected prostheses are performed by general orthopedic surgeons, as in most European countries. Best results are obtained by those, who have some specialization in hip or knee surgery, and who cooperate with a dedicated bacteriologist with good laboratory facilities. In this case, the two-stage treatment is the best choice (Walenkamp, 2001). Two-stage has the following advantages:

1. Tissue cultures can be taken from several places in the deep interfaces.
2. Antibiotics can be chosen for systemic as well as for local application in bone cement or bone graft, based on deep culture results.
3. Local antibiotic treatment with PMMA beads results in much higher concentrations than possible with only the antibiotic-loaded cement used in prosthesis implantation.
4. Strategic decisions can be taken stepwise, based on information of one or more operations and on the clinical parameters.

5. Special prostheses or bone grafts can be ordered and have not to be kept in stock.
6. The success rate is higher.

The disadvantages are:
1. Patients need at least one extra operation.
2. There are more mechanical complications like fractures of a weakened femur.
3. Reimplantation after a short and long-term interval may be more difficult, especially if no spacer is used.

Pharmacokinetic Aspects

The objective of local antibiotic therapy, is to implant antibiotic releasing carriers that will effectively eliminate bacteria in the hematoma and in the adjacent tissues by creating high local antibiotic concentrations. In general, high local concentrations do hardly affect serum levels and, therefore, organs are not exposed to toxicity and systemic side effects can be avoided. Also, higher doses of bactericidal antibiotics can be used in local treatments, so that the resulting tissue concentrations exceed by far the concentrations achievable with systemic therapy.

However, the exact amount of antibiotic concentration, and the ideal duration of treatment is not really known. Animal experiments have shown that a high local antibiotic concentration in a hematoma will decrease after 1–2 weeks following implantation, and that it also decreases significantly with increased distance to the carrier. Effective high concentrations are limited to a distance of 2–4 cms to PMMA beads (Wahlig et al., 1978). This explains why the exsudate concentration should be as high as possible, as in the case of gentamicin even up to a few hundred μg/m. Such high concentrations will also kill moderately resistant bacteria, and may avoid the development of small colony variants (SCV) and other kinds of bacterial resistance (Von Eiff et al., 1997; Neut et al., 2001).

PMMA beads are able to achieve high antibiotic concentrations, because the surface available for elution is relatively large. Exsudate concentrations in patients will increase to a maximum on the second or third day. In gentamicin beads a peak level of 200–400 μg/mL is possible using a proper technique (Walenkamp, 2001) and will decrease in 1 week to a level below 50 μg/mL (Fig. 14.**6**).

Beads are produced commercially and are available on request with gentamicin, vancomycin, clin-

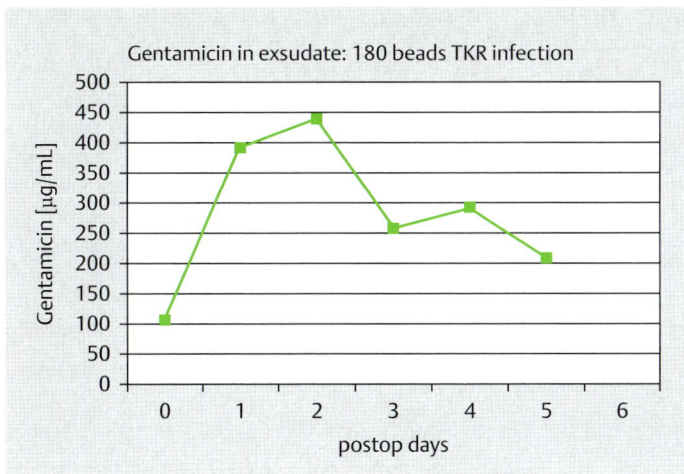

Fig. 14.**6** Local exsudate concentration in a patient after extraction of a total knee prosthesis and implantation of 180 gentamicin beads. The typical increase to a peak level (430 μg / mL) on the second postoperative day is shown.

damycin, or as a combination of these. Resorbable beads are not yet available for clinical use.

Using the proper product, gentamicin collagen fleeces are able to achieve an even higher local exsudate concentration, as the release is generally quicker. In these products the maximum amount of implanted fleeces has to be more strictly taken into account, because nephrotoxicity due to overdoses has been described. The main disadvantage of fleeces is that they have no volume when implanted. In a watery solution, such as a hematoma, they shrink and do not fill the cavity. In prosthesis infection, they are, therefore, very useful at an early stage where the prosthesis still remains in place, but are not suited when it is extracted. They are also available with vancomycin or clindamycin.

Spacers have a smaller surface than beads. If they are prepared by the surgeon in a mold with regular antibiotic-loaded bone cement, there is also less release, because the cement is less porous than PMMA beads. The antibiotic release of spacers may be improved by increasing the amount of antibiotics or by increasing the porosity with additives. A resulting decrease of the cement strength can be disregarded, as it is not required in this particular situation. To avoid fracture of hip spacers at the neck junction, prefabricated spacers with a metal reinforcement have become available. These, however, make an individualized choice of type and dose of the antibiotic more difficult.

The local exsudate concentration achieved with spacers is much lower than with beads (Fig. 14.**7**) and there is no accumulation after a few days.

Moreover, the concentration will immediately decrease after reaching the peak level at the first day, which is not higher then about 30 – 50 μg / mL (Fig. 14.**8**).

Conclusion

The application of local antibiotics is an effective treatment for osteomyelitis and prosthesis infections. For this particular indication, it is advisable to create high local concentrations for several weeks. The use of antibiotic-loaded PMMA beads, is to date still the only effective, reproducible, and safe method – the "gold standard". In general, a two-stage revision will have a higher success rate, especially in more virulent infections and in general orthopedic practice. In addition, this approach offers the advantage of making decisions stepwize.

Spacers facilitate the reimplantation of the prosthesis. For this reason they are useful during the interval – especially in long-term procedures where several months can go by before an infection is cured.

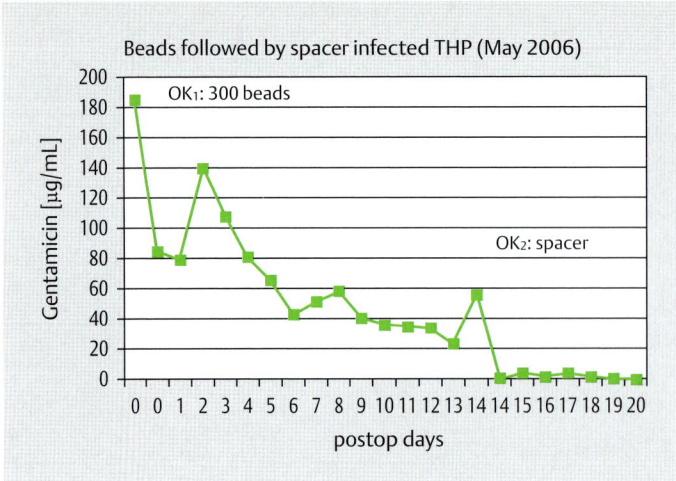

Fig. 14.**7** Exsudate concentration in a patient after extraction of a total hip and implantation of 300 gentamicin PMMA beads (OK$_1$): increase at day 2, afterwards gradual decrease to moderately high levels. At the second operation, the beads are removed and a spacer is implanted: after a moderately high concentration on the first day, no high local antibiotic concentration is achieved.

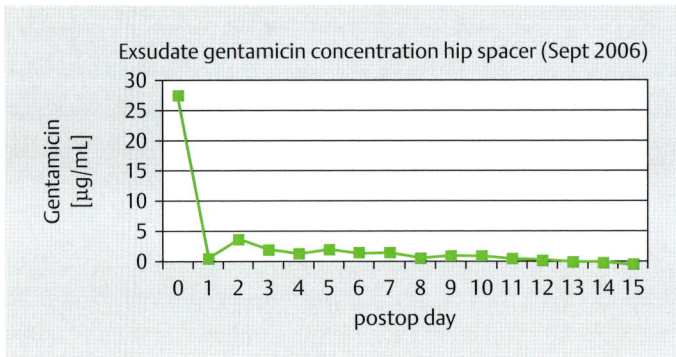

Fig. 14.**8** Exsudate concentration after implantation of a preformed hip spacer treating an infected proximal gamma nail. After the first day, the moderate exsudate concentration decreases rapidly.

References

Anagnostakos K, Fürst OM, Kelm J, Antibiotic-impregnated PMMA hip spacers. Acta Orthop 2006; 77: 628–637.

Buchholz H, Engelbrecht E, Lodenkaemper H et al. Management of deep infection of total hip replacement. J Bonc Jt Surg 1981; 63 B: 342 353.

Eiff von C, Bettin D, Proctor R et al. Recovery of Small Colony Variants of Staphylococcus aureus following gentamicin bead placement for osteomyelitis. Clin Infect Dis 1997; 25: 1250–1251.

Garvin K, Evans B, Salvati E, Brause B. Palacos gentamicin for the treatment of deep periprosthetic hip infections. Clin Orthop Rel Res 1994; 298: 97–105.

Garvin K, Hanssen A. Infection after total hip arthroplasty. J Bone Joint Surg 1995; 77-A: 1576–1588.

Gehrke T. Revision is not difficult. In: Breusch S, Malchau H eds. The well-cemented total hip arthroplasty. Berlin: Springer; 2005: 348–358.

Gillespie W. Infection in total joint replacement. In: Norden C ed. Osteomyelitis. Philadelphia: Saunders; 1990: 465–484.

Hanssen A, Spangehl M. Treatment of the infected hip replacement. Clin Orthop Rel Res 2004; 420: 63–71.

Ipsen T, Jorgensen PS, Damholt V, Torholm C. Gentamicin-collagen sponge for local applications. 10 cases of chronic osteomyelitis followed for 1 year. Acta Orthop Scand 1991; 62: 592–594.

Jackson W, Schmalzried T. Limited role of direct exchange arthroplasty in the treatment of infected total hip replacements. Clin Orthop Rel Res 2000; 381: 101–105.

Kanellakopoulou K, Giamarellos-Bourboulis EJ. Carrier systems for the local delivery of antibiotics in bone infections. Drugs 2000; 59: 1223 – 1232.

Langlais F. Can we improve the results of revision arthroplasty for infected total hip replacement? J Bone Joint Surg 2003; 85-B: 637 – 640.

Neut D, van de Belt H, Stokroos I et al. Biomaterial-associated infection of gentamicin-loaded PMMA beads in orthopaedic revision surgery. J Antimicrob Chemother 2001; 47: 885 – 891.

Raut V, Orth M, Orth MC, Siney P, Wroblewski B. One stage revision arthroplasty of the hip for deep gram negative infections. Int Orthop 1996; 20: 12 – 14.

Sørensen TS, Sørensen AI, Merser S. Rapid release of gentamicin from collagen sponge. In vitro comparison with plastic beads. Acta Orthop Scand 1990; 61: 353 – 356.

Toms A, Davidson D, Masri B, Duncan C. The management of peri-prosthetic infection in total joint arthroplasty. J Bone Joint Surg 2006; 8 (2) 149 – 155.

Trebse R, Pisot V, Trampuz A. Treatment of infected retained implants. J Bone Joint Surg 2005; 87-B: 249 – 255.

Vielpeau C, Lortat Jacob A. Management of the infected hip prostheses. Rev Chir Orthop 2002; 88 (Suppl 1): 159 – 216.

Wahlig H, Dingeldein E, Bergmann R, Reuss K. The release of gentamicin from polymethylmethacrylate beads. An experimental and pharmacokinetic study. J Bone Joint Surg Br 1978; 60-B: 270 – 275.

Walenkamp G. Gentamicin PMMA beads and other local antibiotic carriers in two-stage revision of total knee infection: a review. J Chemother 2001; 13: 66 – 72.

Walenkamp GH, Vree TB, van Rens TJ. Gentamicin-PMMA beads. Pharmacokinetic and nephrotoxicological study. Clin Orthop Relat Res 1986: 171 – 183.

Walenkamp GHIM. Gentamicin PMMA beads. A clinical, pharmacokinetic and toxicological (thesis). KU Nijmegen; 1983.

Walenkamp GHIM. How I do it: Chronic osteomyelitis. Acta Orthop Scand 1997; 68: 497 – 506.

Walenkamp GHIM, Klein LA, de Leeuw M. Osteomyelitis treated with gentamicin-PMMA beads. 100 Patients followed for 1 – 12 years. Acta Orthop Scand, 1998; 69: 518 – 522.

Willenegger H. Therapeutische Möglichkeiten und Grenzen der antibakteriellen Spüldrainage bei chirurgischen Infektionen. Langenbecks Arch Chir 1963; 304: 07.

Revision of Infected Total Hip Prostheses in Norway and Sweden

Eivind Witsø, Lars Birger Engesæter

An Overview

The primary goal when treating an infected total hip arthroplasty (THA) is to relieve pain, eradicate the infection, and to restore a functional extremity. The different treatment options include
- one-stage reimplantation,
- two-stage reimplantation,
- resection arthroplasty (permanent Girdlestone),
- soft tissue debridement with retention of the prosthesis, and
- chronic suppressive antibiotic treatment only.

Several factors have to be considered when determining the optimal surgical treatment for an infected THA. The type of postoperative infection has to be defined. Traditionally, infected arthroplasties have been divided into
- early postoperative infections
  (within 3 months),
- delayed postoperative infection
  (from 3 months to two years), and
- hematogenous infection.

Nowadays the division between early and late infections is usually drawn at 4 weeks (Tsukayama et al., 2005; Masterson et al., 1998).

In cases of a well fixed, stable prosthesis and a short-time history of infection, soft-tissue debridement with retention of the implant is an option (Trebse et al., 2005). However, this treatment strategy should not be employed in cases with poor soft-tissue conditions, drainage sinus tracts, and unknown pathogens (Zimmerli, 2000; Garvin and Urban, 1995). In delayed postoperative infections, two-stage revision has been considered as the standard treatment (Garvin and Urban, 2003). A meta-analysis comparing single and two-stage procedures has shown a success rate of 82% and 91%, respectively (Garvin and Hansen, 1995).

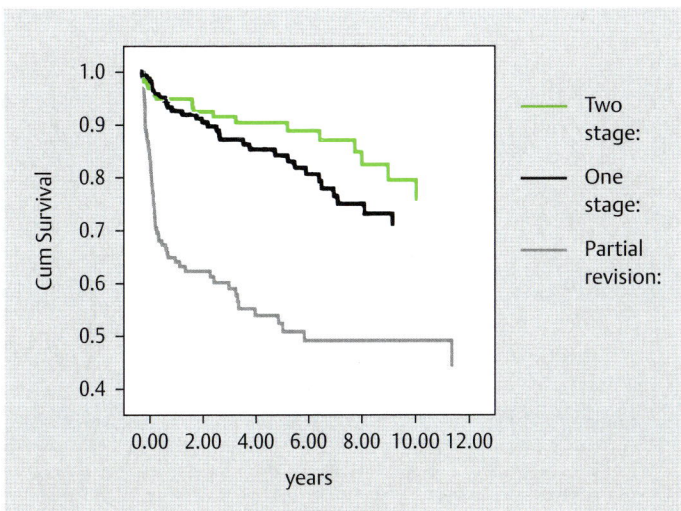

Fig. 15.1 The figure shows the survival after septic THA revision treated with:
one-stage revision (n=429),
two-stage revision (n=709),
and partial revision (n=72).

According to the arthroplasty registers in Norway and Sweden, 506 THA revisions (out of 91 718 primary THAs) were performed due to infection in Norway between 1987 and 2005; and 960 infected THAs were revized in Sweden between 1979 and 2000. The population in Norway and Sweden is 4.6 and 9 million, respectively.

Out of 1466 infected THA revisions in Norway and Sweden, 429 (29%) were treated with one-stage reimplantation, 709 (48%) were treated with two-stage reimplantation, and 256 (17%) were treated with a resection arthroplasty. Due to the design of the registers, patients treated with soft-tissue debridement or chronic antibiotic treatment only, have not been registered.

In addition to the patients treated with one-stage reimplantation, two-stage reimplantation and resection arthroplasty, a fourth group was identified in Norway: 72 (5%) patients with an infected THA were treated with one-stage exchange of just one of the components of a THA – i.e., a partial revision. The results for this group were far inferior to the others and 50% of the prostheses had to be removed during the first six years after the partial revision (Fig.15.**1**).

In conclusion, according to the Norwegian and Swedish arthroplasty registers the best revision results for infected THA are achieved with two-stage procedures, followed by one-stage reimplantation and partial revision.

References

Garvin KL, Hansen AD. Current concepts review. Infection after total hip arthroplasty. Past, present, and future. J Bone Joint Surg Am 1995; 77 (10): 1576 – 1588.

Garvin KL, Urban JA. Total hip infections. In: Musculoskeletal infections (Ed: Jason H Calhoun and Jon T Mader), Marcel Dekker, Inc., New York, USA 2003: 241 – 291.

Masterson EL, Masri BA, Duncan CP. Treatment of infection at the site of total hip replacement. AAOS Instructional Course Lectures 1998; 47: 297 – 306.

Trebse R, Pisot V, Trampuz A. Treatment of infected retained implants. J Bone Joint Surg Br 2005; 87: 249 – 256.

Tsukayama DT, Estrada R, Gustilo RB. Infection after total hip arthroplasty. J Bone Joint Surg Am 1996; 78 (4): 512 – 523.

Zimmerli W. Prosthetic joint infection: Diagnosis and treatment. Current Infectious Disease Reports 2000; 2: 377 – 379.

The Norwegian Hip Register –
The Influence of Cement and Antibiotics
on the Clinical Results of Primary Prostheses

Lars Birger Engesæter

Abstract

Introduction

Antibiotic prophylaxis is used to reduce the revision rate of total hip arthroplasties (THAs). In this paper, the effect of antibiotic prophylaxis, applied both systemically and in bone cement, is studied according to data from the Norwegian Arthroplasty Register (NAR). In addition, the effect of cements as such is explored by comparing the revision rates due to infection in primary uncemented THAs to those of cemented THAs.

Methods

To have comparable groups, only THAs performed for idiopathic osteoarthrosis were included. The data were stratified according to whether or not antibiotic-loaded bone cement was used, whether or not systemic antibiotic prophylaxis was applied, the duration of the systemic prophylaxis, and whether prostheses were cemented or uncemented. Cox-estimated relative risks (RR) of revision are presented with adjustments for differences among groups in gender, age, cement brand, type of systemic antibiotic prophylaxis, type of prosthesis, type of operating theatre, and duration of the operation.

Results

85120 primary THAs were reported to the NAR during the period between 1987 and 2003. Of these, 3.1 % were revized: 2 % for aseptic loosening and 0.5 % for deep infection. The best results for the cemented THAs were obtained when antibiotic prophylaxis was used both systemically and in the cement. Compared to this combined regimen, patients who only received systemic antibiotic prophylaxis had a 1.4 times higher revision rate with all reasons for revision as endpoint in the analyses (p=0.001), a 1.3 times higher revision rate with aseptic loosening (p=0.02), and a 1.8 times higher revision rate with infection as endpoint (p=0.01). For the combined antibiotic regimen, the results were better if antibiotics were administered 4 times on the day of surgery as compared to once (RR=3.5, p<0.001), twice (RR=2.5, p<0.001), or 3 times (RR=1.8, p=0.02).

Compared to the uncemented THAs, the risk for revision due to infection for cemented THAs without antibiotic-loaded cement was increased (RR=1.8, p=0.04), while no difference could be demonstrated when compared to THAs with antibiotic-loaded cement (RR=1.2, p=0.5).

Conclusions

These observational studies reveal best results when antibiotic prophylaxis is given both systemically and in the bone cement, and when the systemic antibiotic prophylaxis is administered four times on the day of surgery. The risk for revision due to infection was the same for uncemented and cemented arthroplasties with antibiotic-loaded cement, but higher for cemented arthroplasties without antibiotic-containing cement.

Introduction

Due to better surgical techniques, stricter routines before and during operation, as well as stricter antiseptic procedures – e.g., antibiotic prophylaxis – the infection rate after THA has been reduced from 5 – 10 % in the late 1960's to less than 1 % today (Lindgren, 2001). The relative importance of each of the improvements is difficult to assess.

In the present paper, data on primary THAs in the Norwegian Arthroplasty Register are analyzed to elucidate the effect on the revision rate of:
❖ antibiotic-loaded bone cement,

❖ systemic antibiotic prophylaxis,
❖ the length of antibiotic systemic prophylaxis, and
❖ uncemented THAs versus cemented THAs with and without antibiotic-loaded cement.

Patients and Methods

The NAR was established in September 1987. Each THA performed in Norway is reported individually to the register by the respective surgeon. For this purpose, standard forms are completed (Havelin et al., 2000) that include information on the identity of the patient, the date of the operation, indication for surgery, the type of prosthesis, type of cement, operation duration, type of operating room, and if systemic antibiotic prophylaxis was used, the type, duration and dosage of the latter. Failure (revision) of the implant is defined as surgical removal or exchange of the whole or part of the implant. Using the personal identification numbers assigned to each Norwegian resident, information on primary THAs is linked to possible revision procedures. From the start of the register in September 1987 to the end of December 2003, 85 120 primary THAs were reported.

For the study on antibiotic prophylaxis in cement and/or in systemic administration, only primary prostheses in patients with idiopathic osteoarthritis of the hip were included. Also, only prostheses and cements with documented, good long-term results in the register were selected. The following 4 most commonly used combinations of cemented cup/stem prostheses were involved: Charnley/Charnley (DePuy, Leeds, United Kingdom), Exeter/Exeter (Howmedica International, Herouville, France), Titan/Titan (DePuy, Chaumont, France) and Spectron/International Total Hip (ITH) (Smith & Nephew, Memphis, TN, United States). In addition, we selected prostheses with high-viscosity cement of the brands Palacos with or without gentamicin (0.5 g gentamicin per 40 g of bone cement) (Schering-Plough International Inc., Kenilworth, NJ, United States) or Simplex with or without colistin/erythromycin (Howmedica International, London, United Kingdom). Finally, only patients who had received systemic antibiotic prophylaxis with either cephalosporin (first-generation cephalotin or second-generation cefuroxime) or penicillin (cloxacillin or dicloxacillin, both semisynthetic penicillinase-resistant) were included (Engesæter et al., 2003).

To investigate the effect of cement on the revision rate, the following three groups of primary THAs due to idiopathic coxarthrosis were compared: uncemented hip arthroplasty, cemented arthroplasty with antibiotic-loaded cement and cemented arthroplasty without antibiotic-loaded cement (Engesæter et al., 2006).

Statistical analyses

Survival analyses were performed using the Kaplan-Meier method and the Cox regression model. Patients, who died or emigrated during follow-up, were identified from files provided by Statistics Norway. The follow-up time for the prostheses in these patients was censored at the time of death or emigration. A Cox multiple regression model was used to study relative revision risks (failure rate ratios) among the different regimens for antibiotic prophylaxis with adjustments for the possible influences of gender, age (< 70, 70 – 75, > 75 years), cement brand (Palacos, Simplex), type of systemic antibiotic prophylaxis (penicillin, cephalosporin), prosthesis type (Charnley, Exeter, Titan, Spectron/ITH), operating theater ("greenhouse", laminar air ventilation, ordinary ventilation), and duration of the operation (< 61, 61 – 120, > 120 min). Estimates from Cox analyses were used to construct adjusted survival curves. For revisions, the surgeon could record one or more reasons for failure, but in combination with infection, this was considered the primary cause of revision.

Results

Antibiotic prophylaxis applied systemically and/or in cement

In total, 22 170 THAs fulfilled the selection criteria for this part of the study. A combined antibiotic prophylaxis, systemic and in cement, was applied in 71 % of the operations, systemic antibiotics alone were used in 27 % of operations, antibiotics only in the cement in 1.1 %, and no antibiotic prophylaxis at all in 1.3 %. A notable change in the use of prophylaxis in the said period was observed, with clear dominance of the combined regimen after 1998 (Fig. 16.1).

With all reasons for revision as the endpoint of a total of 696 revisions, the best results of the

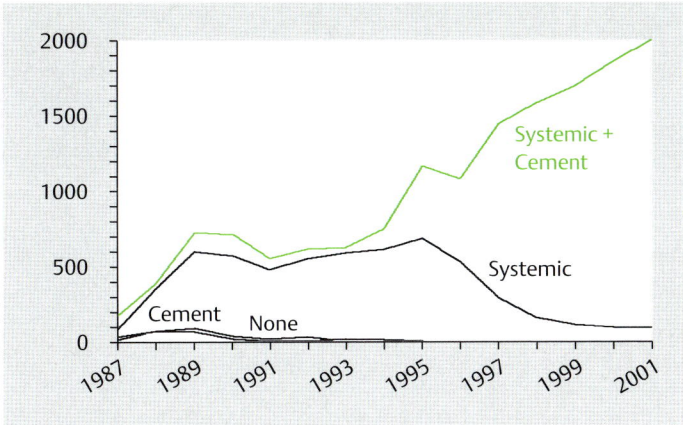

Fig. 16.**1** Number of THAs performed annually from 1987 to 2001 with antibiotic prophylaxis applied both systemically and in cement, only systemically, only in cement, and without antibiotic prophylaxis.

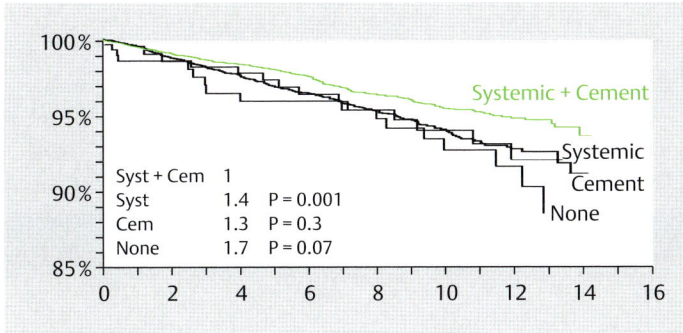

Fig. 16.**2** Cox-adjusted survival curves with all reasons for revision as an endpoint for THAs with antibiotic prophylaxis applied systemically and in cement, only systemically, only in cement, and with no antibiotic prophylaxis.

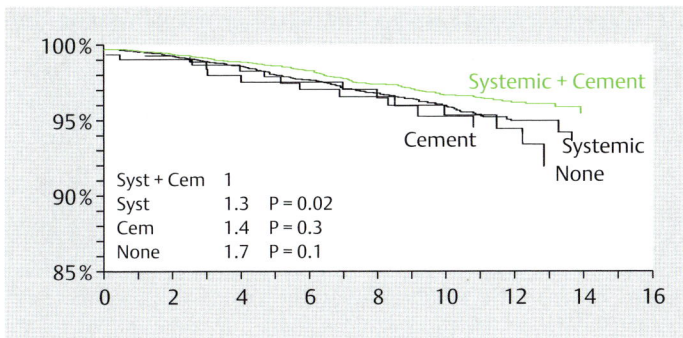

Fig. 16.**3** Cox-adjusted survival curves with aseptic loosening as an endpoint for THAs with antibiotic prophylaxis applied systemically and in cement, only systemically, only in cement, and with no antibiotic prophylaxis.

THAs were achieved with combined antibiotic prophylaxis (Fig. 16.**2**).

Similar results were obtained when the endpoint in the analyses was revision due to aseptic loosening (440 revisions) (Fig. 16.**3**) or infection (102 revisions) (Fig. 16.**4**).

Duration of systemic antibiotic prophylaxis

98% of the patients received systemic antibiotic prophylaxis. Of these, 85% received the prophylaxis only on the day of surgery, 11% for 2 days, 4% for 3 days, and less than 1% for more than 3 days. The length of systemic antibiotic prophylaxis changed from 1987–2001, with 3 or 4 doses

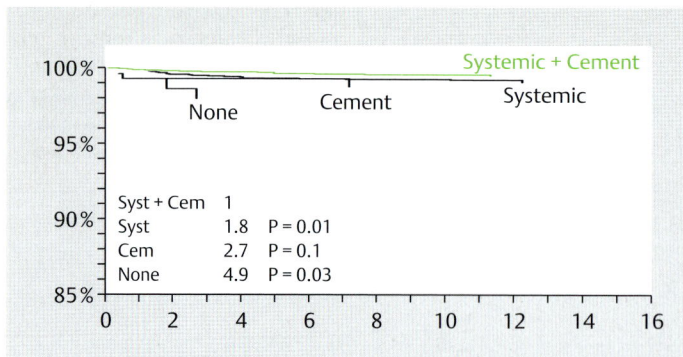

Fig. 16.**4** Cox-adjusted survival curves with infection as an endpoint for THAs with antibiotic prophylaxis applied systemically and in cement, only systemically, only in cement, and with no antibiotic prophylaxis.

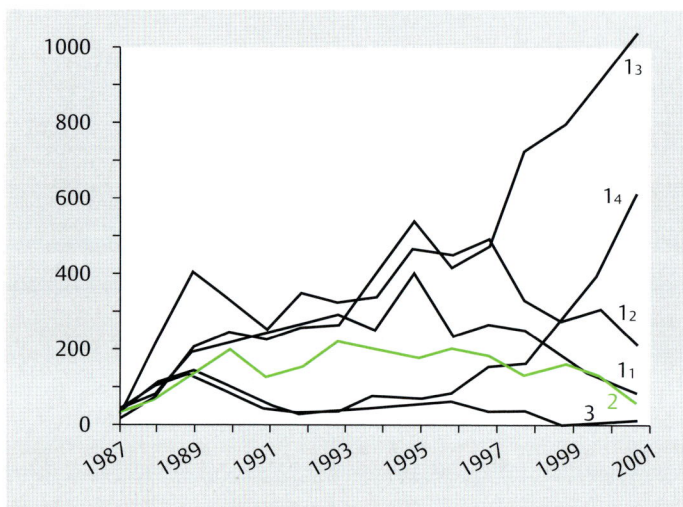

Fig. 16.**5** Number of THAs performed annually from 1987 to 2001 with antibiotic in the cement combined with systemic antibiotic prophylaxis for one day (with the number of doses as subscript, i.e., 1 dose [1_1], 2 doses [1_2], 3 doses [1_3] and 4 doses [1_4]), two days (2) and three days (3).

given only on the day of surgery, as the most dominant regimen in the latter part of the period (Fig. 16.**5**).

In the combined group with systemic prophylaxis only on the day of surgery (11 820 THAs), the effect of the number of antibiotic doses was studied. Compared to systemic prophylaxis with 4 doses on the day of surgery, the revision risk for 3 doses was 1.8 times higher (p=0.02), for 2 doses 2.5 times higher (p<0.001), and for 1 dose 3.5 times higher (p<0.001) with all reasons for revision as an endpoint (total number of revisions was 342) (Fig. 16.**6**). Similar results were obtained with aseptic loosening (219 revisions), (Fig. 16.**7**) or infection (46 revisions) as endpoint (Fig. 16.**8**).

Uncemented versus cemented THA

This study included only primary THAs performed because of primary osteoarthritis, where both the acetabular and the femoral component were either uncemented or cemented (n=56 275). Over the study period, the annual number of uncemented prostheses (9% of the total in this group) remained relatively stable, while cemented THAs with antibiotic-loaded cement (63% of this group) increased, and cemented THAs without antibiotic-containing cement (28%) decreased (Fig. 16.**9**).

With all reasons for revision as endpoint (total number of revisions: 2789) and with uncemented THAs as reference, the revision rates for cemented arthroplasties without antibiotics were reduced to 0.9 times, i.e., reduced by 10% (p=0.01), and arthroplasties with antibiotic-loaded cement were

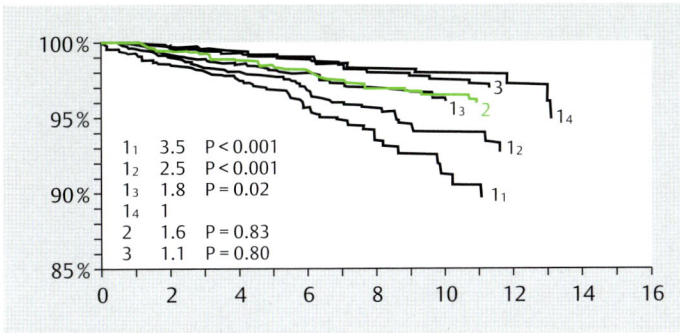

Fig. 16.**6** Cox-adjusted survival curves with all reasons for revision as an endpoint for THAs with antibiotic in the cement combined with systemic antibiotic prophylaxis for one day (with the number of doses as subscript, i.e., 1 dose [1_1], 2 doses [1_2], 3 doses [1_3] and 4 doses [1_4]), for two days (2) and for three days (3).

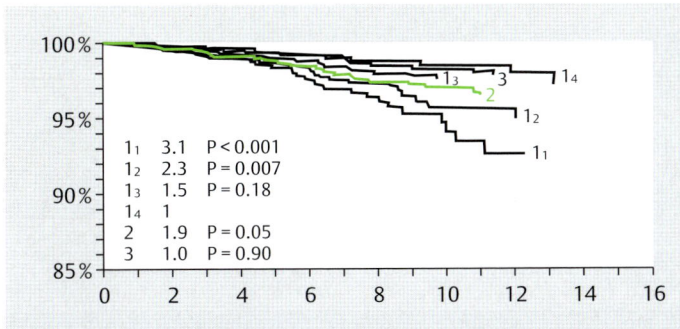

Fig. 16.**7** Cox-adjusted survival curves with aseptic loosening as an endpoint for THAs with antibiotic in the cement combined with systemic antibiotic prophylaxis for one day (with the number of doses as subscript, i.e., 1 dose [1_1], 2 doses [1_2]) 3 doses [1_3] and 4 doses [1_4]), for two days (2) and for three days (3).

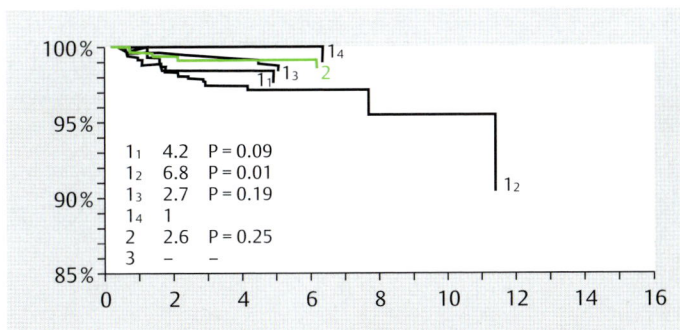

Fig. 16.**8** Cox-adjusted survival curves with infection as an endpoint for THAs with antibiotic in the cement combined with systemic antibiotic prophylaxis for one day (with the number of doses as subscript, i.e., 1 dose [1_1], 2 doses [1_2], 3 doses [1_3] and 4 doses [1_4]), for two days (2) and for three days (3).

reduced to 0.5 times, i.e., reduced by 50% (p<0.001), (Fig. 16.**10**).

With aseptic loosening as an endpoint (1906 revisions) and with uncemented arthroplasties as reference, the risk for revision was 1.3 times higher for cemented arthroplasties without antibiotic cement (p<0.001), but 0.6 lower for cemented hip arthroplasties with antibiotic-loaded cement (p<0.001), (Fig. 16.**11**).

Infection was the reason for revision in 192 THAs. Compared to uncemented THAs, the ce-

mented prostheses without antibiotic cement had a 1.8 times greater risk for revision due to infection (Cox Index [CI] 1.0–3.1, p=0.04), but for the cemented arthroplasties with antibiotic-loaded cement no difference was found (RR=1.2, CI 0.7–2.0, p=0.5), (Fig. 16.**12**).

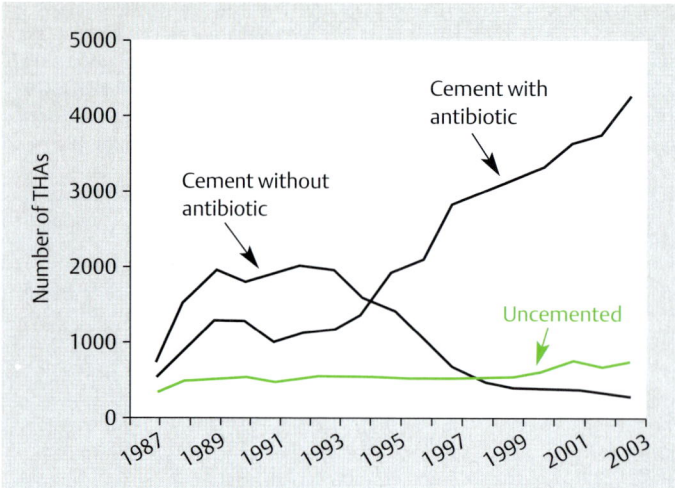

Fig. 16.**9**   Number of THAs performed annually from 1987 to 2003 for uncemented arthroplasties, for cemented hip arthroplasties with antibiotics and for cemented hip arthroplasties without antibiotics.

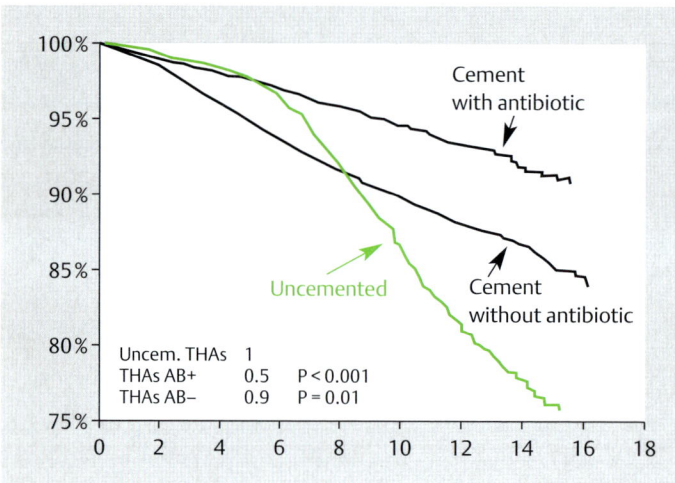

Fig. 16.**10**   Cox-adjusted survival curves with all reasons for revision as an endpoint for uncemented arthroplasties, for cemented hip arthroplasties with antibiotics, and for cemented hip arthroplasties without antibiotics.

Discussion

It is interesting and somewhat surprising to find that the effect of the antibiotic prophylaxis seems to persist 10–14 years postoperatively, not only for revisions, because of infection but also for aseptic loosening. The reduced infection risk with antibiotic prophylaxis is explained by the direct effect on the bacteria and by preventing the bacteria from forming a biofilm on the implant (Van de Belt et al., 2001; Walenkamp, 2001; Kühn, 2000). Low-grade infections are thought to be one of many possible reasons for aseptic loosening (Maathius et al., 2005). Aseptic loosening is a diagnosis of exclusion, which depends on the number of methods available and on the intensity of the search for infection (Neut et al., 2003). In some instances, low-grade infections may be falsely reported as aseptic loosening. This seems to be the most plausible explanation for the reduced rate of aseptic loosening in cemented THAs performed with systemic antibiotic prophylaxis and antibiotic-loaded bone cement in current and previous papers from the our registry (Espehaug et al., 1997; Engesaeter et al., 2003).

Uncemented hip arthroplasties had the same risk for revision due to infection as cemented arthroplasties with antibiotic-loaded cement, but a

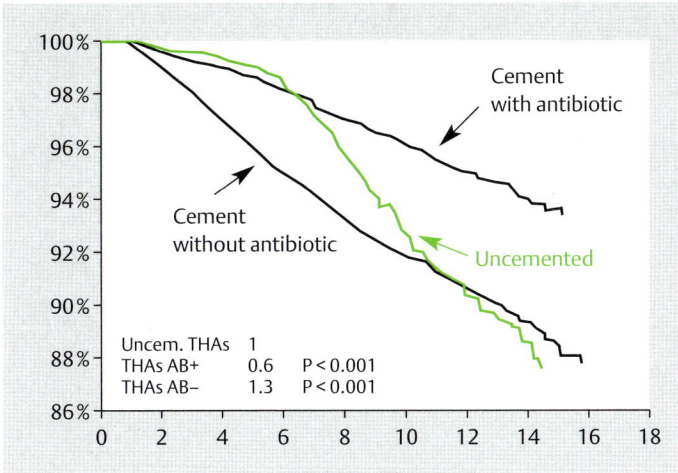

Fig. 16.**11** Cox-adjusted survival curves with aseptic loosening as an endpoint for uncemented arthroplasties, for cemented hip arthroplasties with antibiotic-loaded cement, and for cemented hip arthroplasties without antibiotics.

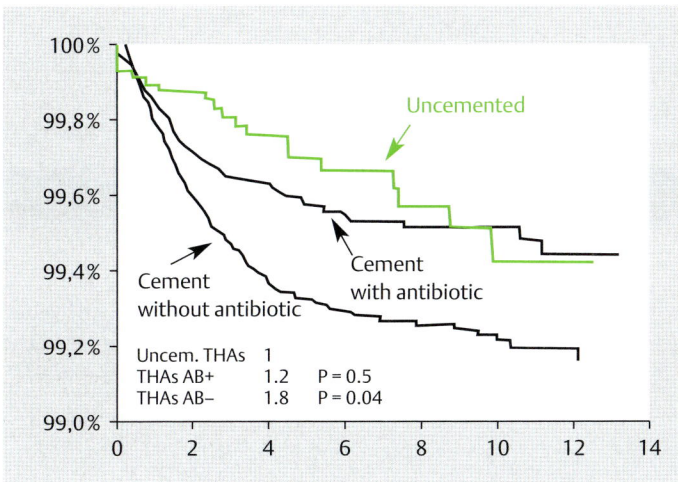

Fig. 16.**12** Cox-adjusted survival curves with infection as an endpoint for uncemented arthroplasties, for cemented hip arthroplasties with antibiotic-loaded cement, and for cemented hip arthroplasties without antibiotics.

reduced risk compared to cemented arthroplasties without antibiotic cement. A possible explanation could be that the cementation as such provides growth conditions for peroperatively unavoidable bacteria. Necrotic bone tissue around the cement, caused by cement toxicity or heat generation during curing of the cement, could be such a potential growth medium. The addition of an antibiotic to the cement may, therefore, offer protection against bacterial growth in this particularly susceptible tissue. The insertion of an uncemented hip prosthesis might cause less tissue necrosis, so that the addition of antibiotics is not required to the same extent.

Conclusion

In conclusion, the best results for primary THAs were seen in patients who received prophylactic antibiotic both in cement and systemically, and where the systemic antibiotic was given 4 times on the day of surgery. Compared to 4 doses of systemic antibiotic prophylaxis only on the day of surgery, no improved results could be detected with a further 1 or 2 days of extended prophylaxis. Based on these findings, and from an economic, microbiological and a clinical point of view, it seems wize to administer the antibiotic prophylaxis only on the day of surgery. Further, compared to cemented arthroplasties with antibiotic-loaded cement, uncemented primary hip arthroplasties reported to the NAR had the same risk for revision due to infection, but a reduced risk compared to cemented arthroplasties without antibiotic cement. Our hypothesis is that the cementation reduces the resistance to infection due to tissue necrosis and that antibiotic in the bone cement partly counteracts this negative effect.

References

Belt van de H, Neut D, Schenk W, van Horn JR, van der Mei HC, Busscher HJ. Infections of orthopedic implants and the use of antibiotic-loaded bone cements. A review. Acta Orthop Scand 2001; 72: 557–571.

Engesæter LB, Lie SA, Espehaug B, Furnes O, Vollset SE, Havelin LI. Antibiotic prophylaxis in total hip arthroplasty. Effects of antibiotic prophylaxis systemically and in bone cement on the revision rate of 22,170 primary hip replacements followed 0–14 years in the Norwegian Arthroplasty Register. Acta Orthop Scand 2003; 74: 644–651.

Engesæter LB, Espehaug B, Lie SA, Furnes O, Havelin LI. Does cement increase the risk for infection in primary total hip arthroplasty? Revision rates in 56275 cemented and uncemented primary THAs followed 0–16 years in the Norwegian Arthroplasty Register. Acta Orthop 2006; 77.

Espehaug B, Engesæter LB, Vollset SE, Havelin LI, Langeland N. Antibiotic prophylaxis in total hip arthroplasty. Review of 10,905 primary cemented total hip replacements reported to the Norwegian Arthroplasty Register, 1987–1995. J Bone Joint Surg Br 1997; 79-B: 590–595.

Havelin LI, Espehaug B, Lie SA, Engesæter LB, Furnes O, Vollset SE. The Norwegian Arthroplasty Register. 11 years and 73,000 arthroplasties. Acta Orthop Scand 2000; 71: 337–353.

Kühn KD. Bone Cements. Up-to-date comparison of physical and chemical properties of commercial materials. Springer-Verlag Berlin Heidelberg, 2000.

Lidgren L. Joint prosthetic infections: A success story. Acta Orthop Scand 2001; 72: 553–556.

Maathuis PGM, Neut D, Busscher HJ, van der Mei HC, van Horn JR. Perioperative contamination in primary total hip arthroplasty. Clin Orthop 2005; 433: 136–139.

Neut D, van Horn JR, van Kooten TG, van der Mei HC, Busscher HJ. Detection of biomaterial-associated infections in orthopedic joint implants. Clin Orthop 2003; 413: 261–268.

Walenkamp GHIM. Prevention of infection in orthopedic surgery. In: European Instructional Course Lectures (Eds Thorngren K-G, Soucacos PN, Horan F, Scott J). The British Editorial Society of Bone and Joint Surgery, London 2001; 5: 5–17.

B Girdlestone Resection Arthroplasty of the Hip – A One-Stage Procedure to eradicate Infection

Michiel Mulier, Jos Stuyck

Abstract

Girdlestone resection arthroplasty is a frequent procedure in the treatment of septic arthritis of the hip, as well as in the management of infected hip replacements. A retrospective long-term follow-up study is presented, in which the curative effect of this procedure for septic conditions and the functional outcomes after hip resection arthroplasty are reviewed.

Between 1976 and 1993, 57 patients aged on average 63 years, underwent a Girdlestone procedure for septic conditions around the hip without further reconversion to total hip replacement (THR). The minimum follow-up was 3 years.

In 49 of 57 cases (86%), the wounds healed completely and there was no further antibiotic therapy. In 8 cases, there was a persisting fistula. On average, wound healing took 3 weeks, which is not significantly longer than in patients with rheumatoid arthritis, or on corticosteroid therapy, or in obese patients. The influence of bacteriology on wound healing was studied: Although *E. coli* and *Pseudomonas* seemed to be associated with longer drainage, this was not found to be significant.

The functional outcome was scored on pain and gait patterns. Pain was seldom a problem. Gait was more problematic, as 63% of the patients had to rely on two crutches. Shortening of the proximal femur and "sub dislocation" or dislocation were correlated with difficulties to walk with one or without crutches. The use of a postoperative hip spica was correlated with a lower incidence of (sub) dislocation of the proximal femur and with a better function.

Introduction

Infections of hip prostheses are difficult to treat with antibiotics, because of the poor bone vascularization. An infected hip prosthesis almost always necessitates a reoperation. There are several options for surgical treatment of late infections of hip prostheses (Table 17.1). The first option is a one-stage revision, whereby the prosthetic mate-

Table 17.**1** Surgical treatment options for late infection of an implant

Revision in one session	This involves taking out the infected implant and suspicious tissues surrounding the infected implant, rinsing the cavities, bone and soft tissues, and then introducing a new implant with or without antibiotic-loaded cement.
Revision in two procedures	This revision can be performed in two stages. First, all the infected material and implants are removed and the wound is debrided. There is the choice of introducing a temporary spacer usually made of antibiotic-loaded cement or beads releasing antibiotics locally. Or one can omit any foreign material and let the wound cavity fill itself with fibrous tissue. In a second stage, the wound is reopened and a new arthroplasty is performed.
Removal of the infected implants and debridement, resulting in a resection arthroplasty (Girdlestone)	The removal of the infected implant and debridement, resulting in a "pseudarthrotic" hip joint, has long been the safest option to eradicate the infection. This method was customary in our department from 1970 to late 1980.

rial is removed, the infected bone is debrided, and a new prosthesis is implanted in one session. The second option consists of the removal of the infected materials followed by appropriate antibiotic treatment. The prosthesis is then replaced in a separate surgical session (two-stage revision), after documentation of complete healing of the infection has been obtained. The third and last option is the Girdlestone hip operation, whereby the infected implant is removed without replacing the prosthesis. Formation of a fibrous joint between the acetabulum and the femoral shaft results in good pain relief and good stability at the cost of reduced mobility. Patients always have a Trendelenburg gait following this operation. It is precisely the reduced mobility that has limited this intervention to a last resort treatment. A review of the literature between 1990 and 2005 shows that it is used in approximately 1% of hip revisions, with a high eradication rate of the infecting pathogens. More than 50% of the patients declare to be satisfied with the results (Stoklas and Rozkydal, 2004; de Laat et al., 1991; Bourne et al., 1984; Rittmeister et al., 2003; Arthursson et al., 2005; Sharma et al., 2005). In our clinical practice, we observe that the age of the first total hip arthroplasty is continuously declining, which directly results in a higher need for reinterventions due to implant wear. Experience, however, shows that reinterventions are more prone to infection. Also, hospital ecology is moving towards a higher incidence of multiresistant pathogens. These observations justify the analysis of the patients treated with a Girdlestone operation in our hospital.

Materials and Methods

In our institution, Girdlestone operations without second revision are the standard procedure for complicated septic conditions of the hip. Since 1993, infected hip arthroplasties have been managed by means of a two-stage revision. Between 1971 and 1993, 57 Girdlestone procedures were performed. The patients' records were retrieved and studied. Besides the analysis of the clinical record only (n=10), patients received a questionnaire (n=10), physical examination was performed on 17 patients, and additional information was come by for 24 patients, by means of a phone interview with the patient or with his relatives. Radiographic imaging was retrieved for all patients. The clinical examination and history were

structured to evaluate pain, gait, and functionality. Gait was rated as poor, difficult, and without problem. Eradication of infection was evaluated in 57 cases and functional outcome was assessed in 49 cases.

Three possible regimens were offered post surgery: skeletal traction, short hip spica cast, or early mobilization. We investigated the infection eradication rate, the factors influencing wound healing, and the factors influencing gait and patients' mobility.

Results

23 of the 57 patients were male. The mean age at time of the intervention was 65 years (range: 33–83). The indications were: sepsis of the THA in 51 patients, septic arthritis in 3, and sepsis after osteosynthesis and repositioning with internal fixation (ORIF) in 3 patients. An abscess or fistula was present in 80% of the cases (45/57). Infectious symptoms were present for a mean period of 36 months (range: 1–240). The last prosthesis was implanted for a mean period of 36 months (range 1–156) prior to the Girdlestone intervention. The mean number of previous interventions was 2.4 (0–11). Classification of the infection type according to Coventry was as follows: type 1 early: wound problem (n=28); type II delayed: l month until 1 year (n=22). These patients had never been free of pain after the initial hip arthroplasty and later developed clear signs of infection; type III hematogenous: >1 year (n=4). Three patients had an infection that could not be classified. At the time of analysis the mean follow-up was 6 years (1–16).

Bacteriology of the infection is illustrated below (Table 17.**2**).

All patients received intravenous antibiotic therapy for 6 weeks, followed by an oral therapy for at least another 3 months. The cultures remained negative in 10 cases, despite the presence of a sinus, which is probably due to previous antibiotic use. Ten patients had multiple infecting organisms. Eradication of the infection and closure of the fistula was achieved in 86% of the cases, without further antibiotic therapy. Persisting fistulas were observed in 8 cases. No difference in infection healing was found between the subgroup with a negative culture and those with multiple infecting pathogens when compared to the group as a whole.

Table 17.**2**   Bacteriology

Acinetobacter 2	MSSE *10*
Clostridium sp 1	*Peptococcus* 1
CNS 3	*Proteus. mirabilis* 5
Escherichia coli 8	*Pseudomonas aeruginosa 3*
Enterobacter 1	Pseudomomas species 5
Enterococcus 1	*Streptococcus viridans* 1
Klebsiella pn 2	*Salmonella* 1
MRSA 5	*Serratia* 1
MSSA 12	No growth 10
MRSE 1	

The factors potentially delaying wound healing are the presence of PMMA cement, bacteriology, and host factors. In our series, 40% of the patients had delayed wound healing if a cement rest was left and in 17% of the cases, where there was no cement left. The difference between the two groups was not statistically significant. Overall, wound healing was not significantly influenced by the type of bacteria isolated prior to Girdlestone operation. However, when *E. coli* was isolated prior to the intervention, 50% of the patients experienced wound healing problems as compared to 28% in the whole group. Host factors such as rheumatoid arthritis, use of corticosteroids, and obesity did not influence wound healing.

The functional outcome can be divided into pain and activities of daily living (ADL), mainly defined by walking abilities.

All patients reported satisfactory pain relief. Functionality was mainly defined by the ability to walk without or with only one crutch or cane,

which was achieved in 37% of the patients. The remaining 63%, who needed two crutches or canes, experienced their functionality as seriously reduced. None of the patients had problems while sitting, even in a car, indicating adequate hip flexion.

Table 17.**3** shows the correlation between gait quality, mean age, and the degree of leg shortening. It can be seen that mean age and degree of leg shortening are important factors influencing gait.

The degree of leg shortening is influenced by the resection level and by proximal subluxation of the femur. As expected, after total hip arthroplasty more than 50% of the patients had a resection in the pertrochanteric area. Gait was judged as without problems in 40% of those patients. The groups with resection at subcapital and subtrochanteric level were smaller. In the subcapital group 75% of the patients were able to walk without problems, while in the subtrochanteric group this was less than 10% (Fig. 17.**1**).

Besides the level of resection, the degree of "dislocation" or partial dislocation of the proximal femur also influences the gait pattern. In this series, a hip was defined as "dislocated" when the lesser trochanter or the subtrochanteric area were at the level of the superolateral border of the acetabulum. Whereas, it was defined as "normal" if the greater trochanter or the intertrochanteric region were at the above mentioned level.

Only 16% of the patients with a "dislocation" had normal gait, while in the "normal" group 60% experienced no problems walking (p < 0.01).

It is clear that dislocation influences shortening and the position of the greater trochanter, and hence the function of the abductors (Fig. 17.**2**).

With a paraarticular ossification index > 2 according to the Brooker classification (Brooker et al., 1973), 75% of the patients had a gait without problems compared to 53% of the patients with a

Table 17.**3**   Gait after Girdlestone

	N	Age (mean) at op.	Age at Fu	Shorter cm
Gait limited	8	70	71	6,4
Gait with two crutches	23	67	72	5,4
Gait without or with one crutch	18	60	64	4,5

The correlation between gait quality, mean age and the degree of leg shortening. Mean age and degree of leg shortening are important factors influencing gait.

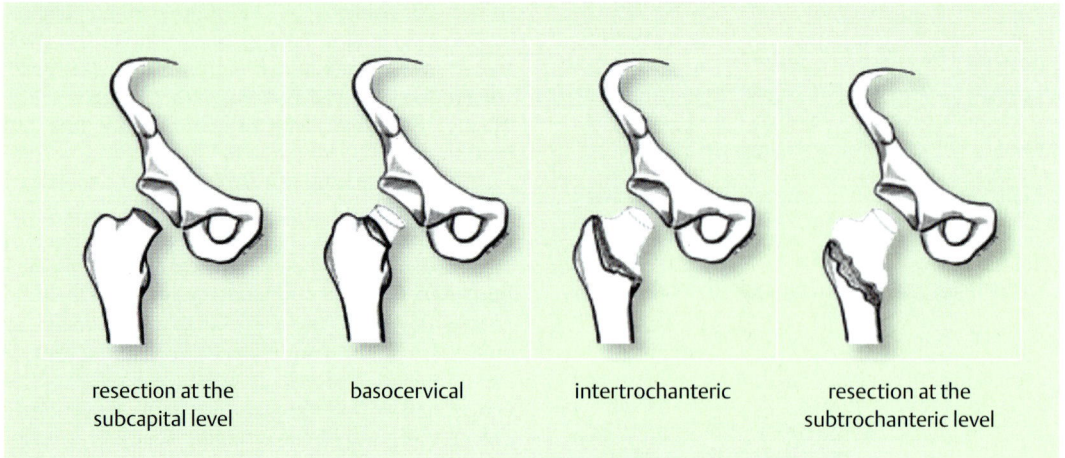

resection at the subcapital level   basocervical   intertrochanteric   resection at the subtrochanteric level

Fig. 17.**1**   In most patients, the resection was performed in the intertrochanteric area, as expected after total hip replacement. After resection at the subcapital level gait is much better and at the subtrochanteric level it is much worse.

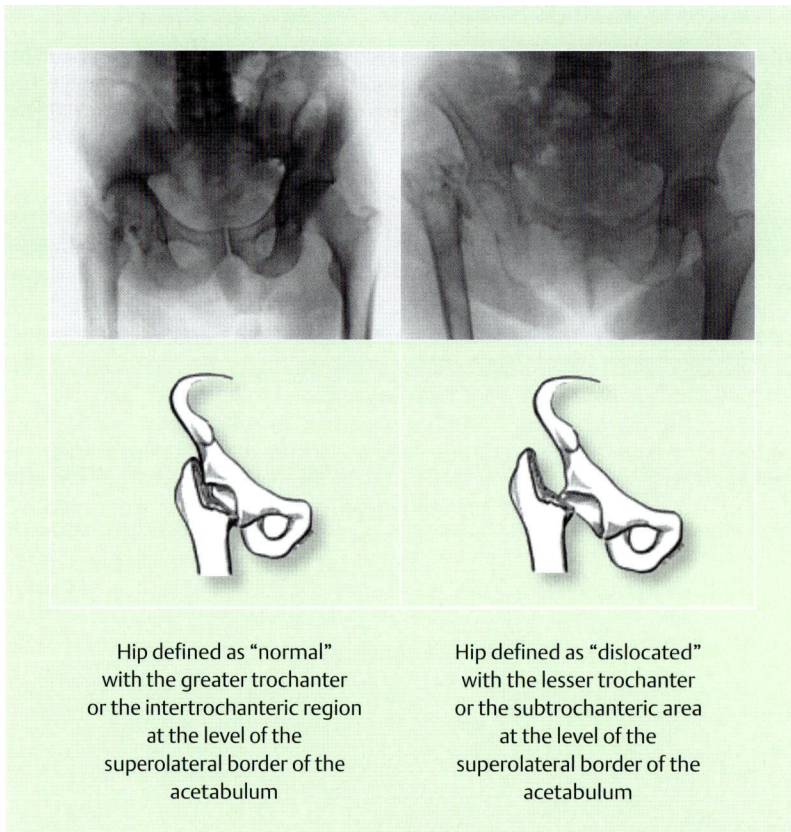

Fig. 17.**2**   The degree of dislocation influences shortening, as well as the position of the greater trochanter and hence the function of the abductors.

Hip defined as "normal" with the greater trochanter or the intertrochanteric region at the level of the superolateral border of the acetabulum

Hip defined as "dislocated" with the lesser trochanter or the subtrochanteric area at the level of the superolateral border of the acetabulum

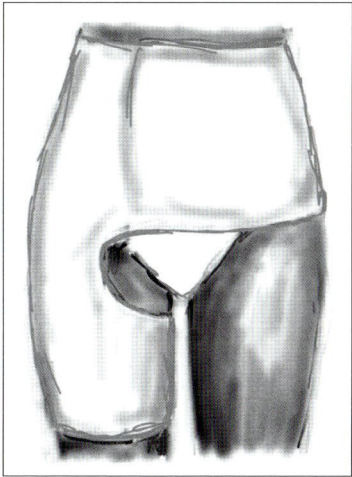

Fig. 17.**3**
A plaster hip spica treatment significantly prevented partial dislocation (p < 0.05), but no correlation between spica and ossification was found.

Brooker index < 2. Thus, paraarticular ossification results in a better gait (p < 005).

Though only a relatively small number of our patients were treated with a hip plaster spica for 3 – 6 weeks after the resection, there is a significant difference between the relative number of patients, who could walk without or with 1 crutch after having had a spica, compared to the group with early mobilization (p < 0.01).

Two potential factors may explain the positive influence of the spica treatment – a higher degree of paraarticular ossification and less dislocation (Fig. 17.**3**).

Discussion

Infection is the complication of a total hip arthroplasty that needs the most rigid treatment. It is managed by eradicating the infection and protecting functionality. Resection arthroplasty of the hip was first reported in 1849 by the English physician White as treatment for septic arthritis. This procedure was named after Gathorne Robert Girdlestone, who used it in 1928 for the treatment of tuberculous arthritis and later for septic arthritis of the hip (Fig. 17.**4**).

It was Taylor, who published a study of 94 patients that had received a Girdlestone procedure for the management of osteoarthritis and ankylosing spondylitis. He concluded that the results were very satisfactory in older patients, providing pain relief and restoration of some mobility and function. With the successful introduction of total hip arthroplasty in the sixties, the "Girdlestone pseudarthrosis" or "Girdlestone resection arthroplasty" was used only as a salvage procedure for an infected arthroplasty.

This seemingly simple treatment, involving debridement and removal of the infected material and implant, deprives the patient of a well functioning articulation. It was initially performed to reduce pain and functional handicap. So the question arises, how a patient could possibly function after a Girdlestone.

In our series of 57 patients, we found that the infection was eradicated in 86 %. All patients had a satisfactory pain relief, but function was judged as

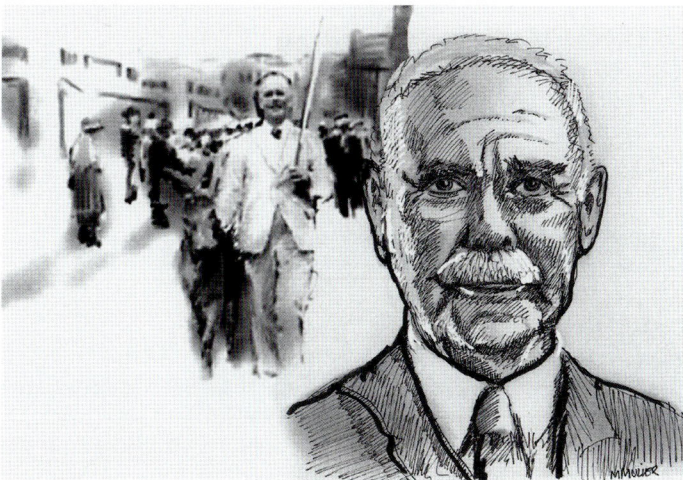

Fig. 17.**4** This figure depicts Gathorne Robert Girdlestone, who was born in 1881 and who died in 1950. Portrait according to old pictures, drawn by M. Mulier.

poor when two crutches were needed for walking, which was the case in 63% of the patients.

The quality of gait proved to be dependent of the patients' age and the shortening of the leg. The latter is related to the level of resection. Gait is less influenced when a subcapital resection is performed, as compared to a subtrochanteric resection. These findings are in accordance with Grauer (Grauer et al., 1989), who stated that "generally walking, function, and the level of activity were better when much of the proximal end of the femur had been retained". The resection level is, however, defined by the degree of infection and the bone condition. The orthopedic surgeon, of course, will always try to preserve as much as possible of the proximal end of the femur. Another factor influencing the shortening of the leg, is the dislocation or partial dislocation. Also, the position of the greater trochanter and the function of the abductors are influenced by the dislocation.

We observed that the use of a spica cast after the intervention might prevent dislocation and improve gait.

Wound healing was delayed when *E. coli* was identified. The ecology of infecting pathogens cannot be controlled and is variable. Other patients' characteristics, such as rheumatoid arthritis, do not have a significant impact on wound healing. It is imperative to remove all PMMA cement during surgery. Debridement should be complete, and if there still is some wound drainage 3 weeks after the resection, a second debridement should be considered.

It has been advocated that local antibiotics may improve healing. Though antibiotic cement beads are specially designed to generate high local antibiotic concentrations, we found that the removal of the supportive wire and the beads may be problematic.

To improve quality of gait, we now advocate the two-step intervention, whereby a new prosthesis is implanted after the infection is completely healed. In a comparative study, Rittmeister (Rittmeister et al., 2004) found a higher patient satisfaction in the group treated with reimplantation after Girdlestone surgery, as compared to the group who had a Girdlestone alone. Sometimes, it is hard for the patient to accept his situation without an artificial articulation, even when the infection is overcome. Also, many patients will readily take the risk of starting it all over again, with the risk of complications of reinfection or with the risks involved with any revision surgery, such as recurrent dislocations.

Given the patient's general good condition and the reintervention being judged as technically possible, this procedure should be proposed and discussed with the patient, thus allowing him or her to make an informed decision (Rittmeister et al., 2004; Rittmeister et al., 2005; Charlton et al., 2003).

In principle, these results are retrospective. The Girdlestone resection arthroplasty has now been reconverted to a new total hip arthroplasty, which has become technically more feasible with the introduction of temporary cement spacers. The latter are used to maintain leg length and to allow the patient to walk, while waiting for the reconversion arthroplasty. In general, the reconversion arthroplasty is performed 6 weeks after the resection arthroplasty, provided the sedimentation rate and the C-reactive protein are back to normal without antibiotic therapy.

In our department, the first cement spacers used in the nineties were home-made with a molding instrument that allowed the surgeon to compose spacers of different dimensions adapting to the individual shape of the femoral cavity (Fig. 17.**5**).

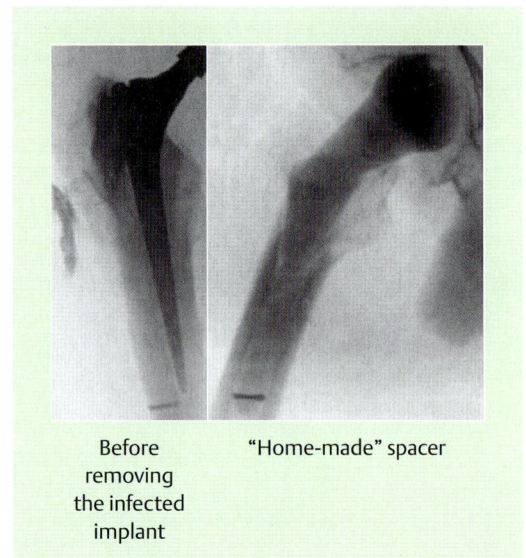

Before removing the infected implant   "Home-made" spacer

Fig. 17.**5** Peroperatively modeleded spacer made by the surgeon adapted to the individual shape of the femoral cavity.

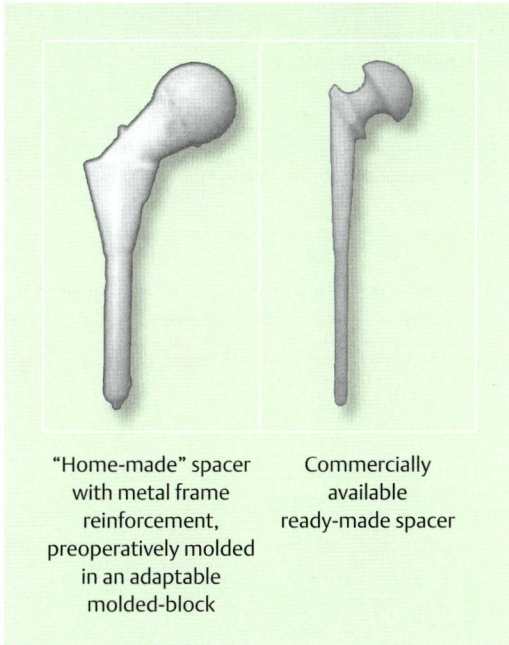

"Home-made" spacer with metal frame reinforcement, preoperatively molded in an adaptable molded-block

Commercially available ready-made spacer

Fig. 17.**6** Home-made adaptable spacer and commercial spacer.

From 2000 onwards, these home-made molds were replaced by commercially available molds (Biomet) and ready-made spacers (Tecres). These provide the advantage of being readily available during surgery, but also have disadvantages. They don't always match the shape of the cavity, and in commercially available spacers the cement cannot be mixed with appropriate antibiotics. The necessity of a CE mark for the metal frame used in the homemade spacers, has forced us to discontinue our own technique of using home-made spacers. According to the peroperative findings, this technique had previously enabled us to make specific adjustments to the geometry of the deformed femoral canal (Fig. 17.**6**).

Conclusion

Infection poses a heavy burden on arthroplasties, in general, and is becoming the most significant complication in implant surgery. As increasing resistance to antibiotics is being observed, the treatment of an infected implant becomes more problematic.

The retrospective study of this series of patients, who had a Girdlestone resection, was intended to evaluate the effectiveness of this procedure in view of ambulation and control of infection.

In our series, we found that the Girdlestone operation alleviated pain and eradicated the infection in 86% of the patients. The main drawback of this intervention was the fact that 63% of the patients needed two crutches to walk, which seriously interfered with their mobility. The use of a spica plaster in the postoperative period enhanced mobility, because of a lower risk of (partial) dislocation.

In accordance with the literature, we can conclude that a Girdlestone resection can effectively relieve pain and control infection, but most patients are limited in their functional capabilities.

In this day and age, a Girdlestone resection is not a readily accepted endpoint procedure anymore, due to the loss of function. Nowadays, most patients prefer a reconversion to a total hip arthroplasty in a second procedure. However, in the past many patients accepted the limitations, as they became free of pain and infection, and also because the Girdlestone procedure finally put an end to their hip problem, after multiple previous surgical interventions and hospitalizations.

References

Arthursson AJ, Furnes O, Espehaug B, Havelin LI, Soreide JA. Validation of data in the Norwegian Arthroplasty Register and the Norwegian Patient Register: 5,134 primary total hip arthroplasties and revisions operated at a single hospital between 1987 and 2003. Acta Orthop 2005; 76 (6): 823–828.

Bourne RB, Hunter GA, Rorabeck CH, Macnab JJ. A six-year follow-up of infected total hip replacements managed by Girdlestone's arthroplasty. J Bone Joint Surg Br 1984; 66 (3): 340–343.

Brooker A, Bowerman J, Robinson R. Ectopic ossification following total hip replacement: incidence and a method of classification. J Bone Joint Surg Am 1973; 551629.

Charlton WP, Hozack WJ, Teloken MA, Rao R, Bissett GA. Complications associated with reimplantation after Girdlestone arthroplasty. Clin Orthop Relat Res 2003 (407): 119–126.

Grauer JD, Amstutz HC, O'Carroll PF, Dorey FJ. Resection arthroplasty of the hip. J Bone Joint Surg Am 1989; 71 (5): 669–678.

Laat de E, van der List J, van Horn J, Slooff T. Girdlestone's pseudoarthrosis after removal of a total hip prosthesis; a retrospective study of 40 patients. Acta Orthop Belg 1991; 57 (2): 109–113.

Rittmeister M, Muller M, Starker M, Hailer NP. Functional results following Girdlestone arthroplasty. Z Orthop Ihre Grenzgeb 2003; 141 (6): 665–671.

Rittmeister M, Manthei L, Muller M, Hailer NP. Reimplantation of the artificial hip joint in girdlestone hips is superior to girdlestone arthroplasty by itself. Z Orthop Ihre Grenzgeb 2004;142 (5): 559–563.

Rittmeister ME, Manthei L, Hailer NP. Prosthetic replacement in secondary Girdlestone arthroplasty has an unpredictable outcome. Int Orthop 2005; 29 (3): 145–148.

Sharma H, De Leeuw J, Rowley DI. Girdlestone resection arthroplasty following failed surgical procedures. Int Orthop 2005; 29 (2): 92–95.

Stoklas J, Rozkydal Z. Resection of head and neck of the femoral bone according to Girdlestone. Acta Chir Orthop Traumatol Czech 2004; 71 (3): 147–151.

Index

A

acrylic
– bone cement (ALAC)
– – – antibiotic-loaded   59 ff
– – – antibiotic requirements   48 f
– – – antibiotics characteristics   61 f
– – – components   31 f
– – – compression   31 f
– – – preparing by hand-mixing   61 ff
– – – static tensile strength   31
– mono- and polymers   31
adherence, biomaterial   95
adhesion, bacterial   1 f, 17
Amikacin
– acrylic bone cement (ALAC)   62
– – requirements   48 f
– efficacy   56
aminoglycoside
– antibiotics   26
– release   41 ff
Ampicillin
– acrylic bone cement (ALAC)   62
– efficacy   56
anaerobes
– acrylic bone cement (ALAC)   62
– antimicrobial treatment   104
antibiotic-cement combination   66
antibiotics
– acrylic bone cement (ALAC)   61 f
– admixture to bone cement   48
– application
– – local   60
– – oral   110
– availability, reduced   59 f
– carrier systems   24 ff
– – polymer layer-forming   24 f
– choice in infected arthroplasty   102 f
– concentration   140
– – local, impregnation of bone graft   43
– customized addition   55
– delivery   114
– distribution in cement powder   55
– elution

– – carrier, antibiotic-loaded   69
– – PMMA bone cement   60 f
– – profile from cancellous bone   42
– Gridlestone resection arthroplasty   156 ff
– high-dose intravenous   134
– industrial addition   55 f
– initiation time   134
– mechanical influence on PMMA bone cement   53 ff
– pharmacokinetics   59 f, 140 ff
– polymer layer-forming carrier system   24 f
– primary prothesis   147 ff
– prophylaxis   147 ff
– – in cement   148 ff
– – cemented versus uncemented prothesis   150 f
– – systemic   148 ff
– quantity per g cement powder   55
– recommended admixture   56
– release
– – bone cement   4 f
– – characteristics   50 ff
– – measurement
– – – dynamic   67
– – – static   66 f
– – mechanism   23
– – PMMA   66
– – time dependence   67
– salts, self-adhesive low-soluble   25 f
– side effects   114
– – – infection after joint arthroplasty   129
– – – revision infected hip prothesis   126
– systemic
– – infected arthroplasty   102 f
– – infection after joint arthroplasty   129
– – septic joint arthroplasty   110 f
– – toxicity   114
antimicrobial
– protection   23 ff
– treatment   104
antiseptics, in polymer layer-forming carrier system   24 f
arthritis and osteomyelitis, recurrence-free period   72
arthrodesis   136 f
arthroplasty
– antimicrobial implant coating   23 ff

arthroplasty
– cemented   23
– cementless   24
– infected   95 ff
– – antibiotic choice   102 f
– – aspiration, preoperative   97 f
– – bacteriology   98 f
– – blood tests   97
– – clinical features   96
– – histological diagnostic techniques   98
– – investigation
– – – experimental   99 f
– – – pathway   101
– – management   100 ff
– – radiographic tests   98
– – revision-related results   96 ff
– – systemic antibiotics   102 f
– registry in Hellenic   116
– septic joint   9 ff
– two-stage revision   7 f
aspiration, preoperative   97 f

B

bacteria
– adherence to biomaterials   95
– antibiotic prophylaxis   152
– colonization, implant surface   13
– inhibited phagocytosis in biofilm   59 f
– orthopedic infection   4
– resistant, two-stage revision   115
– sessile   59 f
bacterial adhesion   1 f
– colonization, coated PTFE vascular prothesis   17
bacteriology
– Gridlestone resection arthroplasty   157
– infected arthroplasty   98 f
beads
– Palasorb G   18
– – gentamicin release   19
– PMMA, gentamicin-loaded s. PMMA beads,
   gentamicin-loaded
– removement   134 f
– versus spacer, comparison   114
benzyl penicillin   105
betalactams release   41 f
biofilm
– bacteria behave   3
– formation   2 f, 13
– – antibiotic prophylaxis   152
– inhibited phagocytosis of bacteria   59 f
– microorganisms   2 f
– production   95
– sesille bacteria   59 f
– Staphylococcus epidermidis   14
biomaterial infection   13

blood test
– arthroplasty, infected   97
– vancomycin concentration   79
bloodstream infection   1
bone
– allograft
– – antibiotic-loaded, toxic serum level   43
– – cancellous   41 ff
– – – antibiotic impregnation   41 f
– cement
– – antibiotic-loaded (ALBC)   1, 47 ff
– – – clinical aspects   5 f
– – – combination   75 ff
– – – commercially available   6
– – – in Italy   122
– – – local antibiotic delivery   114
– – – local therapy   59 ff
– – – studies   5
– – – ultrasound application   7
– – antibiotics
– – – customized addition   55
– – – elution   60 f
– – – industrial addition   55 f
– – – release   4 f
– – difference   31 ff
– – gentamicin-loaded   1
– – high-viscous, gentamicin release   51 ff
– – mechanical properties, admixture of antibiotics
     48
– – mechanical strength   53 ff
– – PMMA, gentamicin release   24
– – tobramycin-loaded
– – – antibacterial activity   78 f
– – – bacteriological properties   77 f
– – – chemical properties   77 f
– – – mechanical properties   75 ff
– – – tensile properties   77
– – use   31
– – vancomycin-loaded   75 ff
– – – antibacterial activity   78 f
– – – bacteriological properties   77 f
– – – chemical properties   77 f
– – – mechanical properties   75 ff
– – – studies   76
– – – tensile properties   77
– cancellous, antibiotics elution profile   42
– graft   65, 114, 124
– – extenders   114
– – substitutes   114
– joint infection center   121 f
– lavage   89
– stock deficiency, two stage revision   115
– substitute, removement   71
– surgery, antibiotic choices   59 ff

C

calcium sulfate, tobramycin-loaded   71
cancellous bone graft   42, 65
carrier
– antibiotic   13 ff
– – cancellous bone allograft   41 ff
– – use   67 ff
– antibiotic-loaded
– – pharmacokinetics   65 ff
– – prophylactic use   71 f
– – release mechanism   69
– – resorbable   135
– – therapeutic use   71 f
– system, polymer layer-forming   24 f
Carynebacterium amycolatum   62
cavity   133
Cefoperazon   62
Cefotaxim   62
Cefperazon, efficacy   56
Cefuroxim
– acrylic bone cement (ALAC)   62
– efficacy   56
– infected arthroplasty   104
cement
– acrylic   31 ff
– application   88
– basic material   31
– beads, antibiotic-loaded   160
– brands
– – powder copolymer classification   32
– – viscosity classification   37
– containment   88 f
– high-viscosity   36 f
– low-viscosity   37
– MA copolymer   33
– medium-viscosity   37
– MMA-MA copolymer   32 f
– polymer type   33
– porosity   4
– powder
– – antibiotics distribution   55
– – component   31 f
– – quantity antibiotics   55
– pressurization   89
– primary prothesis   147 ff
– properties, mechanical   32 f
– properties   32
– – thermal   33 ff
– socket fixation   87 f
– spacer, antibiotic-loaded   121 ff
– styrene-copolymer   33
– technique
– – evolution   89
– – modern   90
– temperature rise   33 ff

– – test   34
– type of copolymer   32
– viscosity   36 ff
– – affected variables   38
cement-antibiotic combination   66
cementing technique   88 f
center specialized for bone and joint infection   121 f
Ciprofloxacin release   42
Clindamycin
– acrylic bone cement (ALAC)   62
– efficacy   56
– release   42
CMW1 bone cement
– – – gentamicin release   24
– – – vancomycin-loaded, in-vivo release   79
– – – vancomycin-/tobramycin-loaded   77 ff
coating
– antibiotic   13 ff
– antimicrobial   23 ff
– method, local   24 ff
– new   13 ff
– porous hydroxyl apatite, antibiotic-loaded   25 f
– process   24 f
– self-adhesive low-soluble antibiotic salts   25 f
– with heavy metal   25 f
collagen   67, 71
– sponge, resorbable   13
complication, postoperative, revision infected hip prothesis   126
copper   26
costs
– annually, infections   75
– total joint replacement   121

D

debridement
– early postoperative infection   134
– late postoperative infection   135
defense, cellular host   59 f
drainage system, with suction   133
drains
– early postoperative infection 134
– hip activity   133
– infection after joint arthroplasty   129
– vancomycin concentration   79
drug
– carrier, resorbable   19 f
– delivery system   13
– level, local   13

E

Edinburgh arthroplasty infection diagnosis study   99 f

Edinburgh Infection Diagnosis Study 98 f
elution 60 f
endoprothesis
– cemented, antimicrobial protection 23
– cementless, antimicrobial protection 24
– gentamicin palmitate-coated 28
– uncoated 27
enoxaparin 124
Enterobacter cloacae 125
Enterobactericeae 62
Enterococci, recommended antibiotics admixture
  56
Enterococcus
– fecalis 62
– species 104
– supp 62
erythrocyte sedimentation rate (ESR) 97
– – – revision infected hip prothesis 124 f
– – – late postoperative infection 135

F

fixation
– cemented 87
– uncemented 87
free radical formation, reduction 13

G

gait, after Gridlestone 157, 160
gentamicin
– acrylic bone cement (ALAC) 62
– beads
– – exsudate concentration 141 f
– – radiographic images 134
– collagen 13, 67
– – fleece 141
– – resorbable 134
– components 50
– concentration 140
– detection methods 50
– efficacy 56
– fatty acid salt 26 f
– – – – synthesis 27
– history of use 65
– infected arthroplasty 105
– infection after joint arthroplasty 129
– in-vitro release from Palasorb G beads 19
– laurate 14, 16
– Palacos R+G cement 102 f
– palmitate 14 ff, 26
– pentakis(dodecylsulfate) 27
– pentakis(myristate) 27
– pentakis(palmitate) 27
– release 26, 28

– – characteristics 51 ff
– – coated titanium plate 28
– – Palacos R 47 f
– – PMMA beads 8
– – PMMA bone cement 24
– – PTFE prothesis 15 f
– resistance 8
– serum concentration 70
– sodium dodecyl sulfate 14
– spacer, exsudate concentration 142
– sulfate, carrier system 26
gentamicin-collagen 71
Gridlestone
– hip 136 f
– – operation 156
– resection arthroplasty 155 ff
– – – bacteriology 157
– – – Brooker index 157, 159
– – – dislocation 157 f
– – – functional outcome 157 f
– – – one-stage 155 f
– – – pain relief 157
– – – resection location 158
gun application 88

H

heavy metal 25 f
– – salts 25 f
hematoma
– early postoperative infection 134
– late postoperative infection 135
hemiarthroplasty, bipolar, chronica open wound
  102
hemocompatibility 17
hip
– activity 133
– arthroplasty
– – infected 80 f
– – total (THA)
– – – antibiotic prophylaxis 147 ff
– – – cemented versus uncemented 150 f
– – – chronically infected 123
– – – primary 147 f
– dislocated 158
– endoprothesis
– – gentamicin palmitate-coated 28
– – uncoated 27
– function test 124 ff
– Gridlestone resection arthroplasty 155 ff
– normal 158
– number of PMMA beads 134
– plaster spica treatment 159
– prothesis
– – infected 145 f
– – – revision 121 ff

– – infection   155 f
– replacement   103
– – total (THR), prevalence   121
– spacer   80 f
– – preformed, exsudation concentration   142
histological techniques, infection diagnosis   98
histology, frozen   98, 101
host defense   13
hydroxylapatite layer   25

I

implant
– coating, antimicrobial   23
– infection, late   155
– orthopedic, infections   4 ff
– surface
– – antimicrobial protection   23 f
– – bacteria colonization   13
– – infection   13
infection
– biomaterial   13
– biomaterial-related   1 ff
– biomaterial-related, incidence   3
– bloodstream related   1
– chronic joint replacement   7 f
– deep   135
– diagnosing difficulties   96 ff
– early postoperative   134 f
– eradication   155 ff
– – Gridlestone resection arthroplasty   156 f, 161
– – rate   128 f
– hip prothesis   155 f
– histological techniques   98
– increase   55
– joint arthroplasty   109 ff
– late   155
– – postoperative   135
– orthopedic
– – bacteria   4
– – device-related, treatment criteria   113
– – implants   1 ff
– – implant-associated, annual costs   75
– pathogenesis   95
– periprosthetic, clinical presentation   109
– prevention with antibiotic-loaded carrier   67
– prothesis-related   7 f
– – treatment   7 f
– rate, postoperative   23
– standard method in diagnosing   3 f
– superficial   134
– surgical procedure related   1

J

joint
– arthroplasty
– – infection
– – – diagnosis   109
– – – management
– – – – nonsurgical   110 f
– – – – surgical   111 ff
– – Pseudomonas aeruginosa   129
– – septic   109 ff
– – Staphylococcus
– – – aureus   129
– – – epidermis   129
– – – Methicillin-resistant   129
– infection, periprosthetic   111 ff
– prothesis, prevention of infection   6 f
– replacement
– – infected, diagnosis   96 f
– – total (TJR), prevalence   121

K

knee
– arthroplasty, infected
– – – management   80
– – – revision strategy   82 f
– joint
– – arthrodesis   116
– – arthroplasty, resection   116
– number of PMMA beads   134
– replacement, total (THR), prevalence   121

L

lavage, pulsatile   89
leg shortening   159
level, antibacterial
– – antibiotic-loaded prothesis   13
– – antibiotic-loaded PTFE prothesis   17 f
local wound compromising factor   112
loosening, aseptic   149 ff

M

material, resorbable suture   13 f
Merle d'Aubigne Score   124 ff
methylacrylate (MA)   32
– copolymer cement   33
methylmethacrylate (MMA)
– bone cement   60 f
– polymer   31
microorganisms, biofilm   2 f

MMA/MA copolymer   32 f
MMA-MA copolymer cement   32 f
multidrug targeting   6

N

new coating technology   19 f
nonfermenters, antimicrobial treatment   104
Norwegian Hip Register   147 ff

O

Ofloxacin
– acrylic bone cement (ALAC)   62
– efficacy   56
one-stage exchange, versus two-stage   101 f
organism adherence, biomaterial   95
orthopaedic implants, infection   1 ff
ossification, heterotopic   125
osteitis, posttraumatic and postoperative   23 f
osteogenesis, antibiotic impregnation of bone graft
   42
osteomyelitis   65
– cement, antibiotic-loaded   66 f
– healing   72
– PMMA beads   69 f
– recurrence-free period   72
– therapy with antibiotic-loaded carrier   71 f

P

pain relief   157, 161
Palacos
– bone cement, different package   49
– history   65
Palacos R
– antibiotic-loaded, first investigations   47
– cement cooling   36
– gentamicin release   47 f
– gentamicin-loaded   103
– temperature rise   35
Palacos R+G cement
– gentamicin-loaded   102 f
– gentamicin release   26, 28
Palasorb G beads   18
– – in-vitro release of gentamicin   19
pathogenes, major bacterial   75
penicillin allergy, infected arthroplasty   104
PMMA   1, 4 f
– antibiotic release   66
– beads
– – antibiotic concentration   140 f
– – application   69 ff
– – gentamicin, release   67 ff

– – gentamicin-loaded   8, 133 ff
– – – exsudation concentration   142
– – number
– – – for hip   134
– – – for knee   134
– – osteomyelitis   69 f
– – use   70 f
– bone cement   31 ff
– – – antibiotic eluation   60
– – – antibiotic-loaded   59 ff
– – – antibiotics
– – – – admixture   56
– – – – as additive   48 f
– – – – mechanical influence   53 ff
– – – as carrier   60
– – – bending strength   54
– – – chemical composition   31 f
– – – compressive strength   54
– – – gentamicin release   24
– – – gentamicin sulfate   26
– – – local antibiotic release   23
– – – production   60
– hip spacer, antibiotic-loaded   123
– synthesis   66
poly-d,l-lactide   19
polyester, biodegradable   24
polyglycolic acid   13 f
polylactic acid (PLA)   13 f
polylactide   24 f
polylactide-gentamicin pellets, in-vitro-release   68
polymer matrix, porosity   4
polymerase chain reaction   100
polymers
– natural   114
– resorbable   13 f
– synthetic   114
polymethylmethacrylate (PMMA) s. PMMA
polytetrafluoroethylene (PTFE) prothesis   14 ff
prophylactic use, antibiotic-loaded carrier   71 f
prophylaxis
– antibiotic-loaded carrier   71 f
– antibiotics   147 ff
– – in cement   148 ff
– – combined   148 ff
– – systemic   148 ff
– – – duration   149 f
Propionibacteriae   56, 62
prosthetic joint infection
– – – staging system   111
– – – treatment duration   105
protection, antimicrobial   23 ff
protein, C-reaktive (CRP)
– – concentration   97
– – late postoperative infection   135
– – revision infected hip prothesis   124 f
prothesis
– cemented versus uncemented   150 f

– cementless, two-stage revision   115
– infected, treatment   133 ff
– polytretrafluorethylene
– – antibiotic-loaded   14 f
– – gentamicin release   15 f
– primary, influences   147 ff
– reimplantation   135 ff
– uncemented, antibiotic prophylaxis   150 f
Pseudomonas aeruginosa
– – acrylic bone cement (ALAC)   62
– – antimicrobial treatment   104
– – joint arthroplasty   129
– – recommended antibiotics admixture   56
– – revision infected hip prothesis   125
– – vancomycin bone cement   75
PTFE vascular prothesis
– – – antibiotic coated   15 ff
– – – hemocompatibility   17
– – – uncoated   15 ff
pulse lavage   134

Q

quinolones   110

R

race for the surface   13
radiographic tests   98
reimplantation   8, 135 ff
– long-term two-stage   138 f
– one-stage versus two-stage   139 f
– short-term two-stage   137
– successful   8
resection arthroplasty   155
resins, fast-curing s. bone cement
resistance, bacterial   5 f
revision
– arthroplasty, cementless versus cemented   128
– aseptic loosening   149 ff
– implant removal   155
– infected
– – hip prothesis   121 ff
– – total hip prothesis   145 f
– one-stage   155
– – infected hip prothesis   155 f
– – survival   145
– – versus two-stage   101 f, 139 f
– partial, survival   145
– prothesis
– – cementless   123 ff
– – dislocation   128
– single-stage   113
– surgery, one-stage   7 f
– two-stage   7 f, 155

– – cementless prothesis   115
– – exchange, concept   114 f
– – hip   123
– – infected hip prothesis   156
– – in Italian center   122
– – length of interval   105
– – long-term   138 f
– – problems   115
– – results   105 f
– – short-term   137
– – survival   145
– – time of second stage   115
rifampicin   110
– release   42

S

Scandinavian arthroplasty register   87, 146
septic joint arthroplasty   109 ff
Serratia marcescens, revision infected hip prothesis   125
serum
– concentration   68 ff
– levels
– – gentamicin   49
– – toxic, antibiotic-loaded bone allografts   43
silver
– ions   26
– nano particle   26
– salt, low soluble   26
sodium salts   27
spacer
– antibiotic-loaded   123, 141
– cement, antibiotic-loaded   121 ff
– dislocation   128
– "home-made"   160 f
– – adaptable   161
– long-stem performed   128
– ready-made, commercially available   161
– temporary   114
– versus beads, comparison   114
spacer G   123 f, 128
staphylococci
– acrylic bone cement (ALAC)   62
– coagulase-negative   95
– – antimicrobial treatment   104
– Methicillin-resistant
– – recommended antibiotics admixture   56
– – antimicrobial treatment   104
– Oxacillin-resistant, recommended antibiotics admixture   56
Staphylococcus
– aureus   3
– – antimicrobial treatment   104
– – biofilm growth   7
– – CMW1 bone cement   79

Staphylococcus, aureus
– – joint arthroplasty   129
– – management septic joint arthroplasty   110
– – multiresistant   116
– – osteitis   23
– – recommended antibiotics admixture   56
– coagulase-negative, revision infected hip prothesis
  125
– epidermidis
– – biofilm   14
– – growth on PTFE prothesis   18
– – human pathogenic germ   15
– – joint arthroplasty   129
– – multiresistant   116
– – osteitis   23
– – recommended antibiotics admixture   56
– – revision infected hip prothesis   125
– – uncoated PTFE vascular prothesis   17 f
– Methicillin-resistant, joint arthroplasty   129
static tensile test, acrylic cement   32
strain, resistant   5 f
strength
– acrylic cement   31 f
– PMMA bone cement   54
– mechanical, bone cement   53 f
Streptococci, acrylic bone cement (ALAC)   62
Streptococcus
– bacteria, recommended antibiotics admixture   56
– spp., antimicrobial treatment   104
suction drainage system   133
Surgical Simplex, temperature rise   35
susceptibility, bacterial   59 f
systemic host compromizing factors   112

technetium isotope scans   98
teicoplanin, infected arthroplasty   105
Temperature rise, cement   33 ff
temperature test   35
– – cement   34
titanium plate
– – coated, gentamicin release   28
– – sandblasted, gentamicin palmitate-coated   26, 28
tobramycin
– calcium sulfate   71
– effect   76

total hip arthroplasty (THA)   87 ff
– – – bone lavage   89
– – – cement application   88
– – – – pressurization   89
– – – cemented   87 f
– – – gun application   88 f
– – – implant survival   90
– – – pulsatile lavage   89
two-stage
– – exchange, concept   114 f
– – results   105 f
– – versus one-stage   101 f
– reimplantation   137
– – long-term   138 f

ultrasound
– antibiotic-loaded bone cement   7
– low-frequency   6 f
urine concentration
– – gentamicin   68 ff
– – vancomycin   79

vancomycin
– acrylic bone cement (ALAC)   62
– bone cement   75 ff
– effect   76
– efficacy   56
– elution rate   78
– infected arthroplasty   104
– infection after joint arthroplasty   129
– perenteral administration   75
– release   41 ff
– side effects   75
viscosity
– affected variables   38
– cement   36 ff
– effect of copolymer percentage   37

wound, chronically open   102